Health Information Science

C000256113

Series Editor

Yanchun Zhang, Victoria University, Melbou

With the development of database systems and networking technologies, Hospital Information Management Systems (HIMS) and web-based clinical or medical systems (such as the Medical Director, a generic GP clinical system) are widely used in health and clinical practices. Healthcare and medical service are more data-intensive and evidence-based since electronic health records are now used to track individuals' and communities' health information. These highlights substantially motivate and advance the emergence and the progress of health informatics research and practice. Health Informatics continues to gain interest from both academia and health industries. The significant initiatives of using information, knowledge and communication technologies in health industries ensures patient safety, improve population health and facilitate the delivery of government healthcare services. Books in the series will reflect technology's cross-disciplinary research in IT and health/medical science to assist in disease diagnoses, treatment, prediction and monitoring through the modeling, design, development, visualization, integration and management of health related information. These technologies include information systems, web technologies, data mining, image processing, user interaction and interfaces, sensors and wireless networking, and are applicable to a wide range of health-related information such as medical data, biomedical data, bioinformatics data, and public health data.

Series Editor:, Yanchun Zhang, Victoria University, Australia;

Editorial Board: Riccardo Bellazzi, University of Pavia, Italy; Leonard Goldschmidt, Stanford University Medical School, USA; Frank Hsu, Fordham University, USA; Guangyan Huang, Victoria University, Australia; Frank Klawonn, Helmholtz Centre for Infection Research, Germany; Jiming Liu, Hong Kong Baptist University, Hong Kong, China; Zhijun Liu, Hebei University of Engineering, China; Gang Luo, University of Utah, USA; Jianhua Ma, Hosei University, Japan; Vincent Tseng, National Cheng Kung University, Taiwan; Dana Zhang, Google, USA; Fengfeng Zhou, Shenzhen Institutes of Advanced Technology, Chinese Academy of Sciences, China

More information about this series at http://www.springer.com/series/11944

Amit Kumar Manocha • Shruti Jain
Mandeep Singh • Sudip Paul

Editors

Computational Intelligence in Healthcare

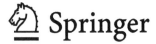 Springer

Editors
Amit Kumar Manocha (iD)
Electrical Engineering
MRS Punjab Technical University
Bathinda, India

Shruti Jain (iD)
Electronics & Communication Engineering
Jaypee University of Information Technol
Solan, India

Mandeep Singh
Electrical & Instrumentation
Engineering
Thapar University
Patiala, India

Sudip Paul (iD)
Biomedical Engineering Department
North Eastern Hill University
Shillong, India

Series Editor
Yanchun Zhang

ISSN 2366-0988   ISSN 2366-0996   (electronic)
Health Information Science
ISBN 978-3-030-68725-0   ISBN 978-3-030-68723-6   (eBook)
https://doi.org/10.1007/978-3-030-68723-6

This Springer imprint is published by the registered company Springer Nature Switzerland AG
The registered company address is: Gewerbestrasse 11, 6330 Cham, Switzerland

Preface

Kirlian photography is a technique based on electrical coronal discharge. In this technique, the photographic plate made of metal is charged with a high-voltage source. The process is also quite simple, and it is recommended to use transparent electrodes instead of the discharge plate. It is an exciting method to capture the corona discharge of individual subjects. Medical image compression finds extensive applications in healthcare, teleradiology, teleconsultation, telemedicine, and telematics. Efficient compression algorithms implement the development of picture achieving and communication systems (PACS). To reduce transmission time and storage costs, efficient image compression methods without degradation of images are needed. In medical image compression techniques, the lossy and lossless methods do not produce optimum compression with no information loss.

The circuit complexity and propagation delay are the primary concern in the design of the digital circuit. In the binary system, as the number of bits increases, the computation speed is limited by carrying. Consequently, it offers low storage density, enormous complexity, and $O(n)$ carry, producing a delay in n-bit base on two application problems. For less complexity and higher information storage density, higher radix number system can be used. Quaternary signed digit (QSD) number system performs carry-free addition and borrows free subtraction. The concept of telemedicine and telehealth is still a novice one to most practitioners. However, the continued advances in technology can demand its usability from a new generation of tech-savvy people due to its convenience, cost-effectiveness, and intelligent features. These include store and forward techniques, real-time interactive modes, remote monitoring, and smartphones for healthcare services like m-health.

In the era of digitization, tracking information on a real-time basis is one of the eminent tasks. Wearable technology involves electronics incorporated into items that can be comfortably worn on a body mainly used to detect, analyze, and transmit contemporaneous information. Wearable technology has applications in many fields, such as health and medicine, fitness, education, gaming, finance, music, and transportation. Wearable devices have become quite inevitable as technology in the medical electronics field advances. These devices are highly cost-effective and portable, making it easy to use, efficient, and safe.

Because people desire a high quality of life, health is a vital standard of living that attracts considerable attention. Thus, the development of methods that enable rapid and real-time evaluation and monitoring of the social health status has been crucial. Moreover, to attain an intuitive insight to detect, monitor, identify, and accuracy is an essential parameter. In this, concerning the characteristics of time-series data acquired using health condition monitoring through sensors, recommendations and bits of advice are provided to apply deep learning (DL) methods to human body evaluation in specific fields.

Emotion detection has been carried out through various techniques such as EEG and image and video recording of facial expressions, body gestures, text-based emotion identification, etc. The non-contact temperature sensor used to detect breathing patterns for various emotions is considered for this to know emotional activities like happiness, surprise, sadness, and anger. Twelve features are taken from the wavelet transformed signal features to get emotional status.

E-health means the availability of various health facilities electronically without going anywhere. There is a tremendous demand for implementing such techniques in rural areas because of the spread of the COVID-19 pandemic. Patients and disabled people from villages faced many difficulties due to the closure of transportation facilities during the lockdown period. There is a significant requirement to develop a connected network that consists of various medical devices like E-health systems to fulfill the needs of those who live in rural areas.

Osteoporosis is a common disease prevalent mostly among elderly individuals. The characteristics of osteoporosis include increased fragility, which is caused due to the reduction of the bone's absorption capability. This leads to an increase in the porosity, reduction in the bone's elastic stiffness, and thinning of the cortical wall. Osteoporosis increases the risk of fractures and hence can cause suffering and also leads to economic loss. The current standard method of detecting osteoporosis is dual-energy X-ray absorptiometry (DXA), which cannot predict whether a person is suffering from porous bones.

Infusion is a mechanism by which an infusion system is used to administer fluids or medications via the intravenous, subcutaneous, epidural, or internal path to the patient in solution. For the healthcare drug delivery devices, exact dosing is crucial. The use of smart pumps can avoid errors resulting from an incorrect dose, dose rate, or solution concentration resulting from the ordering provider, as well as errors resulting from human failures in the programming of pumps.

Cardiovascular diseases(CVDs)are significant reasons for mortality in the world population, and the number of cases is surging every year. Due to coronary artery disease (CAD) and congestive heart failure(CHF), the mortality rate is higher than any other CVD type. Therefore, early detection and diagnosis of CAD and CHF patients are essential. An automated non-invasive approach has been used to detect CAD and CHF patients using attributes extracted from heart rate variability (HRV) signal.

Electrocardiogram (ECG) signal carries the most critical information in cardiology. Care should be taken to avoid interference in the ECG. To avoid too many computations, IIR digital filters have fewer coefficients and the potential of sharp roll-offs, which is acceptable for real-time processing. Coefficients of IIR digital filters are worked out with the genetic algorithm (GA). Using a designed filter, the ECG signal was de-noised by removing the interference. Results indicate that there is noise reduction in the ECG signal.

Heart rate (HR) is one of the essential physiological parameters and acts as an indicator of a person's physiological condition. The algorithm for face detection is used to recognize human faces, and HR information is extracted from the color variation in facial skin caused by blood circulation. The variation in the blood circulation causes changes in the pixel intensity of the live video recorded. The extraction of the specific frequency is achieved by bandpass filtering, and the pixel intensity average is calculated. Finally, the HR of the subject is measured using the frequency-domain method.

Melanoma is the deadlier type of skin cancer. Proper diagnosis and a perfect optimized segmentation methodology rely on thresholding, and watershed algorithms are implemented on dermoscopy images, and the differentiated object is derived for GLCM attributes and qualitative techniques. The attributes are supplied into the support vector machine as a source to identify malignant or benign samples. As perceived by experimental findings, the SVM classification system with watershed segmentation can distinguish benign and malignant melanoma with a higher overall categorization efficiency.

Gastroenterology is a field of medicine that has its roots deeply embedded in the technological revolution of the twenty-first century. It emerges as a specialty dominated by ever-evolving imaging and diagnostic modalities that have surpassed archaic means of diagnosing and treating various gastroenterological disorders. Advancement in cloud computing technology can change healthcare professionals in gastrointestinal (GI) work in the inpatient and outpatient settings.

A coronavirus is a group of infectious diseases that are caused by similar viruses called coronaviruses. The disease's seriousness can vary from mild to lethal in human beings, causing severe illness in older adults and those with health issues like cardiovascular disease, diabetes, chronic respiratory, and cancer. There are a limited number of test kits available in the hospitals as the number of positive cases increases daily. Hence, an automated COVID-19 detection system must be implemented as an alternative diagnostic method to pause COVID-19 spread in the population.

Around 2.1 million women have breast cancer per year globally. The prevalence of breast cancer ranges across nations, but in most instances, the second cause of death for the female population is this form of cancer. Mammography research, which shapes the expert's auto-exploration and manual exploration, is the most powerful technology for the early diagnosis of breast cancer. In the detection of calcifications and masses in the mammography photograph, there is a considerable research effort, apart from other potential anomalies, since these two forms of artifacts are the best markers of a possible early stage of breast cancer.

Artificial intelligence (AI) has solved some of the complex problems virtually in our day-to-day life in today's world. COVID-19, social distancing, and sanitization are new norms of life. The primary diagnostic tool is radio imaging; however, it is much easier to diagnose the disease with artificial intelligence (AI) based deep learning methods. Computer vision is a scientific field that deals with how computers can be made to understand the real world from digital images or videos.

Emerging advances in bioinformatics enable home computers to become powerful supercomputers, reduce research expenses, enhance scientific efficiency, and accelerate novel discoveries. Bioinformatics can be understood as a field of data science based on computers and biology's amalgamation. Hence, to understand the complexity of underlying diseases and its mechanism, bioinformatics can be a fundamental approach to understanding bioinformatics, various omics tools, applications, health informatics, and the healthcare system.

The exponential growth and easy availability of biological and healthcare data have offered a movement in healthcare data science research activity. The traditional methods are incapable of processing and managing enormous quantities of complex, high-dimensional healthcare data in volume and variety. Recently, data science technologies have been increasingly used in the research of biomedical and healthcare informatics.

Bathinda, India   Amit Kumar Manocha
Solan, India   Shruti Jain
Patiala, India   Mandeep Singh
Shillong, India   Sudip Paul

Acknowledgment

We want to extend our gratitude to all the chapter authors for their sincere and timely support to make this book a grand success.

We are equally thankful to all members of Springer Nature's executive board for their kind approval and appointing us as editors of this book. We want to extend our sincere thanks to Susan Evans, Henry Rodgers, Shanthini Kamaraj, and Kamiya Khatter at Springer Nature for their valuable suggestions and encouragement throughout the project.

It is with immense pleasure that we express our thankfulness to our colleagues for their support, love, and motivation in all our efforts during this project. We are grateful to all the reviewers for their timely review and consent, which helped us improve the quality of the book.

We may have inadvertently left out many others, and we sincerely thank all of them for their help.

Amit Kumar Manocha
Shruti Jain
Mandeep Singh
Sudip Paul

Contents

Measurement of Human Bioelectricity and Pranic Energy of Different Organs: A Sensor and CPS-Based Approach   1
Rohit Rastogi, Mamta Saxena, Devendra Kumar Chaturvedi,
Mayank Gupta, Neha Gupta, Umang Agrawal, Yashi Srivastava,
and Vansh Gau

Development of Compression Algorithms for Computed Tomography and Magnetic Resonance Imaging   35
R. Pandian, S. LalithaKumari, D. N. S. RaviKumar,
and G. Rajalakshmi

Realization of Carry-Free Adder Circuit Using FPGA   53
Shruti Jain

Telemedicine and Telehealth: The Current Update   67
Dhruthi Suresh, Surabhi Chaudhari, Apoorva Saxena,
and Praveen Kumar Gupta

Advancements in Healthcare Using Wearable Technology   83
Sindhu Rajendran, Surabhi Chaudhari, and Swathi Giridhar

Machine and Deep Learning Algorithms for Wearable Health Monitoring 105
Chengwei Fei, Rong Liu, Zihao Li, Tianmin Wang, and Faisal N. Baig

Characterization of Signals of Noncontact Respiration Sensor for Emotion Detection Using Intelligent Techniques 161
P. Grace Kanmani Prince, R. Rajkumar Immanuel, B. Revathy,
B. Jeyanthi, J. Premalatha, and A. Sivasangari

Benefits of E-Health Systems During COVID-19 Pandemic 175
Amandeep Kaur, Anuj Kumar Gupta, and Harpreet Kaur

Low-Cost Bone Mineral Densitometer   191
Riddhi Vinchhi, Neha Zimare, Shivangi Agarwal, and Bharti Joshi

Smart Infusion Pump Control: The Control System Perspective   199
J. V. Alamelu and A. Mythili

**Automated Detection of Normal and Cardiac Heart Disease
Using Chaos Attributes and Online Sequential Extreme
Learning Machine**.   213
Ram Sewak Singh, Demissie Jobir Gelmecha, Dereje Tekilu Aseffa,
Tadesse Hailu Ayane, and Devendra Kumar Sinha

**Interference Reduction in ECG Signal Using IIR Digital
Filter Based on GA and Its Simulation**.   235
Ranjit Singh Chauhan

**Contactless Measurement of Heart Rate from Live Video
and Comparison with Standard Method**   257
A. N. Nithyaa, S. Sakthivel, K. Santhosh Kumar, and P. Pradeep Raj

**Automatic Melanoma Diagnosis and Classification
on Dermoscopic Images**   271
Bethanney Janney. J, S. Emalda Roslin, and J. Premkumar

GI Cloud Design: Issues and Perspectives   287
V. Lakshmi Narasimhan, A. K. Sala, and Anne Shergill

**A Hybrid Method for Detection of Coronavirus Through
X-rays Using Convolutional Neural Networks and Support
Vector Machine**.   305
P. Srinivasa Rao

Feature Extraction Using GLSM for DDSM Mammogram Images   317
Neha S. Shahare and D. M. Yadav

**Deep Learning-Based Techniques to Identify COVID-19
Patients Using Medical Image Segmentation**.   327
Rachna Jain, Shreyansh Singh, Surykant Swami, and Sanjeev kumar

Emerging Trends of Bioinformatics in Health Informatics.   343
Mahi Sharma, Shuvhra Mondal, Sudeshna Bhattacharjee,
and Neetu Jabalia

Computational Methods for Health Informatics   369
Jayakishan Meher

**Computational Model of a Pacinian Corpuscle for Hybrid-Stimuli:
Spike-Rate and Threshold Characteristics**.   379
V. Madhan Kumar, Venkatraman Sadanand, and M. Manivannan

Index.   397

About the Editors

Amit Kumar Manocha is presently working as an associate professor of electrical engineering at Maharaja Ranjit Singh Punjab Technical University, Bathinda, India. He is author of more than 50 research papers in refereed journals as well as national and international conferences. Dr. Manocha successfully organized five international conferences in the capacity of conference chair, convener, and editor of conference proceedings and more than 25 workshops and Seminars. He participated in many international conferences as advisory committee, session chair, and member of technical committee in international conferences. Dr. Manocha is member of the editorial boards of many international journals. His area of research includes biomedical instrumentation, remote monitoring, and control systems. He has guided more than 10 master's dissertations and is guiding 5 Ph.D.s at present. Dr. Manocha has been granted 2 patents and Rs. 36 Lacs from the Department of Science and Technology, Government of India, for research project on identification of adulterants in Indian spices.

Mandeep Singh is currently professor and former head of the Electrical and Instrumentation Engineering Department, Thapar Institute of Engineering & Technology, Patiala. Dr. Singh has a Ph.D. in tele-cardiology and is a Master of Engineering in computer science and Bachelor of Engineering in electronics (instrumentation and control). Dr. Singh is a BEE certified energy auditor and an empanelled consultant for PAT Scheme. Dr. Singh has more than 20 years of teaching experience. His current area of research interest includes biomedical instrumentation, energy conservation, alternative medicine and cognition engineering. In addition to his regular responsibilities, he has served Thapar Institute of Engineering & Technology as faculty advisor (Electrical) for more than 8 years. Dr. Singh is currently handling two research projects with DIPAS-DRDO related to fatigue detection and wireless monitoring of ambulatory subjects.

Shruti Jain is an associate professor in the Department of Electronics and Communication Engineering at Jaypee University of Information Technology, Waknaghat, H.P., India, and has received her D.Sc. in electronics and communication engineering. She has a teaching experience of around 15 years. Dr. Jain has filed three patents out of which one patent is granted and one is published. She has published more than 9 book chapters and 100 research papers in reputed indexed journals and at international conferences. Dr. Jain has also published six books. She has completed two government-sponsored projects. Dr. Jain has guided 6 Ph.D. students and now has 2 registered students. She has also guided 11 M Tech scholars and more than 90 B Tech undergrads. Her research interests are image and signal processing, soft computing, bio-inspired computing, and computer-aided design of FPGA and VLSI circuits. She is a senior member of IEEE, life member and editor in chief of Biomedical Engineering Society of India, and a member of IAENG. She is a member of the editorial board of many reputed journals. Dr. Jain is also a reviewer of many journals and a member of TPC of different conferences. She was bestowed with the Nation Builder Award in 2018–19.

Sudip Paul is currently an assistant professor and teacher (I/C) in the Department of Biomedical Engineering, School of Technology, North-Eastern Hill University (NEHU), Shillong, India. He completed his postdoctoral research at the School of Computer Science and Software Engineering, The University of Western Australia, Perth. He was one of the most prestigious fellowship awardees (Biotechnology Overseas Associateship for the Scientists working in the North Eastern States of India: 2017-18 supported by Department of Biotechnology, Government of India). He received his Ph.D. degree from the Indian Institute of Technology (Banaras Hindu University), Varanasi, with a specialization in electrophysiology and brain signal analysis. He has several credentials, one of them is his first prize at the Sushruta Innovation Award 2011 sponsored by the Department of Science and Technology, Govt. of India. Dr. Paul has organized many workshops and conferences, out of which the most significant are the IEEE Conference on Computational Performance Evaluation; 29th Annual meeting of the Society for Neurochemistry, India; and IRBO/APRC Associate School. Dr. Paul has published more than 80 international journals and conference papers and also filed six patents. He has completed 10 book projects with Springer Nature, Elsevier, and IGI Global. Dr. Paul is a member of different societies and professional bodies, including APSN, ISN, IBRO, SNCI, SfN, IEEE, and IAS. He has received many awards, especially the World Federation of Neurology (WFN) traveling fellowship, Young Investigator Award, IBRO Travel Awardee, and ISN Travel Awardee. Dr. Paul also contributed his knowledge in different international journals as editorial board members. He has presented his research accomplishments in the USA, Greece, France, South Africa, and Australia.

Measurement of Human Bioelectricity and Pranic Energy of Different Organs: A Sensor and CPS-Based Approach

Rohit Rastogi, Mamta Saxena, Devendra Kumar Chaturvedi, Mayank Gupta, Neha Gupta, Umang Agrawal, Yashi Srivastava, and Vansh Gau

Abstract The Kirlian photography is one of the most spectacular ways to shoot different subjects. It is a technique based on electrical coronal discharge. It may be quite a mystery for the beginners in the art of photography. It shows the auras of different subjects. In this technique, the photographic plate made of metal is charged with a high-voltage source. It may seem hard to master this, but let me tell you it is still easier to shoot objects using Kirlian photography. The process is also quite simple. All an individual needs is to ready all equipment. It is recommended to use transparent electrodes instead of the discharge plate. It is a very interesting method to capture the coronal discharge of certain subjects. It will surprise you every time! The present manuscript is an effort by the researcher team to discuss the human bioelectricity and measure the different biophysical factors and reasons of different ill symptoms. We have tried to investigate the energy balances, head, and immune and musculoskeletal systems of subjects under study.

Keywords Kirlian photography · Bioelectricity · Covid-19 · Happiness · Radiation · Head · Immune · Musculoskeletal systems

R. Rastogi (✉) · N. Gupta · U. Agrawal · Y. Srivastava · V. Gau
Department of CSE, ABESEC, Ghaziabad, UP, India
e-mail: rohit.rastogi@abes.ac.in; neha.18bcs1006@abes.ac.in;
umang.18bcs1041@abes.ac.in; yashi.18ben1017@abes.ac.in;
vansh.18bcs1158@abes.ac.in

M. Saxena
Ministry of Statistics, Government of India, Delhi, India

D. K. Chaturvedi
Department of Electrical Engineering, DEI, Agra, India

M. Gupta
IT and System Analyst, Tata Consultancy Services, Noida, India

© The Author(s), under exclusive license to Springer
Nature Switzerland AG 2021
A. K. Manocha et al. (eds.), *Computational Intelligence in Healthcare*, Health
Information Science, https://doi.org/10.1007/978-3-030-68723-6_1

1

1 Introduction

1.1 Human Bioelectricity

The electric current continuously flows in the human body (termed as bioelectricity) that plays a vital role in physiological conditions. The human body consists of millions of nerves which transfer information and are responsible for the whole functioning of the body through electrical impulse which is actually bioelectric signals. So we can term bioelectricity as the electric current which is present inside the living body or produced within it. The number of biological processes occurs every second in the human body which leads to formation of bioelectric currents. Bioelectric currents and potential of human cells and tissues are recorded by machines like ECG, EEG, etc., which can be used in making medicines for various organs of human. Consciousness simply means awareness of both internal and external existence of self. Till now, despite of analyses, explanation, and researches, consciousness is still a topic of debate among scientists. Opinions of every philosopher and scientist vary from one to another. In recent days, consciousness is now a significant topic in cognitive science. Even we can measure the degree of consciousness by behavior observation scales. The famous scientist Locke defined consciousness as "the perception of what passes in a man's own mind." Ned Block suggested that there are two types of consciousness named as phenomenal (P-consciousness) and access (A-consciousness).

1.2 Global Understanding on Consciousness

Consciousness can be seen as a role of energy in our brain. Any type of activities requiring energy done by the body involves physical processes leading to biological behavior. This product of energetic activities in our brain is termed as consciousness. The consciousness and functioning of the brain is related to each other in some or other way.

Brain operates on some principles of energy processing, and this presence of energy in the brain with some additional techniques, the presence of consciousness, can be predicted. Thus, the consciousness can be termed as not only presence of mind but presence of some kind of energy that drives various activities taking place in our brain [32].

Meditation refers to a family of techniques which have in common a conscious attempt to focus attention in a non analytical way and an attempt not to dwell on discursive, ruminating thought. The term "discursive thought" has long been used in Western Philosophy and is often viewed as a synonym to logical thought.

1.3 Kirlian Photography

Kirlian photography is contact print photography which is connected with high voltage. In 1939, Semyon Kirlian found that if an object on photographic plate is exposed to strong electric field, an image of object will be created. He claimed that this discovery gives the proof of supernatural auras. These photographs are considered to be mysterious and controversial over the years. Although Kirlian discovered this method in 1939, he didn't make it public till 1958. The machine that was used in this process was a spark generator which works at around 75 kHz. As Kirlian claimed that the images, so produced, showed aura of living entities, his machine trends among the professional scientists [7]. After the success of this experiment, Kirlian became very popular. All magazines and newspaper were flooded with the success story of Kirlian; even a short educational film was produced on this experiment. The physiologist Gordon Stein wrote that Kirlian photography is only a hoax and it had nothing to do with vitality and auras of living being. In order to verify that claims of Kirlian were true, a typical experiment was done on a leaf which is popularly known as torn leaf experiment.

Photography is one of the most visual medium to capture something. There are a wide variety of techniques and aspects used in photography. The right use of these aspects can lead to unexpected results.

A similar technique was accidentally discovered in 1939 by Semyon Kirlian and his wife Valentina and thus given the name Kirlian photography. Once during their visit to a hospital, they noticed a patient receiving high-frequency generator treatment and that sparked in them an idea to conduct an experiment [30].

The Kirlian photography is also known to be as aura photography as it contains different auras/subjects. Their inventors claimed that it can be used to shoot different aura of living beings. The photographs resulted from this experiment also depicted force that surrounds every single being on this planet (Ref.: https://www.pixsy.com/kirlian-photography-image-protection/).

1.4 Energy Measurement

In physics, we define energy as the physical quantity which can only be transferred from one form to other. Energy can neither be created nor be destroyed. The SI unit of energy is joule. There are also other forms of energy such as kinetic energy (moving body), potential energy (position of body), and gravitational energy (gravitational force of earth). The most famous scientist of all time Albert Einstein said that energy and mass are correlated to each other, and he proposed his statement by eq. $E = MC^2$.

Every living organism needs energy to survive, and most of their energy they get from food they eat. James Prescott Joule was the scientist in honor of which SI unit of energy was named as joule. The units of measurement of energy is numerous, among them well-known are tons used for coal, barrel for crude oil, cubic meter for gases, and liters for petrol and diesel. Besides joule, there are many other units of energy measurement such as kilowatt hour (which is widely used to calculate bill of electricity). The most common units measuring heat include the BTU (British thermal unit) and the kilogram calorie (kg-cal) [5].

There are two types of energy, where one is energy in rest and other is energy in motion. Energy is measured in various units. Some of them can be seen as:

- Joule (J)
- Watt which is joule/second
- Their definitions are the following:
- 1 Joule (J) is the MKS unit of energy which is equivalent to force of 1 Newton
- 1 Watt is the power of a Joule of energy per second

1.5 Bioelectricity

The electric current continuously flows in the human body (termed as bioelectricity) that plays a vital role in physiological conditions. The human body consists of millions of nerves which transfer information and are responsible for the whole functioning of the body through electrical impulse which is actually bioelectric signals. So we can term bioelectricity as the electric current which is present inside the living body or produced within it [9]. The number of biological processes occurs every second in the human body which leads to formation of bioelectric currents. Bioelectric currents and potential of human cells and tissues are recorded by machines like ECG, EEG, etc., which can be used in making medicines for various organs of human. All the bioelectric activities associated with the skin and tissue are used to make biomedicines. Till the eighteenth century, European physicians and philosophers believed that nerves transfer the information to the brain through some organic fluid, but later on two Italian scientists demonstrated the concept of bioelectricity. Emil du Bois-Reymond, a very famous scientist of that time, discovered that during any tissue injury a unique electric potential is generated, and he named bioelectric current as "the current of injury" [8].

1.6 Pranik Urja

The life energy which keeps us alive and strong is called prana or ki. The word prana is derived from Sanskrit word and is recognized by most of our ancient culture. It also means the breath of life. The more life energy that one person has, the more energetic and excited that person is. Pranayama is the nutrition of life. It is essential to keep the body healthy and happy. Sun, wind and ground are the major sources of Pranik Urja. The solar prana (or energy) can be obtained by sitting in the sunlight for 5–10 minutes or by drinking water kept under the sun. The air prana is absorbed directly by our energy centers. It is obtained by slow and rhythmic breathing. Color prana or life energy is mostly of six types: red prana, orange prana, green prana, yellow prana, blue prana, and violet prana. And the pranic energy is mainly defined into two types: electric violet pranic energy and golden pranic energy [29]."By remembering you are in an ocean of life energy, your life energy level will automatically increase."

Pranik Urja means pranic energy (feel divinity all around you).

The main sources of these kinds of energy are solar, air, and the ground.

1.7   The Human Body and Seven Chakras

The human body is one of the most complex structures of living beings. It has millions and billions of cells, tissues, RBC, WBC, nerves cells, etc. The human body is the most developed and advanced structure, as it has brain (organ to think, very memory), heart (for blood circulation), lungs (for breathing), kidneys (to filter out toxics from body), etc. The study of the human body involves anatomy, and physiology. The main component of the human body is hydrogen, oxygen, calcium, carbon, and phosphorus. The human body contains several systems like circulatory system, digestive system, immune system, and many more. The human body is like a machine which runs only when energy is provided to it. It is said that there are seven chakras in the human body [15].

First one is root chakra (Muladhara); it represents the foundation of human and is located around spine base. Second is sacral chakra (Swadhisthana) which helps in dealing our emotions with others and located in the lower abdomen. Third is solar plexus chakra (Manipura) which represents our confidence and located around the upper abdomen. Fourth is heart chakra (Anahata); it is located in the chest center. Fifth is throat chakra (Vishuddha) which controls our communication and is located in the throat. Sixth is third-eye chakra (Ajna) and located between the eyes. Last is crown chakra (Sahasrara) which is found on top of our head [1].

Ours mental health depends on our outlook and our attitude toward everything. The way we think and the way we develop rapid thoughts are the reason we grow in life. Hence, there are some energy centers in our soul which give us energy to do anything. They are the following:

- Muladhara chakra – root chakra
- Swadhisthana chakra – sacral chakra
- Manipura chakra – solar plexus chakra
- Anahata chakra – heart chakra
- Vishuddha chakra – throat chakra
- Ajna chakra – third eye chakra
- Sahasrara chakra – crown chakra

All the above chakras lead us to live life and have their own significance [6].

1.8   Aura of the Human Body

The word "aura" means wind or breeze. It is believed that there exists an aura or human energy field. Since ancient times we see many pictures and paintings in which the human body is surrounded by a visible energy field known as aura energy field. The aura represents the mental, physical, and spiritual energy of being, and it also contains a mixture of different color frequencies in which each color has its own significance and characteristics. By scientific researches, scientists came across a conclusion that this aura actually is electromagnetic field of energy which comes out from a body of men and is 4–5 feet tall in the case of healthy person, but its strength reduces in the case of unhealthy person. Studies show that aura is associated with the human health. If a person is healthy in terms of physical vitality, mental clarity, and emotional well-being, then obviously that person will emit a positive spiritual energy. Today all scientists come across a result that the matter which appears to be solid is not real solid. These solids actually are made up of energy which is emitting frequencies; it is also confirmed that whenever there is an electric field, there develops magnetic field around it. So aura is an electromagnetic field of the body [11].

The human aura means energy field of the human body which acts as shield to the human body.

It is directly connected to energy centers of the body, the seven chakras discussed above. It creates an egg-shaped field aura surrounding the human body originating from the chakras. Actually, the truth is we all are interconnected. Still it's our thoughts which make us believe we're different. Actually this interconnectedness can be observed through the term human aura. Some examples of above arguments are feeling of love, anxiety, sadness, and fear [2].

1.9   Yin and Yang Energy

Yin and Yang is related to Chinese philosophy. Actually Yin and Yang is a concept of duality, i.e., the opposite poles. It is related to negative-positive, dark-bright, meaning things that are contrary to each other. Yin is receptive and Yang is active principle, and it is seen in every form such as annual cycle (winter-summer), sexual couples (men-women), etc. In Chinese cosmology, yin and yang are material energy from which the universe has created. Yin and yang are opposite of each other, and both are interdependent on each other. Both of them are necessity of life as they counterbalance each other, but they can't inter-transform each other. It seems that every human has yin and yang energy or good or bad side, and it depends on human to which side they prefer and what they become. Yin and yang is also present in symbol form in which yin represents white area and Yang represents black area. Yang energy is considered to be masculine, very expanding, active, energetic, and light. Some properties of Yang are heaven, sun, light, time, etc. [10].

It is a concept of dualism, meaning that even the forces which seem opposite or contrary can also be complimentary, interconnected, or interdependent in the natural world. These all actually give rise to each other. According to the Chinese cosmology, the reason of this universe is primary material energy which forms all kinds of objects and lives. In the concept of Yin and Yang, Yin is the passive, i.e., receptive, and Yang is the active principle. They can be seen in all forms of change. Some of them are annual cycle, sociopolitical history, sexual coupling, the landscape, and all other different laws of nature [14].

1.10 Quantum Consciousness

It was a failure of classical mechanics which was not able to explain consciousness and derived a group of hypothesis known as quantum consciousness. They proposed quantum-mechanical phenomenon like superposition that plays vital role in brain functioning of human and can easily explain consciousness. Also, it is believed that quantum idea is necessary for the brain to even exist.

There exists a strange link between the human mind and quantum physics. Nobody understands quantum and consciousness. It's because both are somehow related to each other. The classical mechanics cannot explain the human consciousness [16].

The consciousness emerges from complex computation among brain neurons which is similar to digital computing in quantum physics. Same as quantum can be used to understand the two various things at a time, the human mind can contain two mutually exclusive ideas at a time. Just as quantum is mysterious, same as consciousness.

Thus, consciousness is a manifestation of quantum processes in the brain.

Some still thinks consciousness is a mere illusion. Yet, the real origin of this is still unknown.

The famous "double-slit experiment" simply introduces the quantum mechanics in a more fashionable way.

The concept behind the term is that quantum theory may actually explain how the brain really works. Same as quantum objects can be apparently present at two places at a time; similarly, the quantum brain can hold onto two mutually exclusive ideas at the same time [17].

1.11 Science of Meditation and Its Effect on the Human Body

Now discussing about medication, studies show that medication can affect both physical and mental well-being of a person. The main purpose of doing medication is to know what is going on in one's mind. Medication can be useful in many ways, but side by side its harmful too. By taking medication, we get relief from pain, depression, and anxiety. In ancient time many people die as we don't have any cure for it, but now we have medication for almost all the diseases that surround us. From cancer to simple cold, we have medication for everything; from headache to stomachache, all can be cured. Consuming a lot of medicines can have many side effects; it may harm the antibodies, produce many hormones, and/or reduce fertility in both male and females. According to a research by Harvard, there have been a number of key areas like depression, anxiety, etc. where mindful meditation has shown benefits for the patients. Meditation has shown many benefits. Eight weeks of meditation can reduce aging. It can improve memory [18].

Our health has two aspects: physical and mental. When the body is fit physically, it doesn't mean he/she is fit mentally and emotionally. The highest level is spiritual level which is even far higher than soul. It means understanding the real self and the reason for your existence. All these can be achieved by performing meditation which can be said as an exercise for the better mind.

Different types of meditation practices followed are concentration, mindfulness, etc.

The benefits are the following:

- Lower blood pressure
- Less perspiration
- Less stress and anxiety
- Deeper relaxation
- Feeling of well-being [19]

Our mental health is as much important as the body. Meditation helps the mental health in following ways:

- Reduce stress
- Controls anxiety
- Promotes emotional health
- Enhances self-awareness
- Increases concentration
- Reduces memory loss due to aging
- Also reduces bad addictions
- Builds honesty and kindness
- Helps in quick healing
- Improves bad sleeping habits
- Improves blood pressure problems

1.12   Science of Mantra and Its Effect on the Human Body

Yajna means sacrifice, devotion, and offerings. It is the holy work that we do to make our god happy; we offer mantras, japs. It has been seen that in our scriptures, we are doing Yagya for welfare of humanity. Whenever we face a gigantic difficulty, a solution is to make gods happy by doing Yagyas. Its effect is very positive on humanity. The chanting sound of Gayatri mantra and heat from the fire of Yajna is a powerful combination and produces some important effects. We chant the Sanskrit mantras while performing the Yagyas; these send vibrations which ensure proper functioning of our body parts. The cosmic energy associated with the Gayatri Mantra is of the sun. These mantras sooth our mind and calm us. Performing Yagya also helps in removal of insects and bacteria in our environment. The environment becomes light and pleasurable. Not only it makes us happy, but it provides positivity to people who participate in them [12, 13].

This is believed to be another gift of Indian sciences which is for the betterment of us.

In the course of doing this holy Yagya, the two main energies, heat and sound, are released. This, along with the sound of the mantras such as Gayatri Mantra or other Vedic mantras, helps to achieve what we are wishing for. This is mainly done to get some physical, psychological, or spiritual benefits [20].

Yajna literally means devotion, worship, and offering. It is a process of cleaning oneself by invoking fire.

1.13 Science of Yajna (Yagya) and Its Effect on the Human Body

Yagya is a type of Holy Fire Ritual performed by Hindus to destroy the demons (the Asuras).

It is a ritual followed since the Vedic times with fact that it destroys negative energy.

The head and sound are two basic types of energies.

In performing Yajna, these two energies, namely, the heat from Yagya fire and the sound of the chanting of the Gayatri and other Vedic Mantras, are blended together to achieve the desired physical, psychological, and spiritual benefits [21].

The science behind using Ghee in Yagya is that Ghee helps in combustion of wood and keeping fire on. So, it is an important reason to recommend to perform rituals of Yajna in sunlight.

This reason is taken from (https://www.speakingtree.in/allslides/scientific-aspects-of-yagya-the-holy-fire-ritual).

1.14 Artificial Intelligence for Health Informatics

In modern world, which is full of new fresh ideas which are capable of generating innovative technology which has a potential to surprise everyone in this world? This modernization we can see in our medical sciences. Healthcare organizations have adopted new development. Today, machines can act, sense, and behave similar to the brain of the human being which is made possible only because of artificial technologies.

Due to AI, our medical system handles large set of data sets (information overload issue faced by health official is solved), solve complex problems using its analytical skills, and also able to handle administrative functions.

AI is able to handle large data and work efficiently because of machine learning technology which acts as its backbone [33].

1.15 Health Sensor Data Management

With its regular increase in market size, smart devices such as smart watch, smartphone, fit-bit like devices have created its popularity and unique identity.

With their useful features and extra ordinary applications of sensor based gadgets, people love to use these products so that they can keep an eye on data of patients without affecting their personal lives in a convenient way. Smartphone contains many embedded sensors such as microphones, cameras, gyroscopes, accelerometers, compasses, proximity sensors, GPS, and ambient light. Easily wearable and tear-off medical sensors can easily connect with the smartphones and transfer the sensing results directly. This helps a lot in maintaining blood pressure and calories in the body using fit-bit-type smart device.

Newly arising technology like artificial intelligence, internet of things, and data analytics gives an edge in easy and fast approach of data collection and performs certain action on it [22].

1.16 Multimodal Data Fusion for Healthcare

Data Classification is one of the most important area of work for understanding the features and conditions of different objects and data mining is a popular tool regarding this. The medical and healthcare sector handles big data which is available in unstructured form and it generates many difficulties like complexity of characteristics, functional diversity and redundant informations. These problems generated by multimodal unstructured data cannot be directly utilized by traditional machine learning methods. Therefore, some researchers have tried to implement multimodal data fusion using deep learning techniques [23].

Multimodal data fusion-based data processing method has high flexibility. This data processing method has a potential to work upon traditional data processing methods and respond to dynamic data. This method is able to reduce the load of data calculation by combining different fusion methods, but it requires significant effort to fuse data in the right way.

1.17   Heterogeneous Data Fusion and Context-Aware Systems for the Internet of Things Health

The number of internet-connected devices present in our day-to-day life is currently increasing in an exponential way. We use these devices at every place like home, workplace, etc. Even people like to interact with each other using these embedded devices [24].

A quite high number of researches are done on data fusion process using complex algorithms. In this, data is acquired and processed from heterogeneous sources and always centralized on a powerful computing node. We have a method which is based on lightweight service composition model to implement a distributed data fusion acquisition, which is able to ensure the correctness of collaborations without a cyclic behavior. Due to this method, we can work on decentralized and distributed manner and allow developers to use the concept of service and the interaction among services to design the high level of abstraction in IoT scenario [25].

The distributed approach for data fusion makes the service model very scalable and a really important aspect in the development of future applications, which can be deployed in embedded devices.

2   Literature Survey

Paper-1 Starting with some analysis, what we did was, we compared 61 healthy-state people with 256 patient people who had bronchial asthma. The study of the so-called bioelectrograms of those patients had been studied for the same. A widely used technique gas discharge visualization, i.e., GDV, had been employed for all the analysis. It is a type of bioelectrograph technique. Let's have a brief discussion on this technique as how this originated and from where. The GDV-gram taken from the fingertips of the hands of the person being the victim and the method of same is given further.

The main instrument and technology used hereby the team of authors is GDV camera and GDV processor which helps in maintenance of GDI processing and records. The main factors that we have taken into account was organization of data; other than this, the focus was on factors which interfered with our analysis. The main condition was to do registration of subjects to be done on GDV camera to see the Kirlian effects. Also, the mandatory coefficients like integral area, form, and emission are also required as methods of the GDV-gram being taken. Moving further, before giving out the conclusion and result of analysis, an experimental data has been studied. Its application is mentioned herewith.

As mentioned and reported before, GDV-gram of fingertips of both hands are taken separately to be able to differentiate the value of indices of both hands. Then, basically, the average is taken as a final observation. Both fingers' study taken as an individual study is thus obtained by us. Now, moving more further, based on the obtained value, the final evaluation of result is thus done, and the final lines are obtained as a conclusion.

While expanding the discussion a little for clear understanding, GDV (Gas Discharge Visualization) has been accepted and it is a type of bio electro graph technique.

All the data and info is collected in a group of three people, the elaborated types of the three are as follows. First type consisted healthy people, the second including BA victim, and the last one included ulcer and stomach patients. This was done basically to study the results more widely and clearly differentiate them. The main parameters we focused on was on the coefficients like farcicality (FC) , emission (EC), and the integral area as already being mentioned above. Using the calculated values, the results are drawn.

This was just an upgrade of the previous derived techniques, now also known as gas discharge (GDV) bioelectrograph. In this one we added a more wider medical practice, beyond the previous one. Now, it is capable of monitoring clinical trials by clinical acumen and diagnostics. It was thus able to upgrade the previously used practices and tools. Formally, the collection and monitoring of multi-morbid patients can be now more organized with the help of the impact created by medications in comparison with the properties related to energy information. This also made selecting the right therapy simpler and accurate.

For our second-category people comprised of BA victims, this technique can be more widely employed. The biological functions of their body are made more in the course of the treatment process. This can also help in other ways too. Let's talk about them. The indications which are more relevant for medicinal as well as non-medicinal mergers of treatment are drawn now from the GDV-gram.

There can be one disadvantage here in this process. The patients with acute myocardial infarction is not accurate and not allowed as well as it can have side effects on them.

Now conning on the main section of the literature survey, the conclusions are ready to be mentioned. The patterns obtained from those samples of the GDV-gram can be simply and accurately related now with all three different groups of people. The main correlation was obtained by the BE technology with all collected pathogenic information. The result can be categorized into two sections. First, the traditional medical solution and homeopathy which is a collection of strategies, some of which are optional. We are now introduced to a newer technology, GDV-BE, which can study different medicinal solutions and problems such as diseases and infections and allergies by fluid commonly called as auras in vitro which is clearly biological. Also, the more elaborated organism can be studied in the similar way by simple comparison. At last, this can be more used in the fields of sports, business, professions, and other well-known works.

Paper-2 In these series of analysis and studies, the contributors have categorized the conditions into three subsets. First one is orthostatic test followed by deep breathing, second is 10 minutes of serious exercise, and the last one is intake of chocolate, being the most important as it is performed to reduce stress and fear.

Different correlations can be observed in these tests such as the correlation of the sympathetic component of HRV and GDV. As a result of these, the GDV measures can be used as well-being in different physiological conditions.

These physiological conditions are affected by different negative thoughts and emotions such as anger and fear, whereas the positive thoughts will leave a positive and productive effect on the body. This investigation examines as if such correlation between HRV and GDV can measure a well-being. All the cardiovascular activities are regulated by the nervous system; hence, the activities of both branches of the nervous system can be observed or judged by the heart rate variability (HRV) [3].

The methodology used in this paper is the amplifier with time constant (T) = 2.5 and (T) = 10 s. The rheostat and a variable capacitance are connected in parallel in the Wein bridge.

A sinusoidal wave of 1000 cps is used as an alternating current in the process.

For observing galvanization effect, DC is used [31].

Instruments and Data set used were related to traditional electrocardiogram which was equipped with four electrodes which as connected to left and right hands and left and right ankles to measure the HRV (Heart Rate Variability). GDV Compact Device and GDV Processor Software were used for the analysis of those images.

In supine position, the patient was asked to take a deep breath. This was done for a time period of 5 minutes. Also, the subject was asked to resume regular tidal breathing. Then after that, the readings were obtained. Before the GDV and HRV parameters are calculated, a 10-minute exercise was involved. Then, the third condition involved consumption of dark chocolate 3 hours after GDV and HRV parameters were measured [3].

Application of Work

Impedance change during response: On comparing the obtained GRS's, the impedance is observed to vary gradually with lapse of time.

The effect of removal of the epidermis: Two records (lower and upper) are recorded using small and large electrode, respectively. It is performed on the left little finger and right little finger [31].

A comparison of endosomatic and exosomatic method is made, and the changes in the wave form are observed using small electrodes.

Impedance change observed by negative process and sweat gland activities is judged by positive process.

The impedance change is independent of secretary activities. The response always followed a monophasic fashion [31].

Paper-3 In the absence of the epidermis, the galvanic skin reflex can be observed. It can be recorded by impedance change in the presence of current flow. Two processes called as negative and positive can be observed simultaneously using this. Two parts of the body are in connection using a galvanometer in Tarchanoff's galvanic skin response.

Tarchanoff also suggested the involvement of a sweat gland in this reflex. The indication of physiological event is confirmed using the abovementioned methods. It will also help to clarify the quantitative treatment of this galvanic skin reflex [31].

Gas discharge visualization (GSV) and heart rate variability (HRV) are mainly two methods used. The two were used as follows:

- GSV – Image analysis, registering both static and dynamic GDV images, and all the GDV parameters are described using this method.
- HRV – Using R-R time interval variability, the parameters are measured, and peaks in the very-low-frequency range are revealed by the spectral analysis of those time domain parameters [3].

Instruments and data set used: (A) Wein bridge is used as an instrument in the above process. (B) Variable resistance and capacitance are connected to form a parallel circuit. (C) GSR is used to check the balancing of the bridge. (D) The endosomatic and exosomatic methods are used for comparing the GRS [31].

Application of work is that, as discussed above, the cardiovascular activities are centrally controlled by our nervous system; it involves fluctuations in HRV. Hence, these fluctuations provide us a tool to measure the relativeness of both its branches. Also, the correlation between spectral analysis and fetal well-being is allowed by high sensitivity to hypoxia [3].

Future scope and limitations of this paper state that mostly positive deflection is observed in the removal of the epidermis. The negative one can be recorded after a slight regeneration of the same. The positive deflection was less observed with small electrode.

Conclusions of this paper says that the main purpose to establish the correlation was successful. Using those parameters of GDV and HRV, the main conclusions drawn are as follows:

- The study clearly observes a statistical correlation exists between brightness parameters of GDV and HRV (VLF component).

The range of frequency (VLF) is seen as 0.003–0.04 Hz, whereas the upper region can be seen as 0.01–0.04 Hz [3]. Therefore, on seeing the correlation, it can be concluded that "well-being can be measured as resilience to psychophysical stimuli."

3   The Methodology and Protocols Followed

The methodology which was followed during this experiment were based on capturing photos by Kirlian camera. The volunteers had to chant and meditate for 15 minutes daily. Then they also had to perform Yagya. This turned out to be very beneficial for cancer patients. Even the European platform of Cancer and European Organization for Research and Treatment of Cancer supported this research work. It also shows a positive growth toward people's happiness index and quality of life.

3.1 Experimental Setup of an Expert System

The experiment was conducted on almost 20 volunteers for over a month. The research was mainly focused on Kirlian photography, which could analyze the volunteer's organs and brain structure. During this 1 month, they all had to do mantra jap and meditation.

Mr. Jagdish Sharma, Jaipur, 35 years old, and Mr. Manish Lakshar, Noida, 38 years old, participated in it and followed all the protocols and experiment-related disciplines.

4   Results and Discussions

4.1   Results, Interpretation, and Analysis on Healthcare Experiments

In the experiment, two subjects have been taken. These persons were checked for various states of energy before and then 30 minutes after Yagya. Their reports were compared and analyzed.

On a detailed analysis of individual organs, it has been found that before Yagya the energy variation across the organs was more, from 3.795 to 4.920×10^{-2} joule. Energy in the body is not evenly distributed. Some organs on higher side of energy state cause other organs to be on lower energy state. This misbalance in energy states causes unbalanced organs.

It has been clearly seen that the nervous system before Yagya has been found in higher energy side, while the organs like musculoskeletal systems are having lowest energy. But after 30 minutes of Yagya, the energy state has been found more evenly distributed, i.e., from 3.83 to 4.46×10^{-2} joule. This leads to balanced organs in our body that will definitely lead to healthier emotional balance and happy life. The organs of higher energy states moved toward lower energy state, while organs on lower energy state starts moving toward higher energy state, creating overall energy balance across the organs. Let's see each organs analysis individually (as per Fig. 1.1).

On analysis of different organs, the energy distribution before and after has been analyzed, as below.

4.2   Head System

The brain controls all the activity of the human body. It's the brain who sends signal to different body organs and parts. The brain is a large web of connected neurons, called as "connectome." Connectome fires when human senses, feels, sees, and

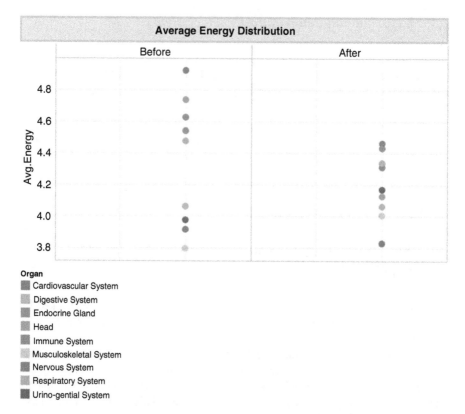

Fig. 1.1 Energy distribution through Kirlian of both subjects for their different organs before and after the Yajna/meditation and mantra protocols

experiences various things around us. By firing, it creates subjective experience for humans. On the other hand, human unconscious brain pays close attention to the nature of what person is focusing on, accordingly, then produced neurotransmitters like dopamine or norepinephrine. Dopamine makes the good motivation and helps remember the things, while norepinephrine is associated with sadness, pain, or bad feelings; thereby, release of it makes people more focused (as per Fig. 1.2).

These neurotransmitters in turn affects energy levels, by triggering the nervous system which in turn increases the blood rate by increasing the heart pumping which improves the blood circulation and muscle tone. All these make humans more switched on and productive.

This is also two-way true, i.e., the change in energy level of the brain will trigger the corresponding sad or good mood swings. So, maintaining the energy level of the brain in the normal range and in sync with other body organs is very much required.

Both the subject reduction in energy of 16.8% and 9% is observed.

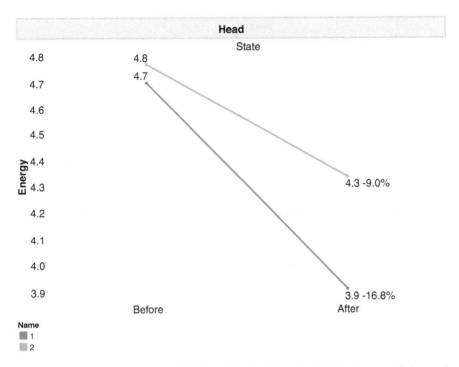

Fig. 1.2 Energy distribution through Kirlian of both subjects for their head systems before and after the Yajna/meditation and mantra protocols

4.3 Immune System

Maintaining good immune system is very much required to safeguard our body from external viruses and bacteria attacks. Immune system is like the doctor within our body which takes care of our body from external attacks. Maintaining the harmonious energy level of immune system is very important for good physical, mental, and emotional health (as per Fig. 1.3).

In the current study, subject 1 immune system energy was on the higher side before the Yagya which reduced by 12.3% and brings toward the mean energy level of other body organs, whereas the other subject's immune system has almost the same energy level as that of the body, so there is no much change in the body.

4.4 Musculoskeletal System

Muscle gets tensed in response to body stress, in order to guard against injury and pain. When the body is not used to muscle tension, eventually atrophy promotes the chronic stress. Yagya helps with relaxation of the muscles which reduces the pain

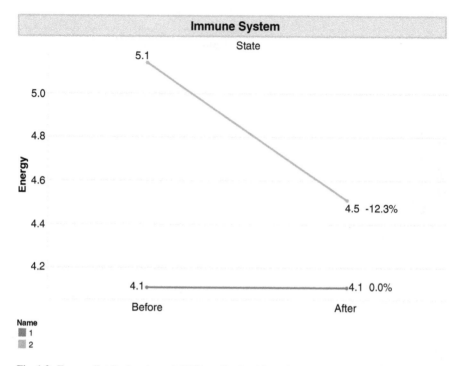

Fig. 1.3 Energy distribution through Kirlian of both subjects for their immune systems before and after the Yajna/meditation and mantra protocols

such as muscle-related pains like headache, migraine pain, etc. In the same way when energy level gets down for muscles, the stress gets induced, due to which maintaining the proper energy of muscles is very important (as per Fig. 1.4).

Subject 1 has reduced 10.4% of energy level to come to mean energy level of the body, while subject 2 has increased 30.2% of energy to reach up to 3.9×10^{-2} joule of energy.

5 Applications of Yagya and Mantra Therapy in Kirlian Captures

5.1 Science of Mantra and Its Effect on the Human Body

Researchers are done on mantras, and the results need to be understood. Mantra is the most powerful tool for human says our culture and beliefs. Mantra empowers us and our mind. Doing jap and mantra reduces fear, suppression, depression, and disappointment in humans. Mantra has a great impact on our body; it keeps us cool, sensible, and confident, and all these are proven in researches. It provides benefit at

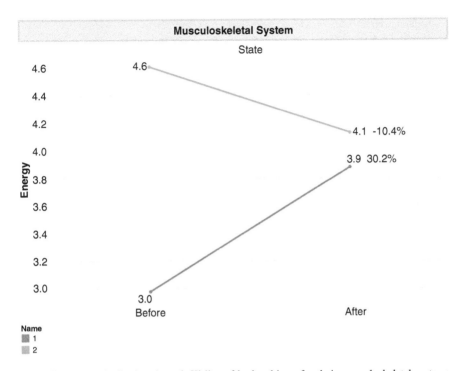

Fig. 1.4 Energy distribution through Kirlian of both subjects for their musculoskeletal systems before and after the Yajna/meditation and mantra protocols

all physical level, mental level, spiritual level, and psychological level. Mantra is also discussed in Geeta, all our Vedas. A study at Duke University showed significant improvement in the moods after practicing 4 weeks of mantra. Mantra connects to our inner soul. When mantra is accompanied with peace and calmness, it helps bring the positive memories. So, it has been proved by research that ancient mantra practice can heal and strengthen our mind and body.

Application of Mantra effectiveness is captured by a sound tool in Sanskrit language and Om is one of the group of syllables applied myriad in all such Mantras. In fact, the sound of the universe is also believed to be Om and also the sound of the human mind. That's why, during yoga, people keep chanting Om. It gives inner feeling of relaxation and peace [28].

Applications in chakra measurements – Illness or bad health of our body is as much dependent on our mind as body. The mental, spiritual, or overall attitude of a person toward life, the thoughts, gestures, communication strategy, and feelings play an integral part in one's growth.

Keeping this in mind, the seven chakras can be classified as:

- Sahasrara: Crown chakra which signifies spirituality
- Vishuddha: Third-eye chakra which depicts awareness
- Ajna: Throat chakra which means communication

- Anahata: Heart chakra which means love and feelings
- Manipura: Solar plexus chakra which means power of wisdom
- Swadhisthana: Sacral chakra which signifies sexual creativity
- Muladhara: Root chakra which contains trust

Applications in Pranik Urja calculations – Pranik is a Hindi word meaning life or pran.

This is a type of energy present all around us in different forms helping us to live life or we can say, because of them we can be alive, e.g., air, water, land, etc.

This is also known as life energy and without which we can't live. The following types of pranic energy are solar prana or solar energy received from sunlight which helps us to energize our cells and keep us in good health. However, it should be taken in limited amount.

Air and water are the two most fundamental requirement of any living organism. The air we breathe in is absorbed by the lungs which is then transferred to main energy centers of our body known as chakras. The third type of energy is absorbed by our feet when we walk. This is ground energy which makes us able to walk.

6 Future Research Perspectives

There exists a clear correlation between normal human adult and the diseased patients with the help of these GDV and HRV parameters. Therefore, any of the GDV or HRV parameters might help us to correlate between the well-beings in a non-disease population also. Also, acute myocardial infarction is followed by the cardiovascular patients in the first 3 days [3].

7 Novelty of the Research

There are millions of behaviors we possess in our day-to-day life. That may be a kind of process or movement taking place in our body. What do you think? What controls them? Yes, you are right. It's the brain that manages all those activities through well-designed nerves. Any animal life is so complex to understand but can be classified into three key components [27].

They are as follows:

- Communication
- Play
- The use of various tools

All these components interact with each other on the basis of anticipatory behavioral control which is common in almost all kinds of life. Thus, consciousness is actually a kind of behavior controlled by the brain. Some of those include awareness, communication, embodiment, objectivity, play, tool use, virtual reality, etc.

This research is very new and unique in all the aspects. Researches on similar fields were carried out on 2002 by the Russian Scientist Konstantin Korotkov. Since then much efforts in this field haven't been witnessed.

The manuscript also deals with the aura, a part of our body, that all living beings have. It is an energy anatomy which surrounds us. This can be understood as the layer or covering to the human body that connects our energy to that of energy of the universe. The one who understands this will get to know the reason of his/her existence. It reveals the real you.

Many religions such as Buddhism and Jainism believed this and can be found there. This interconnects the energy chakra of our body to the central energy which binds all of us.

It has several layers:

- Archetypal
- Spiritual
- Mental
- Emotional
- Imaginal
- Etheric
- Physical (Ref.: https://paranormal.lovetoknow.com/Human_Aura)

8 Recommendations

Om is the most powerful word of this universe. The sound which is inevitable in this universe is sound of Om. Hindus says it as Om, Christians says it as Amen, and different religions call it by different name. In our country we know there is a culture of jap; it is from ancient times. We have many stories of ancient time where sadhus are doing jap to achieve the powers, satisfaction, and self-development and bring pleasure in them. For jap we use mala in hand; this mala has several pearls, and we count each pearl till it counts 108 (it is the minimal count of jap). Talking about the effect of jap on the human body, it's effect is unexpectedly very positive on the human body [26].

By doing jap and chanting Om, the level of stress psychological pressure is reduced. It provides mental strength to fight against odds. It helps the mind and the body to stay wide awake. It removes our negative thoughts and the electric signal through our living cell changes. The harmony of chanting echoes through all our body parts like our heartbeat, breathing, etc. [4].

9   Conclusion

The fundamental phenomenon of life habits parallel to physiology of medicinal activities is termed as bioelectricity. Bioelectricity is the electrical currents and electrical potentials generated by or occurring within living cells, tissues, and organisms. For example, neurons conduct signals by using electrical fields.

It comprises use of active, stimulating, current-carrying electrodes. It is employed through nature for survival produced by differential movement of charged ions across biological membranes.

Bioelectricity is not the kind of electricity that turns on your lights when you flick the switch. That kind of electricity is based on electrons: negatively charged particles flowing in a current. The human body – including the brain – runs on a very different version: the movements of mostly positively charged ions of elements like potassium, sodium, and calcium.

It is a process of quieting and focusing the mind using a sound, word, or phrase known as mantra which is recited repeatedly. It is done for the spiritual growth and relaxing our mind. It builds sense of trust and confidence for the very reason we are performing the mantra, i.e., it makes us feel better and confident.

The main mantra is Om mantra which is said to be the original tone of the universe, i.e., the sound of the universe was found like that of Om. It's really interesting.

Next is Gayatri Mantra which is another most recited mantra in the Hindu scriptures.

Besides all this, it is done to achieve a peaceful mind, leading to a healthy mind, body, and soul with all coherent thoughts.

Acknowledgments The author team would like to extend special thanks to IIT Delhi, IIT Roorkee, Dev Sanskriti Vishwavidyalaya Haridwar, Patanjali Foundation, and Ayurveda Institute, Dehradun, for their guidance and support in completing our project.

We also pay our deep sense of gratitude to the ABESEC College management to provide us all the facility, the direct-indirect supporters for their timely help and valuable suggestions, and the almighty for blessing us throughout.

Key Terms and Definitions

Yajna Yajna literally means "sacrifice, devotion, worship, offering" and refers in Hinduism to any ritual done in front of a sacred fire, often with mantras. Yajna has been a Vedic tradition, described in a layer of Vedic literature called Brahmanas, as well as Yajurveda. The tradition has evolved from offering oblations and libations into sacred fire to symbolic offerings in the presence of sacred fire (Agni).

Mantra A mantra is a sacred utterance, a numinous sound, a syllable, word, or phoneme, or group of words in Sanskrit believed by practitioners to have psychological and/or spiritual powers. Some mantras have a syntactic structure and literal meaning, while others do not.

Jap Jap is the meditative repetition of a mantra or a divine name. It is a practice found in Hinduism, Jainism, Sikhism, Buddhism, and Shintoism. The mantra or name may be spoken softly, enough for the practitioner to hear it, or it may be spoken within the reciter's mind. Jap may be performed while sitting in a meditation posture, while performing other activities, or as part of formal worship in group settings.

Ayurveda Ayurveda system of medicine with historical roots in the Indian subcontinent. Globalized and modernized practices derived from Ayurveda traditions are a type of alternative medicine. In countries beyond India, Ayurvedic therapies and practices have been integrated in general wellness applications and in some cases in medical use. The main classical Ayurveda texts begin with accounts of the transmission of medical knowledge from the Gods to sages, and then to human physicians. In Sushruta Samhita (Sushruta's Compendium), Sushruta has considered the Dhanvantari as Hindu God and pioneer of Ayurveda.

Sanskrit Sanskrit is an Indo-Aryan language of the ancient Indian subcontinent with a 3500-year history. It is the primary liturgical language of Hinduism and the predominant language of most works of Hindu philosophy and some of the principal texts of Buddhism and Jainism. Sanskrit, in its variants and numerous dialects, was the lingua franca of ancient and medieval India. In the early first millennium AD, along with Buddhism and Hinduism, Sanskrit migrated to Southeast Asia, parts of East Asia, and Central Asia, emerging as a language of high culture and of local ruling elites in these regions.

Vedic The Vedic period or Vedic age (c. 1500–c. 500 BCE) is the period in the history of the northern Indian subcontinent between the end of the urban Indus Valley Civilization and a second urbanization which began in the central Indo-Gangetic Plain c. 600 BCE. It gets its name from the Vedas, which are liturgical texts containing details of life during this period that have been interpreted to be historical and constitute the primary sources for understanding the period. These documents, alongside the corresponding archaeological record, allow for the evolution of the Vedic culture to be traced and inferred.

Energy Measurements There are various kinds of units used to measure the quantity of energy sources. The standard unit of energy is known to be joule (J). Also, other mostly used energy unit is kilowatt/hour (kWh) which is basically used in electricity bills. Large measurements may also go up to terawatt/hour (TWh) or also said as billion kW/h.Other units used for measuring heat include BTU (British thermal unit), kilogram calorie (kg-cal), and most commonly ton of oil equivalent. Actually it represents the quantity of heat which can be obtained from a ton of oil.Energy is also measured in some other units such as British thermal unit (BTU), calorie, therm, etc., which varies generally according to their area of use.

Bioelectricity The term bioelectricity is used to define certain electric currents and potential produced by some activities in the living organisms. A living organism involves millions of biological processes which result to these types of currents.Bioelectric potentials are similar to potentials produced by devices such as batteries or generators except that it is produced by living cells. All cells in living beings are electric, and thus this study of electricity in and around living cells is termed as bioelectricity.Different biological phenomenon comprising certain movement of ions leads to generation of electricity that can also help in understanding of this life.

Yin and Yang Energy This term is brought by the Chinese cosmology. All the traditional Chinese medicine, the martial arts, and their existence are believed to be because of this dynamic concept Ying and Yang.Yin is feminine energy and Yang is masculine energy, or passive and active energy, meaning they can't exist without each other. One's presence is because of the existence of the other.The Yang force is expressed by a contrasting opposite quality of energy to Yin, and thus both are said to be complimentary to each other. All types of order and disorder, winter and summer etc. are to balance the Yin and Yang energy.

Annexure

Agreement Letter

I_____son/daughter_____age_____, resident of_____want to do my own clinical examination/examinations and request for necessary medicines from the Yagyopathy Research Centre, essential medical/treatment, etc.

I declare that I am over 18 years of age.

I will follow all the instructions given by the physicians of Yagyopathy Research Centre during the course of treatment.

I give my consent to receive therapy/treatment from the Yagyopathy Research Centre. The nature and purpose of therapy/treatment is explained to me. I have been given due information for all the inherent risks involved in clinical investigation, medicines, and medical/treatment. I have been duly informed, and with a proper understanding of all these risks, I will do my investigation and medicines and give my consent to the necessary medical/treatment. I will be fully responsible for all results of medical/treatment.

I have voluntarily given this consent without any pressure.

Date: _____ Signature of the patient

Consent for Research Purposes

At the beginning of therapy/treatment for medical, scientific, educational, and research purposes, I have no objection to photography and videography of my condition. I along with publishing this information, its scientific observations in scientific journals presenting the data, and using it in conferences/seminars/workshops without using my name, I give my consent for submission.

Patient's signature:

(Agree)/(Disagree)

The Readings Collected for Different Experiments

Happiness Index

The EORTC QLQ (C-30)

EORTC QLQ-C30: **Questionnaire developed to assess the quality of life of cancer patients**

ENGLISH

EORTC QLQ-C30 (version 3)

We are interested in some things about you and your health. Please answer all of the questions yourself by circling the number that best applies to you. There are no "right" or "wrong" answers. The information that you provide will remain strictly confidential.

Please fill in your initials: ⌞⌞⌞⌞⌟
Your birthdate (Day, Month, Year): ⌞⌞⌞⌞⌞⌞⌞⌟
Today's date (Day, Month, Year): 31 ⌞⌞⌞⌞⌞⌞⌞⌟

		Not at All	A Little	Quite a Bit	Very Much
1.	Do you have any trouble doing strenuous activities, like carrying a heavy shopping bag or a suitcase?	1	2	3	4
2.	Do you have any trouble taking a <u>long</u> walk?	1	2	3	4
3.	Do you have any trouble taking a <u>short</u> walk outside of the house?	1	2	3	4
4.	Do you need to stay in bed or a chair during the day?	1	2	3	4
5.	Do you need help with eating, dressing, washing yourself or using the toilet?	1	2	3	4

During the past week:

		Not at All	A Little	Quite a Bit	Very Much
6.	Were you limited in doing either your work or other daily activities?	1	2	3	4
7.	Were you limited in pursuing your hobbies or other leisure time activities?	1	2	3	4
8.	Were you short of breath?	1	2	3	4
9.	Have you had pain?	1	2	3	4
10.	Did you need to rest?	1	2	3	4
11.	Have you had trouble sleeping?	1	2	3	4
12.	Have you felt weak?	1	2	3	4
13.	Have you lacked appetite?	1	2	3	4
14.	Have you felt nauseated?	1	2	3	4
15.	Have you vomited?	1	2	3	4
16.	Have you been constipated?	1	2	3	4

<u>Please go on to the next page</u>

During the past week:	Not at All	A Little	Quite a Bit	Very Much
17. Have you had diarrhea?	1	2	3	4
18. Were you tired?	1	2	3	4
19. Did pain interfere with your daily activities?	1	2	3	4
20. Have you had difficulty in concentrating on things, like reading a newspaper or watching television?	1	2	3	4
21. Did you feel tense?	1	2	3	4
22. Did you worry?	1	2	3	4
23. Did you feel irritable?	1	2	3	4
24. Did you feel depressed?	1	2	3	4
25. Have you had difficulty remembering things?	1	2	3	4
26. Has your physical condition or medical treatment interfered with your _family_ life?	1	2	3	4
27. Has your physical condition or medical treatment interfered with your _social_ activities?	1	2	3	4
28. Has your physical condition or medical treatment caused you financial difficulties?	1	2	3	4

For the following questions please circle the number between 1 and 7 that best applies to you

29. How would you rate your overall _health_ during the past week?

| 1 | 2 | 3 | 4 | 5 | 6 | 7 |

Very poor   Excellent

30. How would you rate your overall _quality of life_ during the past week?

| 1 | 2 | 3 | 4 | 5 | 6 | 7 |

Very poor   Excellent

Data Readings

Name	State before and after Yajna	Stress value	Energy value	Balance value	Organ balance value
Manish Lakshar	Before	3.08	49.46	94.04	3.38
Manish	After	3.45	46.82	96.42	1.87
Jagdish	Before	4.12	46.27	87.67	11.92
Jagdish	After	2.68	46.71	99.62	0

Name	State before and after Yajna	Organ	Energy	Balance %
Manish	Before	Head	4.77	0.9929
Manish	Before	Cardiovascular system	4.01	0.9728
Manish	Before	Respiratory system	4.28	0.8302
Manish	Before	Endocrine gland	4.72	0.9363
Manish	Before	Musculoskeletal system	4.61	0.9226
Manish	Before	Digestive system	4.55	0.9352
Manish	Before	Urinogenital system	4.12	0.9406
Manish	Before	Nervous system	5.17	0.8123
Manish	Before	Immune system	5.14	0.9718
Manish	After	Head	4.34	0.9845
Manish	After	Cardiovascular system	3.91	0.9196
Manish	After	Respiratory system	3.93	0.9692
Manish	After	Endocrine gland	4.43	0.9696
Manish	After	Musculoskeletal system	4.13	0.9295
Manish	After	Digestive system	4.38	0.9655
Manish	After	Urinogenital system	3.75	0.9952
Manish	After	Nervous system	4.63	0.9466
Manish	After	Immune system	4.51	0.9934
Jagdish	Before	Head	4.7	0.8872
Jagdish	Before	Cardiovascular system	3.82	0.8479
Jagdish	Before	Respiratory system	4.67	0.987
Jagdish	Before	Endocrine gland	4.36	0.9353
Jagdish	Before	Musculoskeletal system	2.98	0.4196
Jagdish	Before	Digestive system	3.57	0.6746
Jagdish	Before	Urinogenital system	3.83	0.8295
Jagdish	Before	Nervous system	4.67	0.9268
Jagdish	Before	Immune system	4.11	0.839
Jagdish	After	Head	3.91	0.8849
Jagdish	After	Cardiovascular system	3.75	0.9988
Jagdish	After	Respiratory system	4.19	0.9676
Jagdish	After	Endocrine gland	4.43	0.9318
Jagdish	After	Musculoskeletal system	3.88	0.6998
Jagdish	After	Digestive system	4.29	0.9967
Jagdish	After	Urinogenital system	4.59	0.9557
Jagdish	After	Nervous system	4.29	0.8562
Jagdish	After	Immune system	4.11	0.8283

References

1. Chaturvedi, D.K. "Relationship between Chakra Energy and Consciousness," Biomedical Journal of Scientific and Technical Research, *15(3)*, (2019): pp. 1–3. DOI: https://doi.org/10.26717/BJSTR.2019.15.002705, ISSN: 2574-1241.
2. Chaturvedi, D. K, & Satsangi, R. "The Correlation between Student Performance and Consciousness Level," *International Conference on Advanced Computing and Communication Technologies (ICACCT™-2013)*, Asia Pacific Institute of Information Technology SD India, Panipat (Haryana), (16 Nov. 2013): Souvenir –pp.66, proc. pp. 200–203.
3. Cioca, G.H., Giacomoni, P., Rein, G. "A correlation between GDV & HRV measures for well being," in Konstantin G. Korotkov (eds.), Measuring energy fields. Current Research— Backbone Publishing Co, Fair Lawn, USA, (2004): pp. 59–64.
4. Gurjar, A. A, Ladhake, S. A, Thakare, A.P. "Analysis of acoustic of "OM" chant to study its effect on nervous system," IJCSNS International Journal of Computer Science and Network Security, 9(1), (1 Jan 2009): pp. 363–366.
5. Johnson, R. D., ed. *Computational Chemistry Comparison and Benchmark DataBase*, National Institute of Standards and Technology. https://doi.org/10.18434/T47C7Z. (2002).
6. Kim, K.J. &Tagkopoulos, L. "Application of machine learning rheumatic disease research," Korean J Intern Med., 34, (2019): 708–722
7. Konikiewicz, Leonard W. "Introduction to electrography: A handbook for prospective researchers of the Kirlian effect" *in biomedicine Leonard's Associates*, (1978).
8. Korotkov, K. G. "Bio well: Analysis of personal energetic homeostasis by measuring energy field," MedSci Sports Exerc, (2019): 35, S451–75.
9. Michael, L. "The wisdom of the body: Future techniques and approaches to morphogenetic fields in regenerative medicine, developmental biology and cancer," Regenerative Medicine (2011): 6, 667–73.
10. Mistry, R., Tanwar, S., Tyagi, S., Kumar, N. "Blockchain for 5G-Enabled IoT for Industrial Automation: A Systematic Review, Solutions, and Challenges," Mechanical Systems and Signal Processing, (2020): 135, pp. 1–19.
11. Mouradian, C., Naboulsi, D., Yangui, S., Glitho, H., Morrow, M.J., Polakos, P.A. "A Comprehensive Survey on Fog Computing: State-of-the-Art and Research Challenges," *IEEE, 20, 2017*): 416–464. Available:https://ieeexplore.ieee.org/abstract/document/8100873/authors#authors
12. Nigal, S.G. "Axiological Approach to the Vedas," *Northern Book*, (1986): pages 80–81. ISBN 978-8185119182.
13. Patton, L. "The Hindu World,ed.Mittal, S., Thursby, G., Routledge," (2005): pages 38–39. (Editors:, ISBN 978-0415772273.
14. Pang, Z., Yang, G., Khedri, R., Zhang, Y.T. "Introduction to the Special Section: Convergence of Automation Technology, Biomedical Engineering, and Health Informatics Toward the Healthcare 4.0.," *IEEE, Vol No: 11*, (July 2018): Page No: 249–259. Available: https://ieeexplore.org/document/8421122.
15. Jain, R. "Hatha Yoga For Teachers & Practitioners: A Comprehensive Guide to Holistic Sequencing," (13 June 2020). Reference: https://www.arhantayoga.org/blog/7-chakras-introduction-energy-centers-effect/
16. Rastogi, R., Chaturvedi, D.K., Sharma, S., Bansal, A., Agrawal, A. "Audio Visual EMG & GSR Biofeedback Analysis for Effect of Spiritual Techniques on Human Behaviour and Psychic Challenges," *in Proceedings of the 12th INDIACom; INDIACom-2018;* (14th – 16 March, 2018a): pp 252–258.
17. Rastogi, R., Chaturvedi, D.K.,Satya, S., Arora, N., Sirohi, H., Singh, M., Verma, P., Singh, V. "Which One is Best: Electromyography Biofeedback Efficacy Analysis on Audio, Visual and Audio-Visual Modes for Chronic TTH on Different Characteristics," *in the proceedings of International Conference on Computational Intelligence &IoT (ICCIIoT) 2018*, at National

Institute of Technology Agartala, Tripura, India, ELSEVIER-SSRN Digital Library (ISSN 1556-5068), (14–15 December 2018b).

18. Rastogi, R., Chaturvedi, D.K., Satya, S., Arora, N., Saini, H., Verma, H., Mehlyan, K. "Comparative Efficacy Analysis of Electromyography and Galvanic Skin Resistance Biofeedback on Audio Mode for Chronic TTH on Various Indicators," *in the proceedings of International Conference on Computational Intelligence &IoT (ICCIIoT) 2018,* at National Institute of Technology Agartala, Tripura, India, ELSEVIER-SSRN Digital Library (ISSN 1556-5068), (14–15 December 2018c).

19. Rastogi, R., Saxena, M., Sharma, S.K., Muralidharan, S., Beriwal, V.K., Singhal, P., Rastogi, M., Shrivastava, R. "EVALUATION OF EFFICACY OF YAGYA THERAPY ON T2-DIABETES MELLITUS PATIENTS," *in the proceedings of The 2nd edition of International Conference on Industry Interactive Innovations in Science, Engineering and Technology (I3SET2K19)* organized by JIS College of Engineering, Kalyani, West Bengal, (13–14 Dec. 2019a). https://papers.ssrn.com/sol3/papers.cfm?abstract_id=3514326.

20. Rastogi, R., Saxena, M., Gupta, U.S., Sharma, S., Chaturvedi, D.K., Singhal, P., Gupta, M., Garg, P., Gupta, M., Maheshwari, M. "Yajna and Mantra Therapy Applications on Diabetic Subjects: Computational Intelligence Based Experimental Approach," *in the proceedings of The 2nd edition of International Conference on Industry Interactive Innovations in Science, Engineering and Technology (I3SET2K19)* organized by JIS College of Engineering, Kalyani, West Bengal, (13–14 Dec. 2019b). https://papers.ssrn.com/sol3/papers.cfm?abstract_id=3515800.

21. Rastogi, R., Saxena, M., Sharma, S.K., Murlidharan, S., Berival, V.K., Jaiswal, D., Sharma, A., Mishra, A. "Statistical Analysis on Efficacy of Yagya Therapy for Type-2 Diabetic Mellitus Patients through Various Parameters," *In: Das A., Nayak J., Naik B., Dutta S., Pelusi D. (eds) on Computational Intelligence in Pattern Recognition (CIPR),* Kalyani, West Bengal, Pages 181–197. Adv in Intelligent Syst Comput, *Vol. 1120,* Computational Intelligence in Pattern, Recognition, (13–14 Dec. 2019c). 978-981-15-2448-6, 487895_1_En, (15), doi: https://doi.org/10.1007/978-981-15-2449-3_15.

22. Rastogi, R., Chaturvedi, D.K., Verma, H., Mishra, Y., Gupta, M. "Identifying Better? Analytical Trends to Check Subjects' Medications Using Biofeedback Therapies," *IGL Global, International Journal of Applied Research on Public Health Management (IJARPHM: Volume 5),* Issue 1, Article 2. (2020a): PP. 14–31,ISSN: 2639-7692|EISSN: 2639-7706|DOI: 10.4018/IJARPHM,https://www.igi-global.com/article/identifying-better/240753. DOI: 10.4018/IJARPHM.2020010102

23. Rastogi, R., Gupta, M., Chaturvedi, D.K. "Efficacy of Study for Correlation of TTH vs Age and Gender Factors using EMG Biofeedback Technique," *International Journal of Applied Research on Public Health Management (IJARPHM) 5(1),*Art 4., (2020b): PP. 49–66, DOI: https://doi.org/10.4018/IJARPHM.2020010104.

24. Rastogi, R., Chaturvedi, D.K., Satya, S., Arora, N., Gupta, M., Verma, H., Saini, H. "An Optimized Biofeedback EMG and GSR Biofeedback Therapy for Chronic TTH on SF-36 Scores of Different MMBD Modes on Various Medical Symptoms," *in Studies Comp. Intelligence, Vol. 841, : Hybrid Machine Intelligence for Medical Image Analysis,* 978-981-13-8929-0, 468690_1_En, (8) (2020c): S. Bhattacharya et al. (eds.), https://doi.org/10.1007/978-981-13-8930-6_8.

25. Rastogi, R., Chaturvedi, D.K., Satya, S., Arora, N., Trivedi, P., Singh, A.K., Sharma, A.K., Singh, A. "Intelligent Personality Analysis on Indicators in IoT-MMBD Enabled Environment," *editors: S. Tanwar, S. Tyagi, N. Kumar (EDs), Multimedia Big Data Computing for IoT Applications: Concepts, Paradigms, and Solutions, Springer Nature Singapore,* (2020d): pp. 185–215. https://doi.org/10.1007/978-981-13-8759-3_7.

26. Saxena, M., Sengupta, B., & Pandya, P. "A study of the Impact of Yagya on Indoor Microbial Environments," *Indian Journal of Air Pollution Control,Vol. 7,* issue-1, (2007a): pp. 6–15.

27. Saxena, M., Sengupta, B., & Pandya, P. "Comparative Studies of Yagya vs. Non-Yagya Microbial Environments," *Indian Journal of Air Pollution Control,Vol. VII,* No. 1, (2007b): pp. 16–24.

28. Saxena, M., Sengupta, B., & Pandya, P. "Effect of Yagya on the Gaseous Pollutants, *Indian Journal of Air Pollution Control,*" *Vol. VII,* No. 2, (Sept. 2007c): pp. 11–15.
29. Saxena, M., Sengupta, B, & Pandya, P. "Controlling the Microflora in Outdoor Environment: Effect of Yagya," *Indian Journal of Air Pollution Control, Vol. VIII,* No. 2, (Sept. 2008): pp. 30–36.
30. Saxena, M., Kumar, B., &Matharu, S. "Impact of Yagya on Particulate Matters, *Interdisciplinary Journal of Yagya Research,*" *1(1),* (Oct. 2018): pp 01–08.
31. Takagi, K. & Nakayama, T. "Peripheral Effector Mechanism of Galvanic Skin Reflex," Jap J Physiol 5, (1956): 5–7.
32. Thakur, G.S. "YAJÑA-A VEDIC TRADITIONAL TECHNIQUE FOR EMPIRICAL AND TRANSCENDENTAL AND ACHIEVEMENT," *Indian Streams Research Journal,* vol no 04, (May 2014): page no 5.
33. Yesha, P., Elonnai, H., Amber, S., Udhbhav, T. "Artificial Intelligence in the Healthcare Industry in India," The Centre for Internet and Society, India, (2018).

Additional Readings

Source:-https://qz.com/1630159/bioelectricity-may-be-key-to-fighting-cancer/AND   https://onlinelibrary.wiley.com/doi/abs/10.1111/jtsb.12101
Bansal, P., Kaur, R., Gupta, V., Kumar, S., & Kaur, R.P.(31 Dec. 2015). Is There Any Scientific Basis of *Hawan* to be used in Epilepsy-Prevention/Cure?, *5*(2): 33–45, *doi:* https://doi.org/10.14581/jer.15009.
Source:-https://www.doyou.com/how-mantras-work-39322/
Source:-https://blog.sivanaspirit.com/sp-gn-scientific-benefits-chanting/
Source:- https://www.worldpranichealing.com/en/energy/what-is-pranic-energy/AND.
Sui,C.K., The Ancient Science and Art of Pranic Healing &Advanced Pranic Healing.
Source:-https://www.encyclopedia.com/medicine/encyclopedias-almanacs-transcripts-and-maps/bioelectricity.
Source:-Williams, M. (McGraw-Hill, 2006). Nutrition for Health, *Fitness and Sport, 8th Ed.*
Ferrera, L.A., (Nova Publishers, 2006). Focus on Body Mass Index And Health Research.
Source:-Mills, A.(29 June 2009). Kirlian Photography, *History of Photography,33*(3).
Source:- Wikipedia (https://simple.wikipedia.org/wiki/Chakra).
Source:-https://www.chakra-anatomy.com/human-aura.html
Source:-Prabhat S., (January 7, 2010). (http://www.differencebetween.net/miscellaneous/difference-between-yin-and-yang/).
Source:-https://rationalwiki.org/wiki/Quantum_consciousness
Source:-gaiam.com/blogs/discover/how-does-meditation-affect-the-body
Varman H. (2014), Five important levels of the human consciousness, BSIIJ.
Grujin J. (2016), What is Kirlian Photography? Aura Photography Revealed, *light stalking.*
Buelteman R. (2012), Shocks Flowers With 80,000 Volts Of Electricity, *BSIIJ.*
4 Grimnes S., Martinsen G. (2015), Bioimpedance and Bioelectricity Basics, *ResearchGate*(3).
Sui C. K. (2012), Pranic Energy: Feel Divinity All Around You, *IJITEE.*
Wisneski, Leonard A., (2010). The Scientific Basis of Integrative Medicine, *IJITEE.*
Chhabra G. (2015), Human Aura: a new Vedic approach in it, University of Petroleum and Energy Studies.
Chig T. T. (1998), What is Yin Yang? Always Dream Even When Awake, Taoist Articles.
Sia P. D. (2016), Mindfulness: Consciousness and Quantum Physics, University of Padova.
Smith J. A., Suttie J., Jazaieri H., Newman K. M. (2018), Things We Know About the Science of Meditation, *Mindfulness Research.*
Dudeja J. (2017), Scientific Analysis of Mantra-Based Meditation and its Beneficial Effects: An Overview, *ResearchGate.*
Acharya S. S. (2001), The Integrated Science of Yagna, *IIT Bombay.*

Rohit Rastogi received his B.E. C. S. S. Univ. Meerut, 2003, Master's degree in CS of NITTTR-Chandigarh from Punjab University. Currently he is getting a doctoral degree from the Dayalbagh Educational Institute in Agra, India. He is an associate professor in the CSE department of ABES Engineering College, Ghaziabad, India. He has won awards in a various of areas, including improved education, significant contributions, human value promotion, and long-term service. He keeps himself engaged in various competition events, activities, webinars, seminars, workshops, projects, and various other educational learning forums.

Dr. Mamta Saxena is Director General in Ministry of Statistics, GoI, and has completed her PhD in Yajna Science with CPCB (Central Pollution Control Board). She has keen interest to revive our ancient culture and science through modern instruments. She is a scientist by thought and working on the study of effect of Yajna, mantra, and yoga on mental patients, patients suffering with various diseases like diabetes, stress, arthritis, lever infection, and hypertension, etc., with joint collaboration with different organizations, AIIMS, NIMHANS, NPL, etc.

Dr. D.K Chaturvedi is working in the Dept. of Elect. Engg., Faculty of Engg., D.E.I., Dayalbagh, Agra, since 1989. Presently he is a professor. He did his B.E. from the Govt. Engineering College Ujjain, M.P., and then he did his MTech and PhD from D.E.I. Dayalbagh. He is a gold medalist and received Young Scientists Fellowship from DST, Government of India, in 2001–2002 for post-doctoral research at the University of Calgary, Canada. Also, he had research collaboration with different organizations at national and international level. He is a fellow of the Institution of Engineers (India), fellow of Aeronautical Society of India, fellow of IETE, Sr. member of IEEE, USA, and member of many national and international professional bodies such as IET, UK; ISTE, Delhi; ISCE, Roorkee; IIIE, Mumbai; SSI, etc. The IEE, UK, recognized his work in the area of power system stabilizer and awarded honorary membership to him in 2006. He did many R&D projects of MHRD, UGC, AICTE, etc. and consultancy projects of DRDO. He contributed in the national mission of ICT of the Government of India as virtual power lab developer. He has guided 10 PhDs, 65 MTech dissertations, and published more than 300 international and national papers. He has chaired and co-chaired many international and national conferences. He is referee of many international journals including IEE Proceedings and IEEE Transactions. He is Head of the Dept. of Footwear Technology, Convener, Faculty Training and Placement Cell, and Advisor, IEI Students' Chapter (Elect. Engg.), D.E.I., Dayalbagh, Agra.

Vansh Gaur is an engineering student in AKTU. Presently he is BTech second-year student of CSE in ABESEC, Ghaziabad, India. He is working presently on Yagya and mantra therapy and its analysis by machine learning. He has keen interest in YouTube surfing. His hobbies are playing badminton and reading books. He is young, talented, and dynamic.

Mayank Gupta is acting as system and IT analyst in Tata Consultancy Services, Noida, and expert of data sciences and business analytics. He has skill to visualize the situations from different perspectives and explore the real facts through critical analysis. He has deep interest in human health domains. Currently he is working on Japan projects on life sciences.

Neha Gupta is a student of BTech (CSE) in ABESEC which is affiliated to AKTU. She is currently working on yagyopathy where she is analyzing the data and translating them. She has a keen interest in coding and cyber security. Her hobby is to watch movies. She wishes to do something for her society in the coming future with her all resources.

Umang Agrawal is an engineering student in AKTU. Presently he is BTech second-year student of CSE in ABESEC, Ghaziabad, India. He is working presently on Yagya and mantra therapy and its analysis by machine learning. He has keen interest in Google surfing. His hobbies are playing badminton and reading books. He is young, talented, and dynamic.

Yashi Srivastava is an engineering student in ABESEC Ghaziabad from AKTU Lucknow, UP, India. Presently she is in second year of ECE branch of BTech. She is working as a content writer and a researcher on Yagya and Mantra therapy and its analysis by machine learning. She enjoys designing and loves playing with the concept of mathematics but remains attached to her life roots. Apart from studying, she likes to play chess, visit different places with friends, and hunting for new shows on Netflix.

Development of Compression Algorithms for Computed Tomography and Magnetic Resonance Imaging

R. Pandian, S. LalithaKumari, D. N. S. RaviKumar, and G. Rajalakshmi

Abstract Medical image compression finds extensive applications in the fields of healthcare, teleradiology, teleconsultation, telemedicine, and telematics. The development of picture archiving and communication systems (PACS) is implemented by efficient compression algorithms. The medical imagery also needs to be compressed to obtain optimum compression with high diagnostic quality. In order to achieve reduction of transmission time and storage costs, efficient image compression methods without degradation of images are needed. In medical image compression techniques, the lossy and lossless methods do not produce an optimum compression with no loss of information. The high compression and without loss of diagnosis ability for the medical image should only be aimed at developing an optimum image compression techniques. Medical image compression algorithms developed so far focused toward only on space reduction and did not concentrate much on the characterization of the images and the effects of compression on the image quality.

Keywords Compression · CT · MRI · PSNR · CR · MSE · PACS

1 Introduction

The enormous quantity of data as medical images demands extensive data storage capacity, data processing, and data analyzing as they are difficult to transfer. Even though latest developments in the storage systems are available, the digital communication system needs larger data storage capacity and data transmission bandwidth which exceeds the capabilities of available technologies. It is advantageous to represent with smaller storage bits; whenever there is a need for the original image to be reconstructed, it is transferred as compressed image information. Image compression is a minimized graphics file without significant degradation in the quality of the image. In the image decompression, the images are converted back to the original one, or the best approximation of the original images. Digital image is a

R. Pandian (✉) · S. LalithaKumari · D. N. S. RaviKumar · G. Rajalakshmi
School of EEE, Sathyabama Institute of Science and Technology, Chennai, India

© The Author(s), under exclusive license to Springer
Nature Switzerland AG 2021
A. K. Manocha et al. (eds.), *Computational Intelligence in Healthcare*, Health Information Science, https://doi.org/10.1007/978-3-030-68723-6_2

two-dimensional array of picture elements called pixels which represents the intensity at specific points in an image. Nowadays medical imaging generates images in the digital format for easy access, storage for future retrieval, and transmission from one location to another. As these imaging techniques produce a high volume of data, compression becomes mandatory for the storage and reducing transmission time. Digital images can be classified into different types, e.g., binary, grayscale, color, false color, multispectral, and thematic [1, 2].

1.1 Image Compression

The process of representing the image with less number of bits by removing the redundancies from the image is called compression (Gonzalez and Woods 2002) which is described in terms of compression ratio (CR) or the number of bits per pixel (bpp) termed bit rate. CR and bit rate are determined using the following formula [3]:

$$CR = \frac{\text{Original image size in bits}}{\text{Compressed image size in bits}}$$

$$\text{Bit rate} = \frac{\text{No of bits transmitted}}{\text{seconds}}$$

In general, three types of redundancy can be identified [4].
There are three types of redundancies:

- Coding redundancy
- Inter-pixel redundancy
- Psycho-visual redundancy

1.2 Coding Redundancy

In images, some gray values appear more frequently than others. By assigning less number of symbols (bits) to more probable ones and a number of symbols (bits) to less probable ones, coding redundancies can be effectively reduced. A variable length coding is a commonly used technique which explores coding redundancy to reduce the redundant data from the image [5]. The most accurate and popular coding techniques of variable length are Huffman and arithmetic coding.

1.3 Inter-pixel Redundancy

This method is used to remove the inter-pixel correlation of images [6].

1.4 Psycho-visual Redundancy

The natural eye doesn't have equivalent affectability to all or any visual detecting data. Certain data might be a littler sum huge than other data in typical visual handling. This data is named as psycho outwardly excess data. It's frequently wiped out without changing the visual nature of the image as such an information isn't urgent for ordinary visual preparing. The end of psycho-visual excess information is alluded as quantization, since it brings about loss of quantitative information [7].

1.5 Image Compression Model

The image pressure framework is presented in Fig. 1. The source encoder that is presented in Fig. 1a lessens redundancies of the information image. The mapper changes the information image into a variety of coefficients to diminish between pixel redundancies which is a reversible cycle. The image encoder makes a fixed or variable length code to speak to the quantizer yield.

The source decoder is presented in Fig. 1b. It contains two squares, namely, image decoder and reverse mapper. These squares play out the converse activity of image encoder and mapper individually. The recreated image could conceivably be an accurate copy of the information image [8, 9].

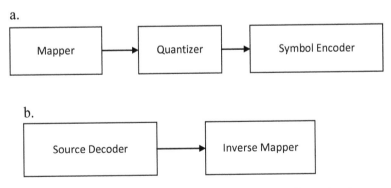

Fig. 1 Block diagram of image compression. (**a**) Source encoder. (**b**) Source decoder

1.6   Classification of Image Compression

Comprehensively the image pressure is separated into two sorts: lossless image pressure and lossy image pressure. In lossless image pressure, the remade image is practically like the first image. The degree of image pressure accomplished can be spoken to by CR. The CR showed for lossless strategies is regularly around 2:1 to 3:1. The pressure proportion of lossy image pressure is consistently higher than that of lossless pressure methods. However, the reproduced image contains corruptions, comparative with the first image. A lossy compression method is called visually lossless. The loss of information caused by compression method is invisible for an observer.

1.7   Quality Measures for Image Compression

Quality measures are evaluated on the grounds that the quantitative proportions of attributes or properties of the outcome. Quality measures are the estimation devices which might not decide the norm of the outcome. Quality measures additionally choose how legitimate the calculations are in conceiving the predefined results. The quality estimates utilized for assessing the pressure are top sign to commotion proportion (PSNR), compression ratio (CR), mean square error (MSE), and bits per pixel (bpp). During this PSNR and compression proportion are valuable for pressure and information transmission. Mean square mistake is useful for imagining the blunder. PSNR gauges the norm of a remade image contrasted and a smart image. The basic thought is to register one number that mirrors the norm of the packed image. Customary PSNR measures probably won't acknowledge as obvious with human abstract recognition. A few examination bunches are performing on perceptual measures, yet PSNR is utilized in light of the fact that they're simpler to figure. Likewise note that various measures don't generally mean better quality.

The mean square error (MSE) of the reconstructed image is computed as follows:

$$\text{MSE} = \frac{1}{n} \sum_{i=1}^{n} \left(y_i - \overset{-}{y}_i \right)^2 \tag{1}$$

where Eq. (1) is the sum over i and j denotes the sum of all pixels in the images. The PSNR relates the MSE to the maximum amplitude of the original image. PSNR is measured in decibels and is defined as

$$\text{PSNR} = 10 \log_{10} \left[\frac{\max\left(r(x,y)\right)^2}{\frac{1}{n_x n_y} \sum_{0}^{n_x-1} \sum_{0}^{n_y-1} \left[r(x,y) - t(x,y) \right]^2} \right] \tag{2}$$

where in Equation (2) 255 is the maximum possible intensity for 8-bit grayscale image. In image compression, acceptable values of PSNR are in between 30 dB and 50 dB; the higher is better [11].

1.8 Lossless Compression

In lossless weight methodologies, the reproduced picture after weight is a lot of equivalent to the principal picture. Generally, lossless weight is gotten by coding strategies. Entropy coding encodes the genuine game plan of pictures with the less number of pieces expected to address them using the probability of the pictures. Weight is procured by giving variable size codes to pictures. The shorter codeword is given to more potential pictures. Huffman coding and arithmetic coding are the chief recognized entropy coding methods. Lossless weight systems are regularly realized using Huffman coding and arithmetic coding. Huffman coding may be a most picked prefix code. It consigns a social event of prefix codes to pictures set up on their probabilities. Pictures that happen more consistently will have shorter code-words than pictures which happen less generally. Also two pictures having code-words with same most extraordinary length happens once in a while. Huffman coding is insufficient when the letter set size is almost nothing and a probability of happening of pictures is very skewed. Calculating coding is more capable when the letter size all together is near nothing or the picture probabilities are outstandingly skewed. Making codewords for plans of pictures is viable than conveying an extraordinary codeword for each picture during a string. A specific number related code could be created for a specific progression without making codewords for all game plans of that length. This is routinely unprecedented for Huffman codes. One marked regard is allotted to a square of pictures, which is especially decodable. Calculating coding gives higher weight extents than Huffman coding. Run-length encoding strategy is the most un-irksome weight methodology. It's profitable when the information to be compacted contains long runs of repeated characters or pictures [12].

1.9 Lossy Compression

Lossy compression can be implemented by transform and encoding methods. The transform will decompose the image and encoder will remove the repeated data. This method will give high amount of compression.

Table 1 Image compression algorithms

Algorithms	Methodologies
Lossless compression	The lossless compression is used, where there is no compromise on high quality of output image
Lossy compression	Transform methods provide higher image compression DCT- wavelet method lacks from blocking facts at low bitrates Wavelet-based compression methods have various levels of wavelet decomposition leading to difficulty
Medical image compression	All the methods delineated above include various degrees of wavelet decay bringing about the high computational complex at the more elevated level of disintegration which brings about more subtleties that can be of limit to get bigger pressure proportions but leads to energy loss
Hybrid algorithms	All the hybrid algorithms are based on transform method The transform-based algorithm falls under the category of lossy compression

1.10   Medical Image Compression

Several analysts inside their investigations have shown the novel advance in the field of clinical pressure in both lossless and lossy classifications [13]. Lossless compressions can do a high pressure proportion of 3:1, restoring the image without loss of information. As advanced images include a sweeping proportion of room for putting away, the more prominent aspect of the investigation is focused on lossy pressure that clears irrelevant information sparing all the appropriate and crucial image information. All the methods include different degrees of wavelet deterioration prompting the high computational intricacy at the upper degree of disintegration more subtleties which will be an edge to ask bigger pressure proportions yet brings about energy misfortune. Energy held will be more if the image is decayed to less levels; however pressure accomplished is a littler amount [14, 15].

Table 1, the development of medical image compression algorithms concern only on space reduction and does not concentrate much on the characterization of the images after compression [16]

2   Wavelet Transform

The wavelet transform is very important for image compression. This will decompose the images. There are many transforms available. Based on their characteristics, we can select suitable transform for particular applications. There are Daubechies, Haar, Symlet, Coiflet, and biorthogonal transforms available. Wavelet transform is used in this work to decompose the images. The basic wavelet is Daubechies wavelet. The Haar wavelet is given below [17–19]:

$$\psi(t) = \begin{cases} 1 & 0 \leq t < 1/2, \\ -1 & 1/2 \leq t < 1, \\ 0 & \text{otherwise.} \end{cases} \quad (3)$$

Its scaling function $\phi(t)$ can be described as

$$\phi(t) = \begin{cases} 1 & 0 \leq t < 1, \\ 0 & \text{otherwise.} \end{cases} \quad (4)$$

2.1 Wavelet Transform-Based Compression

In lossy pressure, the reproduced image after pressure is a guess of the primary image. A lossy pressure technique is entitled outwardly lossless when the loss of information brought about by pressure strategy is undetectable to a spectator. Lossy pressure is frequently characterized into two classes, namely, spatial space methods and change area procedures. In spatial area methods, the pixels inside the image are utilized, whereas in change space procedures, the image pixels are changed over into a substitution set of qualities, as change coefficients, for additional preparing. Prescient coding might be a recognizable spatial space strategy that works explicitly on the image pixels. Transform technique is a widely utilized technique in lossy pressure. An image is compacted by changing the corresponding pixels to a totally novel portrayal (change space) where they're de-related. The change coefficients are free of one another, and the vast majority of the energy is stuffed during a couple of coefficients. The change coefficients are quantized to downsize the measure of pieces inside the image, and accordingly the piece of quantized nonzero coefficients must be encoded. This is frequently a many-to-one planning. Quantized coefficients are additionally compacted utilizing entropy coding procedures to an obviously flexible and better by and large pressure. The change used in the change area might be a direct change. It gives more effective and direct method of pressure. Lossy pressure comprises of three sections. The essential part might be a change to downsize the between pixel excess of image. At that point a quantizer is regularly applied to dispose of psycho-visual repetition to speak to the information with less number of pieces. The quantized pieces are then productively encoded to ask more pressure from the coding excess. In lossy pressure the information misfortune is because of quantization of the image co-production. Quantization is frequently measured in light of the fact that the way toward arranging the image into various pieces and speaking to each piece with a value. A quantizer fundamentally decreases the measure of pieces important to store the changed coefficients by lessening the precision of these qualities. Scalar quantization (SQ) is frequently performed on every individual coefficient and vector quantization (VQ) on a gaggle of the coefficient. Numerous scientists are attempting to improve pressure plans utilizing modern vector quantization yet setting apportioning in various leveled tree accomplished better outcomes utilizing uniform scalar quantization. During this pressure uniform scalar quantization is frequently utilized for improving pressure efficiency [20, 21].

2.2 Significance of Wavelet Analysis

In compression it is ought to be underlined that Fourier change includes averaging of the sign with a period direction which brings about a misfortune inside the nitty gritty transient data of the sign. Fourier change likewise includes a fixed goal for all frequencies. Conversely, wavelet examination changes an image inside the time area into a recurrence space with various goals at various sign frequencies. As such, it gives a multi-goal way to deal with image investigation. Inside the wavelet-based methodology, the higher the sign recurrence, the better the goal and the reverse way around. The wavelet approach gets a period scale deterioration of the sign into account utilizing an interpretation (time) boundary and a scale boundary. There are two methodologies: persistent wavelet changes (CWT) and discrete wavelet changes (DWT). In both CWT and DWT approaches, the understanding boundary is discrete; though the size boundary is permitted to fluctuate consistently in CWT [22], it is yet discrete in DWT. So as to beat impediments in pressure, a few methodologies are proposed which upheld time-recurrence confinement, similar to envelope examination: Gabor windowed Fourier transform (GWFT) and wavelet investigation techniques. Generally, the Fourier change (FT) is broadly used in image handling. Since it doesn't give time confinement, it's seldom suitable for non-fixed cycles. Along these lines it's less valuable in breaking down non-fixed information, where there's no reiteration inside the district sampled [23]. Furthermore, one among the limitations of Fast Fourier transform (FFT) in image investigation is the nonappearance of worldly data. The short-time Fourier transform (STFT) confines time by moving time window. The width is fixed of as far as possible the high-recurrence run. Wavelet changes permit the segments of a non-fixed sign to be investigated, permit channels to be built for both fixed and non-fixed signals, and have a window whose transmission capacity shifts in relation to the recurrence of the wavelet. The wavelet modifies down the image into different scales inside the time area, while the Fourier change presents an image in light of the fact that the total of sinusoidal elements of single recurrence. The wavelet change removes image highlights and non-fixed aggravation highlights in an image over the whole range without a prevailing waveband. The arrangement of wavelets would characterize a base from which a symmetrical deterioration of the main image is regularly made with similarity to the Fourier examination. Symmetrical wavelet changes catch free data. That measures a full decay of the image was done the measure of wavelet coefficients was an equal on the grounds that the first image and will be recombined to recreate the main image. It's accepted that wavelet investigation can assume a major part in pressure research and for diagnostics device. Wavelet transform is a broadly received strategy for pressure. Essential pressure plot during this strategy is actualized inside the accompanying the request the relationship, quantization, and encoding. The DCT and DWT are well-known changes wont to de relate the pixels. The wavelet change deteriorates the image into various recurrence subgroups, to be specific lower-recurrence subgroups and better-recurrence subgroups, by which smooth varieties and subtleties of the image are frequently isolated. The majority of the energy is compacted into lower-recurrence subgroups. The greater part of the coefficients in higher-recurrence subgroups are little or zero and have a twisted to be assembled and furthermore are situated inside a similar relative spatial area inside the subgroups. Hence pressure strategies utilize wavelet changes that are effective in giving high paces of pressure while keeping up great image quality and are better than DCT-based techniques. In DCT a large portion of the energy is compacted into lower-recurrence coefficients to quantization [23]; the vast majority of the upper-recurrence coefficient become little or zero and have a twisted to be assembled. DCT is performed on 8x8 non-covering blocks, and along these lines the DCT coefficients of each square inside the image are quantized. Yet, at higher pressure proportions, hindering antiques are obvious utilizing JPEG strategy. Each degree of deterioration makes low-recurrence parts (estimation sub-band LL) and high-recurrence segments (three detail subgroups LH, HL, and HH) utilizing low-pass and high-pass channels (hL(k) and hH(k), individually. LL sub-band is frequently additionally disintegrated for ensuing degree of decay. On the off chance that the degree of disintegration expands, the better subtleties are caught all the more effectively. The image subtleties are pressed into a little number of coefficients, which are decreased to less number by following a quantization. The blunder

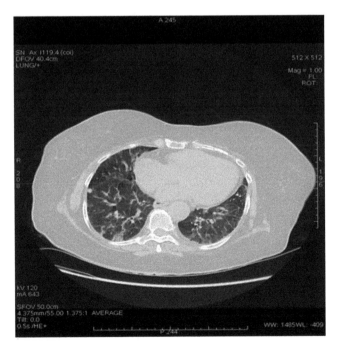

Fig. 2 Original image (512 × 512)

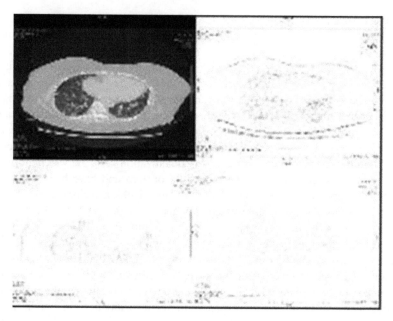

Fig. 3 DWT-based decomposed image (level 1)

or misfortune in data is on account of the quantization step. This results in a mark-down in the pieces with various probabilities and entropy. Figures 2 and 3 show the primary image and hence the 1-level wavelet decay of dark-scale CT lung image which is of size 512×512 [24, 25].

2.3 Selection of Decomposition Level Based on Quality of Image Compression

It is important to choose an appropriate number of decay levels dependent on the idea of the image or on a reasonable model. In this examination, the most extreme incentive for the nature of pressure has been considered as a standard for choice of disintegration level. The utilization of wavelet change to investigate or break down the image is called decay. Wavelets are two sorts of channels. The technique to register the wavelet change by recursively averaging and separating coefficients is known as the channel bank, which initially is a low-pass channel (lpf) and subsequently a high-pass channel (hpf). Every one of the channels is down inspected by two. Every filter of those two yield images can be further [26, 27].

Practically speaking, it's important to pick a suitable number of deterioration levels that will uphold the personality of the image, or on a proper measure. During this investigation, the most extreme incentive for the norm of pressure has been considered as a model for choice of decay level. The utilization of wavelet change to explore or disintegrate the image is named deterioration. Wavelets are two kinds of channels. The strategy to process the wavelet change by recursively averaging and separating coefficients is named the channel bank, which initially might be a low-pass channel (lpf) and subsequently might be a high-pass channel (hpf). Every one of the channels is down inspected by two. Every one of these two yield images is regularly additionally changed. Correspondingly, this cycle is regularly rehashed recursively a few times, prompting a tree structure called the decay tree. Wavelet decay creates a group of progressively composed disintegrations. It breaks down an image into a progressive arrangement of approximations and subtleties. The sum inside the progressive system regularly compares to a dyadic scale. The decision of a fitting degree of the progressive system will rely on the image. At each level j, an estimate at level j or Aj and a deviation image or Dj are manufactured. Figure 4 presents a graphical portrayal of this progressive three-level decomposition [29, 30].

In wavelet-based image coding, differing types of orthogonal and bio-orthogonal filters are designed by researchers for compression. The choice of wavelet filters plays a crucial role in achieving an efficient compression performance, since there's no filter that performs the simplest for all sort of images. The Haar wavelet isn't suitable for compression, thanks to its property of discontinuity, and it yielded the worst performance in compression. The Daubechies wavelet may be a continuous orthogonal compactly supported wavelet, but it's not symmetric. The prevailing compression method uses the biorthogonal wavelet rather than orthogonal. The Daubechies, Symlet, and Coiflet filters have a singular property of more energy conservation, more vanishing moments, and regularity and asymmetry than bio-orthogonal filters. The second-order wavelet was chosen because the mother

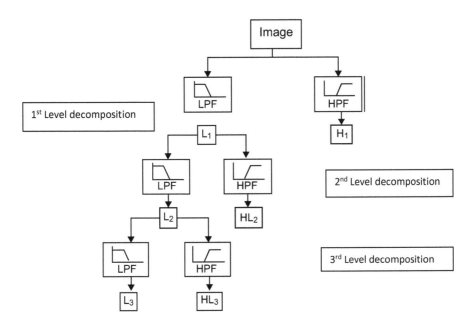

Fig. 4 Graphical representation of three-level decomposition

wavelet has advantages for solving local performance of two-dimensional images. Biorthogonal wavelet of order 1.1, Symlet wavelet of order 2, and Coiflet wavelet of order 2 because of the mother wavelet are chosen for compression. The wavelet transform is employed in compression, for the decomposing of the pictures into low-frequency and high-frequency coefficient. The varied mother wavelets like Symlet, Coiflet, and biorthogonal wavelet transform are utilized in this work, their effectiveness of compression is evaluated, and optimum mother wavelet is additionally chosen from the results.

3   Encoding

3.1   Encoding the Images

This is the method to apply the images after decomposition by transform. Here the following methods are applied and performance is measured.

3.2   Types of Encoding

3.2.1   Embedded Wavelet

The EZW is simple, yet amazingly powerful, image pressure calculation, having the property that the pieces in the spot stream are created arranged by centrality, yielding a totally implanted code. The installed code speaks to a succession of paired choices that separate an image from the "invalid" image. This calculation applies a spatial direction tree structure, from which noteworthy co efficient can be removed in the wavelet domain. EZW encoder doesn't really pack any image. It organizes just the wavelet coefficients so that they can be compacted in the most ideal way.

3.2.2   SPIHT

This algorithm adopts a spatial orientation tree structure, from which significant coefficients can be extracted in the wavelet domain.

The SPIHT algorithm is unique in that it does not directly transmit the contents of the sets, the pixel values, or the pixel coordinates.

The SPIHT coder incorporates a grouping of arranging and refinement passes applied with diminishing greatness limits. In the arranging pass, the coefficients that surpass and equivalent to the current size limit are named as noteworthy and inconsequential assuming in any case. At the point when a coefficient is right off the bat named as noteworthy, the indication of the coefficient is quickly yielded. In the event that the indication of the critical coefficient is positive, SPIHT coder yields

"1." Then again, it communicates "0" to the touch stream. At the point when the unimportant hubs are coded, SPIHT coder examines the coefficient in the fixed request, which spares a ton of pieces by parceling the hubs in the subsets that contain numerous immaterial coefficients for the current size limit. After all the coefficients are examined in the arranging pass, SPITH coder at that point begins to deal with the refinement pass and halves the quantization threshold for the next pass until the magnitude threshold equals to 0.

3.2.3 Spatial Orientation Tree Wavelet

The STW is similar to SPIHT. STW applies the variation in encoding the zero tree information. The locations of transformed values undergo state transitions, from one threshold to the next.

3.2.4 Wavelet Difference Reduction

The WDR gives a lesser PSNR. SPIHT encoding method codes the individual bits of wavelet transform coefficients after decomposing the image in a bit-plane sequence. Thus, it is capable of achieving high compression at higher decomposition level when compared with other encoding methods.

4 Lossless Compression

In lossless compression techniques, there is no loss of information in the reconstructed image after compression. In general, high quality is achieved by this method. This method can be performed by encoding method. The amount of compression of this method is less when compared with lossy method.

Lossless image compression techniques can be implemented using Huffman coding and arithmetic coding.

4.1 *Huffman Coding*

Huffman coding is the most chosen prefix coding technique. It allocates a gathering of prefix codes to images established on their probabilities. Images that happen more regularly will have shorter codewords than images which happen less often. Likewise two images having codewords with same greatest length is less likely to happen. Huffman coding is ineffectual when the letter set size is close to nothing, and along these lines the likelihood of event of images is slanted.

4.2 Arithmetic Coding

Number juggling coding is more productive when the letters in order size are close to nothing or the image probabilities are exceptionally slanted. Creating codewords for successions of images is productive than producing a different codeword for each image during a grouping. A solitary number juggling code are frequently acquired for a particular succession without creating codewords for all groupings of that length. This is regularly inconceivable for Huffman codes. One label esteem is allocated to a square of images, which is solely decodable. Number juggling coding

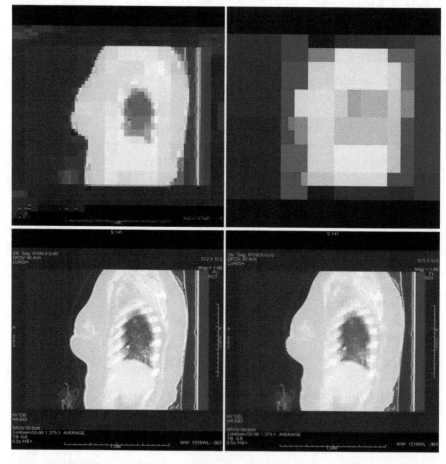

Fig. 5 (**a**) Compressed image of CT cancer lung sagittal view using bio-orthogonal with EZW, (**b**) compressed image of CT cancer lung sagittal view using bio-orthogonal with EZW, (**c**) compressed image of CT cancer lung sagittal view using bio-orthogonal with EZW (**d**) compressed image of CT cancer lung sagittal view using bio-orthogonal with EZW

might be such a variable-length entropy encoding. A string is changed over to number-crunching encoding; as a rule characters are put away with less number of pieces. Number-crunching coding does an identical entire message into one number, a part n where $(0.0 \leq n < 1.0)$.

Figures 5a–d and 6a–d show the compressed image of cancer-affected CT lung sagittal view using biorthogonal wavelet. The numerical results seen from Table 3.15 indicate that the SPIHT yields better results compared to other compression methods.

From the table, it is often inferred that the PSNR is suffering from an outsize marginally with the rise in CR. The choice of wavelet plays an important part in achieving an efficient compression performance because there's no filter that can

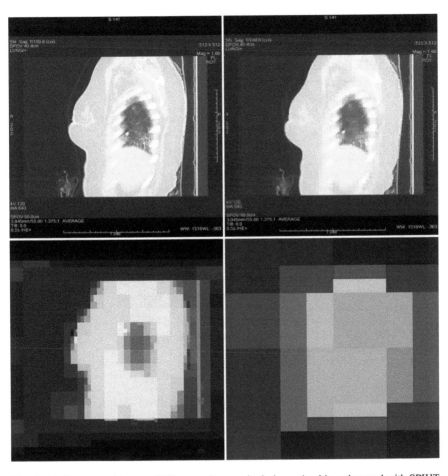

Fig. 6 (**a**) Compressed image of CT cancer lung sagittal view using bio-orthogonal with SPIHT (CR = 85.24%, PSNR = 41.84), (**b**) compressed image using bio-orthogonal with SPIHT (CR = 19.26%, PSNR = 44.24), (**c**) compressed image using bio-orthogonal with SPIHT (CR = 5.9%, PSNR = 36.95), (**d**) compressed image using bio-orthogonal with SPIHT (CR = 1.71%, PSNR = 29.10)

perform the simplest for all images. The main objective of this work is to realize a high compression ratio, which is achieved with a better level of decomposition. The number of filter banks used is high at higher decomposition level. Some information will be lost.

5 Conclusion

In the lossy compression, the decomposition levels and vanishing moments are varied in the different compression algorithms. It is observed that all the mother wavelets performed well at first level of decomposition, irrespective of their types and image formats. The increment in the decomposition level produced a less PSNR value and more compression ratio increase irrespective of the wavelet type used for compression. The bits per pixels are same as PSNR value, since both are related. The minimum errors are obtained by decomposition level one.

References

1. Adler D C et al. (2004), "Speckle reduction in optical coherence tomography images by use of a spatially adaptive wavelet filter", Optics Letters, Vol. 29.
2. Ahmed (1974),"Discrete cosine transform", IEEE Transaction on Computer, Vol. C-23, No. 1, pp. 90–93.
3. Ahmed Al-Gindy (2017), "Digital image watermarking technique for big size watermarks and high-resolution images using discrete cosine transform", International Journal of Signal and Imaging Systems Engineering, Vol 10(6).
4. Akshay Kekre and Dr Sanjay Pokle (2013), "Improved Image Compression Using Wavelet Transform and Differential Pulse Code Modulation Technique" International Journal of Engineering Research & Technology (IJERT) Vol. 2(7).
5. Antonini M et al. (1992),"Image Coding Using Wavelet Transform", IEEE Transaction on Image Process, Vol. 1, No. 2, pp. 205–220.
6. Archana and Deshlahra et al. (2010) "A Comparative Study Of DCT, DWT & Hybride (DCT-DWT) Transform". IEEE Transaction on Image processing.
7. Aree Ali Mohammed and Jamal Ali Hussian (2011), "Hybrid Transform Coding Scheme for Medical Image Application" 2011 IEEE Transaction on image processing.
8. Ashraf et al. (2006), "Compression strength of stainless steel cross- sections", Journal of Constructional Steel Research Vol. 62(1), pp. 105–115.
9. Banafa A Y (1993), "A comparative study of image compression techniques within a noisy channel environment", Ph.D. Thesis, Lehigh University, Bethlehem.
10. Bhatia S K (2006), "Visual Data Processing", Lecture note.
11. Bhavani S and Thanushkodi K (2010), "A survey on coding algorithms in medical image compression", International Journal on Computer Science and Engineering Vol. 2(5) pp. 1429–1434.
12. Boleik (2000), "JPEG2000 next generation image compression system features and syntax", in Proc. International Conference on Image Processing, Vol. 2, pp. 45–48.
13. Bryan E. Usevitch (2001), "A Tutorial on Modern Lossy Wavelet Image Compression: Foundations of JPEG 2000", IEEE Signal Processing Magazine.

14. Cadder Bank A R (1997), "Loss less image compression using integer to integer wavelet transforms", International Conference on image processing, Vol. 1, pp 596–599.
15. Carlos et al. (2007), "Classification of Real Flaws Using Ultrasonic Signals", ndt. Net.
16. Chen and Yen-Yu. (2007) "Medical image compression using DCT-based subband decomposition and modified SPIHT data organization", International Journal of Medical Informatics Vol.76 (10), pp. 717–725.
17. Chenwei Deng and Weisi Lin (2012), "Content-Based Image Compression for Arbitrary-Resolution Display Devices", IEEE Transactions on Multimedia Vol. 4, pp. 1127–1139.
18. Choong et al. (2007) "Cost-effective handling of digital medical images in the telemedicine environment", International Journal of Medical Informatics, Vol. 76(9), pp. 646–654.
19. Christos Stergiou and Dimitrios Siganos D (2007), "Neural Networks", (http://www.docstoc.com/docs/15050/neuralnetworksby-Christos-Stergiou-and-Dimitrios-Siganos) online.
20. Cobas and Carlos J (2008), "Compression of high resolution 1D and 2D NMR data sets using JPEG2000." Chemometrics and Intelligent Laboratory Systems Vol. 91(2), pp. 141–150.
21. Cosman P C et al. (1994), "Evaluating quality of compressed medical images: SNR, subjective rating, and diagnostic accuracy", in of the Proceedings IEEE, Vol. 82(6), pp. 919–932.
22. Davis L and Johns S J (1979), "Texture analysis using generalized co-occurrence matrices", IEEE Transactions on Pattern Analysis and Machine Intelligence, PAMI-1, pp. 251–259.
23. David Bethel (1997), "Optimisation of still image compression techniques", Ph.D. Thesis, Bath University, U.K
24. Dhawan and Sachin (2011), "A review of image compression and comparison of its algorithms", International Journal of Electronics & Communication Technology 2(1), pp. 22–26.
25. Dragan and Dragan Ivetic (2009), "An approach to DICOM extension for medical image streaming", DAAAM international scientific book, pp. 25–35.
26. El-Maleh et al. (2000), "Speech music discrimination for multimedia application", IEEE International Conference on Acoustics, Speech, and Signal Processing, Turkey, pp. 2445–2448.
27. Erickson and Manduca B J (1998), "Wavelet compression of medical images", Radiology, Vol. 206, pp. 599–607.
28. Geeta Kaushik and Lillie Dewan (2016), "Analysis of DWT signal denoising on various biomedical signals by neural network", International Journal of Signal and Imaging Systems Engineering, Vol. 9(6), pp. 342–356.
29. Ramandeep Kaur and Navneet Randhawa (2012), "Image Compression Using Discrete Cosine Transform & Discrete Wavelet Transform", International Journal of Computing & Business Research, pp. 2229–6166.
30. Gemma piella (2005), "Adaptive lifting schemes combining semi norms for lossless image compression", IEEE International conference on image processing. Vol. 1, pp. 753–756, 2005.

Realization of Carry-Free Adder Circuit Using FPGA

Shruti Jain

Abstract The circuit complexity and propagation delay are the main concern in the design of the digital circuit. In the binary system, as the number of bits increases, the computation speed is limited by the propagation of carry. Consequently, it offers low storage density, large complexity, and $O(n)$ carry producing delay in n-bit base 2 application problems. For less complexity and higher information storage density, higher radix number system can be used. Quaternary signed digit (QSD) number system performs carry-free addition and borrows free subtraction. The QSD number system requires a various set of prime modulo-based logic elements for each arithmetic operation. Arithmetic operations on a large number of bits (64, 128, 256, 512, or more) can be implemented with less complexity and constant delay that increases linearly. The data processing speed is limited in the base 2 number system because of the generation of carry peculiarly as the number of bits keeps on increasing. The QSD addition eliminates carry from addition and delayed addition. The authors have also worked on minimizing the delay at a particular frequency. For all these designing and calculations, Xilinx 14.7 software has been used. In this paper, authors have designed the ripple carry adder, carry-save adder, and carry-free adders and achieve 1.075 ns, 1.673 ns, and 1.878 ns delay, respectively.

Keywords QSD · Carry-free adder · Carry-save adder · RCA · Delay

1 Introduction

Operations involving addition, subtraction, and multiplication form the basic arithmetic operations which are extensively used and thus perform a significant part in many digital electronic devices such as signal mainframes and computers [1, 2]. The arithmetic units employing quaternary signed digit (QSD) number system have been a topic of great interest for many researcher scholars [3, 4]. High-performance arithmetic is very crucial as the adders used in the system decide the pace of the data

S. Jain (✉)
Jaypee University of Information Technology, Solan, Himachal Pradesh, India
e-mail: shruti.jain@juit.ac.in

© The Author(s), under exclusive license to Springer
Nature Switzerland AG 2021
A. K. Manocha et al. (eds.), *Computational Intelligence in Healthcare*, Health
Information Science, https://doi.org/10.1007/978-3-030-68723-6_3

processing machine. It also handles a component for amalgamation rest of the calculation assignments [5, 6]. Digital signal processing is the main application of adder where it is used for the execution of FIR and IIR algorithms [7, 8]. Arithmetic operations still experience problems like the number of bits are limited, delay in producing time, and complication of the circuit. The time lag in an adder is established through the carry chain. Some of the drawbacks of BSD number systems are its computational speed that constraints generation and production of carry peculiarly when the number of bits is extended. Accordingly, it contributes to large complications and less cache denseness. Arithmetic which removes carry can be accomplished using a number system with higher radix such as (QSD) [9–11]. In QSD, there is a reduction of computational time due to the elimination of the carry propagation chain; this enhances the speed [12–14]. The QSD subtraction/addition operation utilizes a fixed number of operand size [15, 16]. Signed integer portrayal can be used to conclude the fast addition of integers because it can eradicate carry. The portrayal of a signed-integer QSD number is expressed by using Eq. (1):

$$D = \sum_{n-1}^{i=0} X_i 4^i \tag{1}$$

Authors in [17] reviewed VHDL for quaternary signed adder system. Authors in [18] designed and implemented QSD adders for arithmetic operation. In [19], implementation of large digits of digital like 64, 128, or large numbers can be implicated with the same amount of delay. Authors in [20] explained that with the increase of the radix, the redundancy usually increases in the quaternary (base 4) number system. In [21], multivalued logic is used, design of a paradigm of digital to analog converter circuit using an operational amplifier to substantiate the approach. An author in [22] designed the QSD cipher notation system addition using delayed addition technique.

Earlier, the other number systems were propagating chains, and thus the speed was limited. A lot of research was done on higher number systems, authors in this paper work on the quaternary signed digit. Considering digital logic in the field of VLSI, an optimal solution for the problem in which carry and borrow free addition and subtraction respectively of the quaternary signed digit can be calculated. Using QSD, propagation chains are eliminated and also prevent rippling of carry. QSD numbers are less complex and use 25% less space than binary signed number systems to store numbers. QSD number systems offer not only simple logic but also higher storage density. This paper proposes a tremendous productive QSD adder accomplished of addition and subtraction without the involvement of carry and borrows, respectively, which was simulated in Xilinx using Verilog HDL. In this paper, authors have also designed RCA, carry-save adder, and carry-free adder, and the results are compared with the existing state-of-the-art technique.

Section II of this paper explains the design of the QSD adder, and Section III explains the results of the proposed QSD adder and design of different adders, namely, RCA, carry-select adder, and carry-free adder followed by conclusion and future work.

2 Proposed Methodology

Arithmetic operations have a vital role in several digitized systems like process controllers, computers, image/signal processing, and computer graphics [23, 24]. The latest improvisations in the techniques of integrated circuitries made the bigger circuits based on arithmetic functions to be implemented over VLSI, although such arithmetic functions are still dealing with issues like limited bits, time delay in propagation, and complicacy in the circuit. The flexibility in FPGAs has also supported enhancement in customized hardware giving a high ratio of performance. By choosing arithmetic algorithms that suit FPGA technology and implementing optimal mapping techniques, a high-performance FPGA application can be produced. High-speed QSD arithmetic and a logical unit have the capability of doing various operations like carry-free addition, borrow-free subtraction, multiplication functions, and up-down count. The operation of addition and subtraction by QSD incorporates a defined number for any size of an operand [25, 26]. QSD adder is designed to execute arithmetic functions at a high speed as shown in Fig. 1. In the QSD number system, carry chain propagation is eliminated that further leads to the minimization of computational time. It further improvises the speed of the machine [27].

Quaternary is taken as a base-4 number system [4, 5]. The numbers 0, 1, 2, and 3 are used to present any of the numbers. The number 4 is the maximum digit in subsidizing range and one of the number which is a highly composite number and a square as well, that makes quaternary as a rational selection as a base over this scale. Since it is double in the size than binary, still radix economy of both is the same, although it doesn't work fine in localizing prime numbers. There are two different approaches to convert a decimal number to QSD: long division method and base 2 signed digit (2's complement form). One digit QSD number can be portrayed using a 3-bit base 2 proportionate shown in Table 1.

To novitiate n-bit base 2 data into its proportionate q-digit QSD information, this comprises of the n-bit base 2 information that should be translated into $3q$-bit base 2 information. For a change from base 2 to QSD, the required cardinal portrayal of base-2 bits is shown in Eq. (2):

$$n = 3q - \{1 \times (q-1)\} \tag{2}$$

To attain this, odd bit from LSB to MSB (3rd, 5th, 7th bit, etc.) is split into two different parts, but the MSB bit cannot be divided. Algorithm 1 shows the steps for finding the QSD number from a negative decimal number.

Algorithm 1: QSD number from a negative decimal number Input: Any decimal number

Output: QSD number

Step 1: Consider a negative number $(-109)_{10}$.
Step 2: Convert into base 2 signed bit representation $(1101101)_2$.
Step 3: Conversion in its QSD proportion by considering an odd bit.

Fig. 1 Flow chart showing
QSD addition

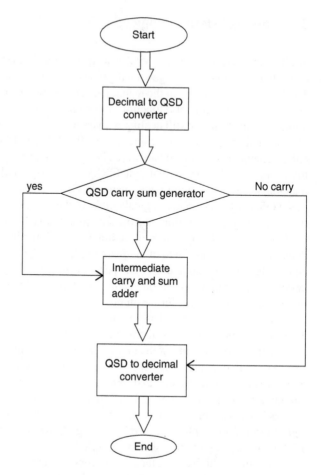

Table 1 Signed digit (2's
complement form)

One digit QSD number	3-bit base 2 proportionate
$\overline{3}$	101
$\overline{2}$	110
$\overline{1}$	111
0	000
1	001
2	010
3	011

Step 4: If the odd bit is 0, then it is divided into 0 and 0, and if it is 1, then it is divided into 1 and 0 as illustrated:

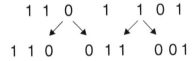

Step 5: Conversion of binary into QSD by making a group of three. Final QSD number $(631)_4$.

More than one QSD representation can be used to represent the same decimal number. The number is chosen to avoid the fluctuation of the carry. The addition of the two QSD integers without carry can be done in the following two different tracks [5]:

1. In step 1, carry (intervening) and sum (intervening) are generated by the adder from the input digits.
2. In step 2, adder sums up the sum (intervening) of an ongoing integer with the carry (intervening) of a reduced indicative integer.

The fluctuation of carry can be removed by performing the following two rules in QSD addition [1]:

Rule 1: It states that the significance of the sum (intervening) must vary from −2 to +2.
Rule 2: It states that the significance of the carry (intervening) must vary from −1 to +1.

From the first step, the intervening sum and the intervening carry are obtained from the QSD adder whose province is from −6 to +6 as mentioned in the above rules. But using redundancy trait of QSD numbers, 655 is selected which satisfies the above-stated rules. When the intermediate sum whose range is from −2 to +2 as obtained in the second step of QSD adder is added with the lower significant digit intermediate carry whose province is from −1 to +1, the output of the addition cannot be larger than 3, i.e., it must lie in the province of −3 to +3; hence, there is no further requirement of carry as the addition output in this province can be depicted by an integer QSD [8–9].

Consider two inputs a_i (a_2, a_1, a_0) and b_i (b_2, b_1, b_0) considering the product yielding the intervening carry (IC as IC_2, IC_1, IC_0) and the intervening sum (IS: IS_2, IS_1, IS_0). The equations for the intervening sum (IS_2, IS_1, and IS_0) are expressed by Eqs. (3, 4, and 5), respectively:

$$IS_0 = a_0 \oplus b_0 \tag{3}$$

$$IS_1 = (a_0.b_0) \oplus a_1 \oplus b_1 \tag{4}$$

$$IS_2 = \left(IS_0.(a_1 \oplus b_1)\right) + \left(\overline{a_1.\overline{b_0}.b_2}\right) + \left((a_0.b_0).\left(\overline{a_1.\overline{b_1}}\right).(a_2 + b_2)\right)$$
$$+ (a_0.b_0.a_1.b_1.a_2.b_2) \tag{5}$$

The equations for intervening carry (IC_2, IC_1, IC_0) are represented by Eqs. (6 and 7), respectively:

$$IC_2 = IC_1 = (a_2.b_2).\left(\overline{a_0.b_0.a_1.b_1}\right) + \left(\overline{a_1 + b_1}\right).\left(a_2.\overline{b_0} + \overline{a_0}.b_2\right) \tag{6}$$

$$IC_0 = IC_2 + \left(\overline{a_2.b_2}\right).(a_1.b_1 + b_1.b_0 + a_1.b_0 + a_0.b_1 + a_1.a_0) \tag{7}$$

The final sum (S_0, S_1, and S_2) is calculated by using Eqs. (8, 9, and 10), respectively:

$$S_0 = IC_0.\overline{IS_0} + \overline{IC_0}.IS_0 \tag{8}$$

$$S_1 = IC_1 \oplus IS_1 \oplus (IC_0.IS_0) \tag{9}$$

$$S_2 = IC_2 \oplus IS_2 \oplus \left((IC_1.IS_1) + ((IC_1 + IS_1).(IC_0.IS_0))\right) \tag{10}$$

The QSD integer ranges from −3 to +3, and when the two QSD integers are added, the result varies from −6 to +6. The product of all the feasible combinations of two numbers is illustrated in Table 2. If the range is exceeded by the decimal number, then there is a requirement of one more QSD digit. In the addition of two-digit QSD outcome, LSB is represented by the sum bit, and MSB bit is represented by carry.

Table 2 Intermediate sum and carry from −6 to +6

Sum	Possible QSD representations	QSD number	
		IC	IS
−6	$\overline{1}\,\overline{2},\overline{2}2$	$\overline{1}$	$\overline{2}$
−5	$\overline{1}\,\overline{1},\overline{2}3$	$\overline{1}$	$\overline{1}$
−4	$\overline{1},0$	$\overline{1}$	0
−3	$\overline{1}1,0\overline{3}$	$\overline{1}$	1
−2	$\overline{1},2,0,\overline{2}$	0	$\overline{2}$
−1	$0\overline{1},\overline{1}3$	0	$\overline{1}$
0	$0\,0$	0	0
1	$0\overline{1},\overline{1}3$	0	1
2	$1\overline{2},02$	0	2
3	$03,1\overline{1}$	1	$\overline{1}$
4	$1\,0$	1	0
5	$11,2\overline{3}$	1	1
6	$12,2\overline{2}$	1	2

By scaling the two digits into intervening sum and intervening carry in such a way that the nth intervening sum and the $(n-1)^{th}$ intervening carry will not at all generate any propagating carry pair so that the rippling of the carry can be eliminated. Confining the representation of the QSD number according to the rules as defined above, the endmost addition will have no carry in the end.

3   Results and Discussion

In this paper, the QSD adder is designed and simulated in Verilog HDL of Xilinx Software 14.7. The circuit is implemented on the FPGA using the VIVADO tool. An FPGA is IC, a semiconductor device which can be reprogrammed by the customer according to his requirement after manufacturing. It comprises of an array of configurable logic blocks (CLBs) and switches (which form a connection between CLBs) [28, 29]. FPGA gives high-speed clock, good performance, and high bandwidth and facilitates simultaneously multiple operations. The FPGA is advantageous for implementation in real-time processing systems. The FPGA can remodel the digital design straight to ASICs. An FPGA consisting interconnections, I/O blocks, and reconfigurable logic, that differs from DSP and microcontroller processors. It is a better implementation solution in the latest digital systems due to its low NRE cost, radiation effects, power consumption, reconfigurable architecture, better performance, and ease of design. The design and architecture of the programmable routing circuit is the main issue and demand in FPGAs. Before the use of FPGA in portable electronic devices, various issues like static power consumption should be addressed. In recent years, FPGA is widely used in medical-related applications because of its flexible programming, low power consumption, easy transfer, and short development cycle.

Using the QSD adder, carry-free QSD adder, ripple carry adder (RCA), and carry-save adder are designed. The circuit is designed as shown in Fig. 2.

Results for ripple carry adder: RCA is considered the basic approach amid all the addition algorithms. An N bit RCA requires N number of full adders in series cascading. RCA and ripple carry subtractor are designed using the proposed QSD adder. The simulation results of the RCA and ripple carry subtractor are illustrated in Figs. 3 and 4, respectively.

In figures, a_0, a_1, a_2, b_0, b_1, b_2, and c_{in} are the inputs; s_3, s_2, and s_1 are the final turnouts; and c_{out1}, c_{out2}, and c_{out3} are the trajectory final turnouts. This result has been obtained by changing the C_{in} value from 0 to 1 in the test bench of the Xilinx code. The synthesis report shows the total number of LUTs and slices used during the simulation of the RCA circuit as tabulated in Table 3. The three different time lags total delay, the logic delay, and the route delay of the circuit are calculated. Table 3 shows the comparison of ripple carry adder with other existing work in terms of different parameters like LUT, slices, gates, and delay.

It has been observed that the design of the ripple carry adder by Prabha et al [16] shows 44.366ns delay. But the calculated delay of our proposed circuit is 1.075ns.

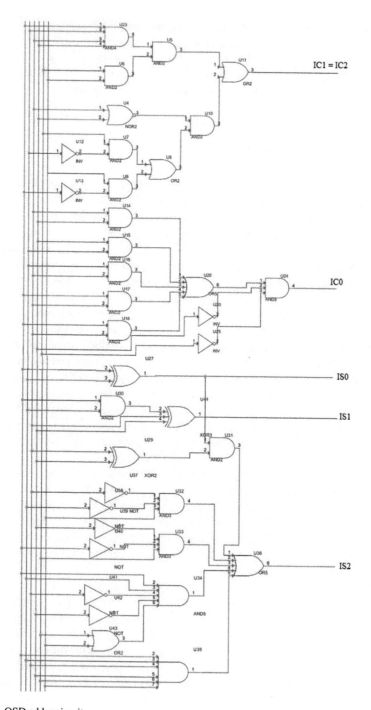

Fig. 2 QSD adder circuit

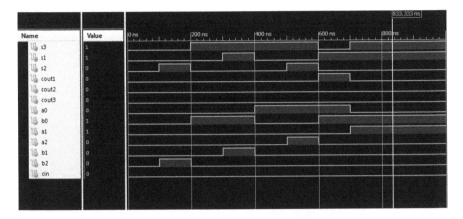

Fig. 3 Simulation result of RCA

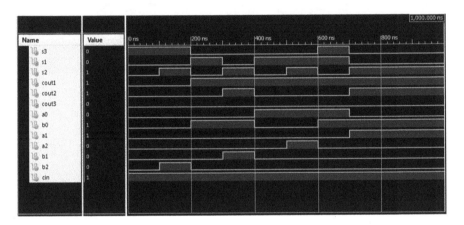

Fig. 4 Simulation result of ripple carry subtractor

Results for Carry-Save Adder: Carry-save adder is used for the fast calculation of addition. For getting sum bit and carry bit, bitwise XOR and bitwise AND operations, respectively, are performed. Finally, add them by shifting carry bit left by one place to sum bit up to produce the final answer. Carry-save adder is designed using the proposed QSD adder. The simulation results of the carry-save adder is shown in Fig. 5.

In figure, a_0, a_1, a_2, b_0, b_1, b_2, and c_{in} are the inputs; s_3, s_2, and s_1 are the final turnouts; and c_{out1}, c_{out2}, and c_{out3} are the trajectory final turnouts. This result has been obtained by changing the C_{in} value from 0 to 1 in the test bench of the Xilinx code. The synthesis report shows the total number of LUTs and slices used during the simulation of the CSA as tabulated in Table 4. Table 4 explains the different values obtained from the synthesis report which have been compared with various other results obtained after studying various research papers.

Table 3 Comparison table for ripple carry adder

Authors	LUT	Slices	Gates	Delay (ns)	Logic delay (ns)	Route delay (ns)
Prabha et al. [16]	11	4	15	44.366	11.28	45.393
Our work	5	5	15	1.075	0.98	0.977

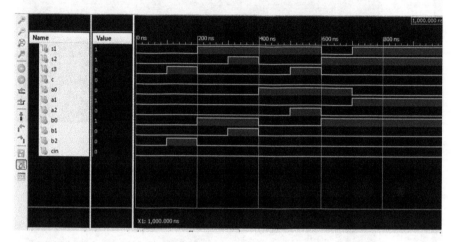

Fig. 5 Simulation result of carry-save adder.

Table 4 Comparison table for carry-save adder

Authors	LUT	Slices	Gates	Delay (ns)	Logic delay (ns)	Route delay (ns)
Kumar and Punniakodi 2013 [30]	13	9	20	1.433	0.289	1.144
Our work	5	5	20	1.673	0.195	1.478

It has been observed that the design of the carry-save adder by Kumar and Punniakodi (2013) [30] shows 1.433 ns delay. But the calculated delay in our proposed diagram is 1.673 ns.

Results Using Carry-Free Adder: The carry-free adder is designed and simulated. The simulation result is illustrated in Fig. 6. The performance parameters were calculated which are tabulated in Table 5.

In Table 5, different values obtained from the synthesis report have been compared with various other results obtained after studying various research papers. It has been observed that the design of the carry-save adder by Hussain and Rao (2014) [31] shows a 2 ns delay. But the calculated delay in our proposed diagram is 1.878 ns resulting in a 6.1% improvement than the other state-of-the-art technique.

This data is processed by FPGA, and the program is burned as shown in Fig. 7. Finally, the carry-free adder output is sent from FPGA to the PC for display.

Carry-free adder, RCA, and carry-save adders are designed, and the results are compared with other state-of-the-art techniques as tabulated in Table 6.

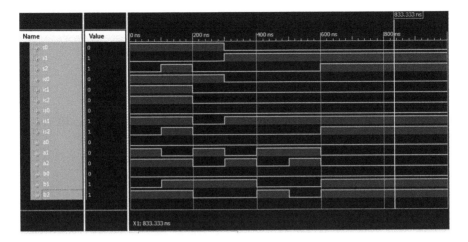

Fig. 6 Simulation result of carry-free adder (QSD)

Table 5 Comparison table for carry-free adder

Authors	LUT	Slices	Gates	Delay (ns)	Logic delay (ns)	Route delay (ns)
Hussain and Rao 2014 [31]	28	47	38	2	0.268	2.257
Our work	9	7	38	1.878	0.195	1.638

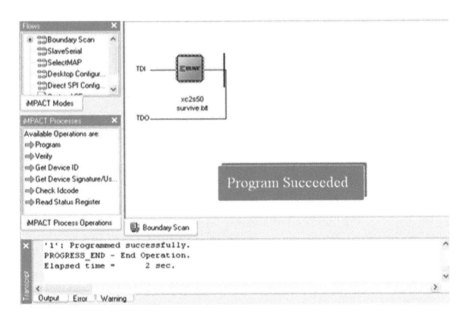

Fig. 7 Implementation of the proposed algorithm on FPGA

Table 6 Delay (ns) calculation

Authors	RCA	Carry-save adders	Carry-free adder
Prabha et al. [16]	44.366	–	10.113
Mitra et al. [32]	3.71	3.09	–
Proposed work	**1.075**	**1.673**	**1.878**

It has been observed that our circuit's results in 71% improvement in RCA circuit and 45.85% improvement in carry-save adder circuit with Mitra et al.

4   Conclusion

In this paper, authors have compared carry-free adder, RCA, and carry-save adders in terms of different performance parameters like delay, LUTs, slices, and gates. The suggested design of QSD generates a time delay of 1.878 ns. The proposed circuit consumes less energy and reduces time lag leading to better performance. It has been observed that our circuit's results in 71% improvement in RCA circuit and 45.85% improvement in carry-save adder circuit with other state-of-the-art techniques. As a result of which, this structure is applicable to be adapted for the implementation of a highly fulfilled multiprocessor which may consist of many processing components. This work can be counterfeited in the transistor level to minimize the delay and optimize the power by considering numerous low-power techniques.

References

1. K. Hwang, Computer Arithmatic Principles Architecture and Design. New York: Wiley.
2. Koren, Computer Arithmetic, New Jersey, Englewood Cliffs: Prentice Hall.
3. S. Dubey, R. Rani, S. Kumari and N. Sharma, "VLSI implementation of fast addition using quaternary Signed Digit number system," *2013 IEEE International Conference ON Emerging Trends in Computing,* Communication and Nanotechnology (ICECCN), Tirunelveli, 2013, pp. 654–659, https://doi.org/10.1109/ICE-CCN.2013.6528581.
4. J.U. Ahmed, A.A.S. Awwal, "Multiplier design using RBSD number system", Proceedings of the 1993 National Aerospace and Electronics Conference, pp. 180–184, Vol. 1, 1993.
5. A. N. Nagamani and S. Nishchai, "Quaternary High Performance Arithmetic Logic Unit Design," 2011 14th Euromicro Conference on Digital System Design, Oulu, 2011, pp. 148–153, doi: https://doi.org/10.1109/DSD.2011.23.
6. S Jain, P.K. Naik, R Sharma, "A Computational Modeling of cell survival/ death using VHDL and MATLAB Simulator", Digest Journal of Nanomaterials and Biostructures (DJNB), 4 (4): 863–879, 2009.
7. N Prashar, M. Sood, S. Jain, "Design and Performance Analysis of Cascade Digital Filter for ECG Signal Processing", International Journal of Innovative Technology and Exploring Engineering (IJITEE), 8(8), 2659–2665, 2019.
8. Kirti, H. Sohal, S. Jain, "FPGA implementation of Power-Efficient ECG pre-processing block", International Journal of Recent Technology and Engineering, 8(1), 2899–2904, 2019.

9. R. Rani, U. Agrawal, N. Sharma and L.K Singh, "High Speed Arithmetic Logical Unit using Quaternary Signed Digit Number System", *International Journal Of Electronic Engineering Research*, vol. 2, pp. 383–391, Number 2010, ISSN 0975-6450.

10. P. K. Dakhole and D.G. Wakde, "Multi Digit Quaternary adder on Programmable Device: Design and verification", *International Conference on Electronic Design*, pp. 1–4, 2008, 1–3 Dec.

11. M. W. Allam and M. I. Elmasry, "Low power implementation of fast addition algorithms," *Conference Proceedings. IEEE Canadian Conference on Electrical and Computer Engineering (Cat. No.98TH8341)*, Waterloo, Ontario, Canada, 1998, pp. 645–647 vol.2, doi: https://doi.org/10.1109/CCECE.1998.685579.

12. R Thakur, S Jain, M. Sood "FPGA Implementation of Unsigned Multiplier Circuit Based on Quaternary Signed Digit Number System" , 4th IEEE International Conference on signal processing and control (ISPCC 2017), Jaypee University of Information technology, Waknaghat, Solan, H.P, India, pp 637–641, September 21-23, 2017.

13. W. Clark, J. Lian, "On arithmetic weight for general radix representation of integers". IEEE Trans. Inform. Theory, Vol. 19, pp. 823–826, 1973.

14. H. Shirahama and T. Hanyu, "Design of High Performance Quaternary Adders Based on Output-Generator Sharing", Proceedings of the 38th International Symposium on Multiple Valued Logic, pp. 8–13. 2008.

15. S.A.Dakhane, A.M.Shah, "FPGA Implementation of Fast Arithmetic UnitBased on QSD", International Journal of Computer Science and Information Technologies, Vol. 5(3), pp: 3331–3334, 2014.

16. A.Divya Prabha, V.Murali Dharan, M.Varatharaj, "Accomplishment of Formidable Agility QSD Adder for VLSI Application", IJRE, Volume 3, Issue 3, pp. 11–13, 2016.

17. P. S. Kamble, Suman M. Choudhary, "Review of VHDL Implementation of Quaternary Signed Adder System" 2012.

18. R. K. Kothuru, P. V. Ramana, "Design and Implementation of QSD Adders for Arithmetic Operation", International Journal of Professional Engineering Studies, Volume II/Issue 3/June2014.

19. S. Kaur, S. Singh, "Design of Hybrid Quaternary Signed Digit (QSD) based divider Using VHDL", International Journal of Engineering Sciences & Research Technology,4(8), August, 2015.

20. K.Kuntal, S.Kumari, R.Rani, N.Sharma, "Implementation of QSD Adder using VLSI", Proceedings of IRF International Conference, 5-6 February 2014, Pune India. ISBN: 978-93-82702-56-6.

21. T Chattopadhyay and T Sarkar, "Logical Design of Quaternary Signed Digit Conversion Circuit and its Effectuation using Operational Amplifier", Bonfring International Journal of Power Systems and Integrated Circuits, Vol. 2, No. 3, December 2012 .

22. S.Mallesh, C.V.Narasimhulu, "Design of QSD Cipher notation System Addition using Delayed Addition Technique", International Journal of Ethics in Engineering & Management Education, Volume 1, Issue 10, pp: 1–4, October 2014.

23. J. Millman, C. Halkias, Integrated Electronics: Analog and digital circuits and systems. New York: McGraw-Hill, Inc.

24. V Patel, K.S. Gurumurthy, "Arithmetic operations in multivalued logic." International Journal of VLSI Design & Communication Systems (VLSICS), Vol. 1, No. 1, March 2010.

25. A. Leela Bhardwaj Reddy, V. Narayana Reddy, "VLSI Implementation of Fast Addition Subtraction and Multiplication (Unsigned) Using Quaternary Signed Digit Cipher notation System", 2(12), pp: 2061–2074, December 2015.

26. P.K. Dakhole, D.G. Wakde, "Multi Digit Quaternary adder on Programmable Device: Design and verification", International Conference on Electronic Design, pp. 1–4, Dec 2008.

27. T. Chattopadhyay, J.N. Roy, "Easy conversion technique of binary to quaternary signed digit and vice versa." Physics Express, Vol. 1, No. 3, pp. 165–174, 2011.

28. Sonal Pokharkar, Amit Kulkarni, "FPGA Based Design and Implementation of ECG Feature Extraction", International Journal of Advance Foundation and Research in Science & Engineering (IJAFRSE) Volume 1, Issue 12, May 2015.
29. A. Armato et al., "An FPGA Based Arrhythmia Recognition System for Wearable Applications," 2009 Ninth International Conference on Intelligent Systems Design and Applications, Pisa, 2009, pp: 660–664. https://doi.org/10.1109/ISDA.2009.246.
30. M.S. Kumar, S. Punniakodi, "Design and Performance Analysis of Various Adders using Verilog", International Journal of Computer Science and Mobile Computing Vol.2, Issue. 9, pp: 128–138, September 2013.
31. S.J.Hussain, K. S. Rao, "Design and Accomplishment of Fast Aggregation Using QSD for Signed and Unsigned Cardinal depictions", International Journal of Engineering Research, Volume No.3 Issue No: Special 2, pp: 52–54, 22 March 2014.
32. A.Mitra, A.Bakshi, B.Sharma, N.Didwania, "Design of a High Speed Adder", International Journal of Scientific & Engineering Research, 6(4), pp: 918–921, April-2015.

Telemedicine and Telehealth: The Current Update

**Dhruthi Suresh, Surabhi Chaudhari, Apoorva Saxena,
and Praveen Kumar Gupta**

Abstract Telemedicine is considered as a tool that is accessible and cost-effective and increases patient engagement. Since its birth in the early 1900s, it has only evolved and grown to be a boon for everyone. Patients can share their medical history, attend virtual health checkups, and have follow-up appointments with their respective medical practitioners. The most benefitted of all would perhaps be the people living in remote and rural areas that have little or no access to proper healthcare facilities. The concept of telemedicine and telehealth could still be a novice one to most practitioners. However, the continued advances in technology can demand its usability from a new generation of tech-savvy people due to its convenience, cost-effectiveness, and intelligent features. There are different methods by which patients can interact with their doctors. These include store and forward techniques, real-time interactive modes, remote monitoring, and the use of smartphones for healthcare services like mHealth. The application of telemedicine in healthcare services is extensive and includes but is not limited to teleradiology, telesurgery, telepsychiatry, etc. As beneficial as it can get, telemedicine also poses some risks to its users. Security breaches, false documentation, and data privacy risks are a few of the concerns that need to be addressed. This review article aims to make people aware of the concept of telemedicine, how it came into existence, its features, and its drawbacks. It will also touch upon the evolution of telemedicine in India and its application in the COVID-19 pandemic that the world is currently facing.

Keywords Telemedicine · Virtual health checkups · Medical practitioners · Technology · COVID-19 pandemic

D. Suresh · S. Chaudhari (✉) · A. Saxena · P. K. Gupta
Department of Biotechnology, R.V. College of Engineering, Bangalore, India
e-mail: praveenkgupta@rvce.edu.in

© The Author(s), under exclusive license to Springer
Nature Switzerland AG 2021
A. K. Manocha et al. (eds.), *Computational Intelligence in Healthcare*, Health
Information Science, https://doi.org/10.1007/978-3-030-68723-6_4

67

1 Introduction to Telemedicine and Telehealth

Telehealth is the dissemination of healthcare services through electronic means as well as telecommunication technologies. Through telemedicine, patients can contact their healthcare providers over long distances and acquire care, monitoring, intervention, medical advice, and admissions, remotely [1]. Telehealth can be a boon in cases of rural settings, lack of mobility and transport, reduced funding, and lack of emergency staff. In addition to this, it also helps in conducting meetings, presentations, and exchange of information among practitioners and helps in data management and integration of healthcare systems [2, 3].

Telehealth and telemedicine are sometimes interchanged (Fig. 1). However, the Health Resources and Services Administration differentiates telehealth and telemedicine in their scope. Telemedicine can be interpreted as clinical services executed remotely, for example, monitoring and diagnosis, whereas, on the other hand, telehealth incorporates promotive, preventative, and curative delivery of care. It also includes nonclinical applications like provider education and administration.

The American Telemedicine Association (ATA) defines telemedicine as: "Telemedicine is the natural evolution of healthcare in the digital world." The World Health Organization (WHO) has provided its definition of telemedicine to be "the delivery of healthcare services, where distance is a critical factor, by all healthcare professionals, using information and communication technologies for the exchange

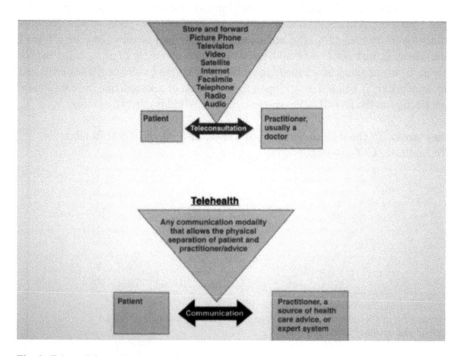

Fig. 1 Telemedicine and telehealth flowchart [4]

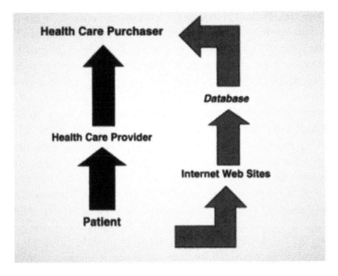

Fig. 2 The flow of information from patient to purchasers of healthcare using the internet [4]

of valid information for the diagnosis, treatment, and prevention of disease and injuries, research and evaluation, and for the continuing education of healthcare providers, all in the interests of advancing the health of individuals and their communities" (Fig. 2). The literal translation of telemedicine is "healing at a distance." It is frequently used as an umbrella term for healthcare delivery, research, health surveillance, education, and promotion of public health.

2 Birth of Telemedicine

Instances in applications of telemedicine technologies can be trailed back to the pre-television era. For example, in the early 1900s, medical service providers communicated through the radio in Antarctica. In the year 1910, the first-ever electrical stethoscope that was trans-telephonic had been demonstrated in England. Scientists started illustrating the possibility of a "remote radio doctor" in early 1924, which could both see and be seen by its patients. Radiological images were believed to be broadcasted for the first time between Philadelphia and West Chester, in Pennsylvania, in the year 1950 [4].

The use of video communications for interactive sessions can be traced back to the late 1950s, when the Nebraska Psychiatric Institute had made use of a two-way television system for teleconsultations in psychiatry with another hospital situated 112 miles away, the Norfolk State Hospital [4]. This connection was established to develop education and carry out specialized consultations and treatments among practitioners and specialists. Another instance of an experimental demonstration came into limelight in the year 1959, when a Canadian-based radiologist had used images that were transmitted coaxially for a diagnostic consult. In the late 1960s, a demonstration project for teleconsultation in dermatology established a link between Massachusetts General Hospital and a polyclinic from Logan International Airport, Boston [4]. Doctors were able to effectively deliver healthcare services through an interactive session that enabled both audio and video modes to communicate degrees of erythema.

Another major organization that played a key role in the early development and growth of telemedicine was the National Aeronautics and Space Administration (NASA). NASA had its objectives to achieve. It was worried about the effects of zero gravity on the physical conditions of astronauts during space missions and needed to monitor their vitals. Powered by its success, NASA established an extensive testbed system. It was called the STARPAHC (Space Technology Applied to Rural Papago Advanced Health Care), and its incubation center was situated on the Tohono O'odham reservations in Arizona [4]. The duration of the program was approximately 20 years, and the program aimed to provide astronauts with a wide range of medical devices through satellite-based communications. NASA had also distributed telemedicine technology following the catastrophic earthquake that had struck Mexico in 1985 [4]. NASA had also granted the Advanced Technology-3 communications satellite (ATS-3), which enabled the Pan American Health Organization and the American Red Cross to communicate and coordinate rescue operations within a short period after there was a disruption of virtual land-based communications [4].

Space Bridge to Russia was the earliest telehealth program conducted internationally by NASA in 1988 [4]. Its objectives were to help the earthquake victims in Armenia by providing medical consultation, although it was originally developed for astronauts. Satellite-based communications were used to deliver medical care services through facsimile, voice, and video. Consultants used it to deliver services in domains like neurology, psychiatry, infectious disease, orthopedics, and general surgery from the United States to a health center in Armenia.

In 1985, a program called SatelLife/HealthNet was launched to provide healthcare services in developing countries [4]. It helped in providing a link between medical centers located in the urban to remote clinics in nine African nations, three countries in America, and the Philippines. It provided email-based communications and the availability of CD-ROM via the HealthSat satellites. These were relatively cheaper than the geostationary satellites conventionally used.

These various programs elucidated that telemedicine could overcome political, economic, cultural, and social barriers, and they set a stage for many similar experiments performed in subsequent years. Dozens of similar projects have since surfaced throughout the world, assimilating these basic concepts into many other applications. However, despite their many successes, most of these projects have been suspended. Their demise was not the result of a lack of efficacy or patient satisfaction. The main reason for failure was their impotence to sustain financially upon withdrawal of funding from an external source. Although these early ventures were not accepted as an effective alternative to the then standard modes of healthcare delivery, they did provide rich evidence for the clinical effectiveness of remote education, training, and consultation.

2.1 Rebirth of Telemedicine

The beginning of the 1990s saw the rebirth of telemedicine [4]. It brought about advances in image digitization and data compression technology that enabled videoconferencing over lower bandwidth lines. The telemedicine renaissance in the United States was brought about with the recognition that there was unequal access to medical care in remote rural areas. It saw an increase in federal funding for such projects. A state-wide telemedicine program was developed by Dr. Jay Sanders of the Medical College of Georgia that became the first of its kind and gained much enthusiasm [4]. By 1993, there were ten programs launched, and it has doubled each year since. The Norwegian Telemedicine Project was probably the most active program in the world and is being developed since 1988 with strong federal support [4].

2.2 Modern Telemedicine

As telemedicine evolved through the years, the real boost in this concept occurred after the inventions of the radio, telescope, and devices as such. Radiology was the first medical field that was able to fully function using telemedical methods, as it involved the transmission of X-ray images, fluoroscopy images, and electrocardiograms [5]. The advent of wireless broadband connectivity greatly impacted the rise of telemedicine as we see today. This enables patients to learn through texts, images, and videos and engage in real-time audio and video consultations with doctors and healthcare providers. The invention of wearable health devices made viewing and digitalization of healthcare records easier. While the advantages of modern telemedicine are immense, it also came with an ability to store huge amounts of data, which if not protected and encrypted according to the HIPAA (Health Insurance Portability and Accountability Act) 1996 can lead to debatable security breaches and data theft [6].

Overall, telemedicine in the age of internet and wireless connectivity has helped humanity have easier and accessible healthcare, using easily available devices like smartphones, wearable health devices, etc. without requiring specific training or visiting the doctor's clinic. Travel expenses, medical costs, and even effort to maintain a file containing all medical prescriptions have been greatly reduced, because of the electronic medical/health records (EMRs or EHRs) which are an essential part of an efficiently functioning telemedical system [7]. Even for healthcare providers, telemedicine comes as a boon, as it increases revenue, fewer cancellations are seen in appointments, increases following, and maintenance of records has become easier [8].

These immense advantages of telemedicine have forced several countries to conduct projects that made use of telemedicine exclusively, such as Uttarakhand Telemedicine and the Kumbh Mela Project in India, the Maternal Care Project and the Xiamen Demonstration Project in China [9], and the dedication of a separate government body to oversee telemedicine provisions, the American Telemedicine Association.

3   General Architecture of Telemedicine

Telemedicine systems follow a structured hierarchical and tiered system (Fig. 3). This broadly includes the following:

Level 1: Remote or Local Center. Primary healthcare units are located in rural areas [10].

Level 2: City and District Hospitals. Rural health centers are connected to district/ city hospitals. Optionally, district hospitals may be connected to state hospitals [10].

Level 3: Specialty Centers. City hospitals may be connected to specialty hospitals for assistance in disease-specific cases [10].

A patient that needs medical attention can visit a nearby local healthcare center where a professional, not necessarily a certified doctor, carries out a complete health checkup. The unit includes basic diagnostic equipment and other teleconsultation devices linked via personal computer and the internet to the nearest city hospital. The job of the healthcare professional is to collect all the vital statistics of the

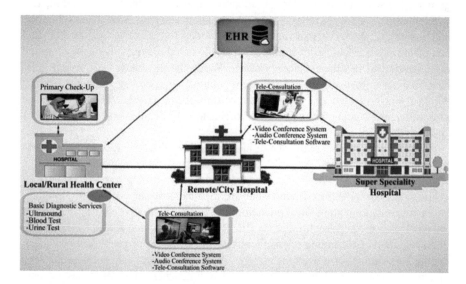

Fig. 3 General architecture of telemedicine [10]

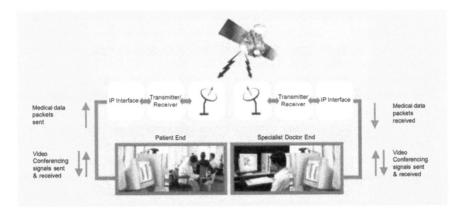

Fig. 4 SATCOM-based telemedicine connectivity [11]

respective patient like blood and urine samples, ultrasound images, blood pressure, etc. This data is then transmitted to the city hospital. These city hospitals may also be connected to specialist hospitals. All the reports are then received by the doctor and analyzed before proceeding to have a live interaction with the patient through video conferencing and automation live feeds. All the recordings of the interaction, vital statistics, and analysis report are stored in a centralized database. This information can be accessed through a web-based interface and mobile apps. A satellite-based communication system is also widely followed by space research organizations like NASA in the United States [4] and the ISRO in India [11] as seen in Fig. 4. In this method, the medical images and other related information are sent to a specialist doctor in a real-time connection using a satellite link (in the form of digital data packets).

4   Methods and Modalities of Telemedicine [12, 13]

The following are the different modalities of telemedicine:

1. Store-and-Forward Mode: It is also called as asynchronous telemedicine. Store-and-forward is a transmission to a healthcare provider, who uses the information to treat the patient outside of real time through an electronic communication system. Across remote regions, this approach is also used by primary care physicians or nurses who prefer to seek consultation from a physician in another location. This is a perfect opportunity to boost quality in treatment as a provider; patient and specialist need not be in the same place, at the same time. In general, this means lower waiting times for patients, better access to medical attention, improved patient outcomes, and optimized physician schedule. Here, the term "store and forward" typically means to store patient's medical data (like a patient portal) to forward or share across providers at different locations. This is a secure

and sophisticated platform like email. The best application of this type of tele-medicine is for the exchange of information between medical professionals (doctors talking to doctors) where a primary care doctor can take inputs from a specialist. The primary care doctor can send patient data like lab results, history, X-ray, or other images to the specialist for review (Fig. 5). The specialist may respond virtually with his/her review. Such virtual appointments will minimize unwanted visits, reduce waiting time, and help avoid unnecessary travel.

2. Real-Time Interactive Mode: Also called as synchronous telemedicine. It is a two-way interaction between a patient and a healthcare provider using audio and visual technology (Fig. 6). This type is commonly used to treat common illness or minor illness and to decide if a patient should head to an emergency room or just care about it at home. It is the best alternative for in-person doctor visits and far more sophisticated and secure than the usual videoconferencing platforms. Doctors are rapidly adopting real-time telemedicine to carry out convenient vir-tual doctor visits for patients and enhance their treatment, facilitate work-home balance, and save time. The only requirements to avail of this service are com-patible devices, internet connection, webcam, and a microphone.

3. Remote Monitoring: RPM means personal health and medical information is collected from a patient or resident of one place and then electronically trans-ferred to a nurse, healthcare provider, or doctor at another location for monitor-ing purposes. This makes it easier to monitor warning signs and quickly intervene who are at health risk or have undergone surgery recently. Successful remote

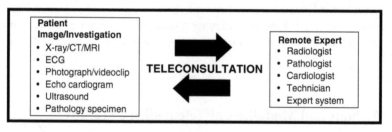

Fig. 5 Store-and-forward mode where the patient images like X-rays, MRIs, and other diagnostic images are sent to healthcare experts for review [4]

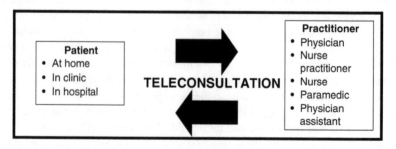

Fig. 6 Real-time interaction between the patient and the practitioner [4]

patient monitoring takes place only when there are right health monitoring devices present in the patient's home. This is getting easier with the rapid growth of human wearable devices. These devices are cheap, fast, and easy to access for track signs and reporting medical data. They are also used for regularly monitoring senior citizens' health. For example, a patient with diabetes can regularly check his glucose level at home and transmit the report to the doctor. If the level seems to be normal, it is simply stored as a record, but if there seems to be something off, the doctor can call in the patient for a consult. Another example would be to monitor the cardiac events using a device that records arrhythmia in patients when they experience dyspnea, angina, palpitations, or unexplained syncope. This data is transmitted to the doctors when an abnormal rhythm is detected.

4. Mobile Health or mHealth: This type of telemedicine uses various kinds of mobile communication devices like smartphones or tablets to provide healthcare services. This kind of telemedicine particularly needs specialized software applications that are user-friendly and organize medical information in one secure place. Some important features include storing personal health information, recording vital signs, scheduling reminders for medicine intake, recording daily activities like step count or calorie intake, and many more.

5 Categories of Telemedicine

1. Teleradiology: Teleradiology enables us to send radiographic images such as X-rays, CT scans, MRIs, etc. from one location to another [14]. The three main components include an image sending station, a transmission network, and an image receiving station. In simpler words, it's two computers connected via an internet connection. Teleradiology begins at the image sending end where the image is generated, scanned, and sent to the image receiving station over a network. The computer at the image receiving end has a high-definition display to review the images. Often, a printer is connected to printing out the images. This enables the patient's X-rays to be analyzed by a qualified radiologist from another location.

2. Telepathology: Telepathology is widely used in diagnosis, research, and education. It is a type of telehealth where the high-resolution pathology data can be transmitted from one location to another [15]. The data can be in the form of images or videos which are used for diagnostic purposes that are commonly practiced in histopathology. Often, the store-and-forward method is used in telepathology.

3. Teledermatology: It allows dermatology consultations over a distance. It allows patients to send images or videos of skin anomalies, rashes, or moles to the healthcare provider for remote diagnosis. Teledermatology has been proved to improve efficiency, save time, and result in satisfaction among patients.

4. Telepsychiatry: Telepsychiatry provides psychiatric services for patients such as consultation with psychiatrists for diagnosis and assessment, medical treatment, educational clinical programs, and routine checkups. It utilizes videoconferencing which means that it happens in real time (synchronous).

5. Telecardiology: The most important application is the transmission of ECGs (electrocardiographs) over the telephone or wirelessly. Another application is monitoring patients with pacemakers to detect arrhythmia if it occurs.

6. Telesurgery: Telesurgery enables patients to undergo surgeries without the surgeons being physically present in the same location. Robotic surgery is the key element in telesurgery where the surgeons control the robots during the surgery.

7. Telerehabilitation: Telerehabilitation delivers rehabilitation services which can include clinical assessment and a clinical therapy. It can be conducted in many ways such as videoconferencing, audiotapes, webcams, etc.

8. Telenutrition: Telenutrition enables clients to consult a nutritionist/dietician from anywhere across the globe. It involves clients uploading their vital statistics, diet charts, or food images. This helps nutritionists/dieticians to set a goal for the patients and can regularly have follow-ups to check the progress. It is most helpful for bedridden or elderly people as they can consult their dieticians from their houses.

9. Telenursing: Telenursing provides a link between the patient and the nurses without the physical presence of the nurse. It helps overcome the problem of shortage of nurses. It helps to increase healthcare coverage in rural, underserved, and sparsely populated areas. It is distinctively used in the monitoring of chronically ill or elderly patients who often find difficulty in traveling.

10. Telepharmacy: Telepharmacy is provided by telecommunication to patients when direct contact with a pharmacist is not feasible. Telepharmacy services include drug therapy monitoring, patient counseling, prior authorization and refill authorization for prescription drugs, and monitoring of formulary compliance with the aid of teleconferencing or videoconferencing.

11. Teledentistry: Teledentistry is provided by telecommunication for basic dental care, awareness, education, and consultation for patients with minor dental problems.

12. Teleneurology: Teleneurology uses technology to monitor patients for the care of strokes, disorders like Parkinson's disease, seizures, etc. It saves time and is cheaper than in-person visits especially in the case of patients with Parkinson's disease [16].

13. Teletrauma care: Teletrauma is widely used to deliver care during the trauma environment. It is used by trauma specialists to interact with personnel or mass affected by casualties or disasters to determine the severity of the injuries and to take necessary clinical steps.

14. Teleophthalmology: Teleophthalmology allows ophthalmologists to check patient's eyes using telecommunication technology. A few applications include routine checkups, diagnosing eye infections and eye diseases, prescriptions for lenses or glasses, and teaching programs. It saves a lot of time and reduces the cost of travel.

6 Risks Involved with Telemedicine

1. Data privacy risks: Telehealth privacy risks involve lack of controls or, in other words, limitations on sensitive information collection, application, and disclosure. Inadvertently, sensors in the home of a patient or interface with the body of a patient to detect safety issues or medical emergencies can collect sensitive household activity information. For example, home sensors to detect falls can also transmit information like spousal or religious interactions or indicate if no one is home. Sometimes, personal information is transmitted to not just the healthcare providers but the manufacturer as well. A mobile health app can be financed by the exchange of third-party advertisers that target advertisements to patients based on the usage of possibly confidential data in the device [17].
2. Standard of care: Many telemedicine practices have distinctively defined various rules about the patient-physician relationship, routine follow-ups, or providing e-prescriptions. However, for various practices and services, the standard of care rules are not legally approved yet. This arises a question on the legitimacy of the telemedicine system [18].
3. Documentation: Documentation is an essential part of the patient-physician interaction. All the patient's details like patient history, prescriptions, and clinical/diagnostic test results should be included in health records. The main challenge here is the access, maintenance, privacy, and security of these health records in telemedicine technology [18].
4. Lack of technical skills in patients and staff: Most of the time, the patient lacks technical knowledge of using the telemedicine services. This usually hampers the accessibility and utilization of these services. Similarly, telemedicine staff also need to undergo technical training which includes training in each type of telemedicine modality, documentation, troubleshoot, and equipment purchase to assist the patients [18].
5. Expensive technology: Equipment used for telemedicine must be required to have high-quality audio-video capacities and up-to-date operating systems and should be secure. Similarly, regular maintenance of equipment is another necessity. So, when the cost of the equipment and the cost of services is added up, physicians and hospitals often find it expensive.
6. Reduced care continuity: If a patient receives telemedicine service from one healthcare provider but later chooses different healthcare providers for his/her subsequent e-visits, then the healthcare providers might not have sufficient patient history to precisely diagnose the problem. This leads to reduced care continuity. One of the main reasons for this is the lack of documentation and electronic health records (EHRs).
7. Patient-physician relationship: It is important to have a positive patient-physician relationship. Physicians are expected to have strong communication skills and good listeners to answer all patient's questions and understand their concerns. Physicians also need to ensure that the diagnosis and the course of treatment are well understood by the patient. For successful interaction, a strong

patient-physician relationship is required which is often missing in telemedicine services due to the artificiality in digital environments and not being physically present in the room.

7 Telemedicine in India

India is a country with an enormous population and majority residing in rural areas. The rural population of India does not receive adequate attention from the healthcare perspective, as most doctors and well-equipped hospitals and nursing centers are concentrated in the cities [7]. The stalwart of telemedicine in India is the Indian Space Research Organisation (ISRO) which has notably initiated and expanded the reach of telemedicine and telehealth services in India. They began with the Telemedicine Pilot Project in 2001 (in partnership with Apollo telemedicine services) which was aimed at connecting urban super specialty hospital services to rural/district hospitals through its INSAT satellites [11, 19]. This project then expanded to the Village Resource Centre (VRC), which is an ISRO-based concept that provides various teleservices and acts as learning centers and connecting centers to urban hospitals. Almost 500 such VRCs are established in India [7]. Recently, the Ministry of Health in the Government of India has undertaken several projects like the OncoNET (National Cancer Network), Integrated Disease Surveillance Project (IDSP), National Rural Telemedicine Network, and National Medical College Network [20]. Government bodies like the ISRO, Ministry of External Affairs, Department of Information and Technology, and Ministry of Health and Family Welfare have overseen many such initiatives that have led to the advancement of telemedicine services in India. Currently, several private organizations are a part of the telemedicine network in India, including Apollo Telemedicine Enterprises, Narayana Hrudayalaya, Aravind Eye Care, etc. These organizations are making active efforts toward the betterment of public health management. Many rural areas and remote localities in Jammu and Odisha have been impacted by them.

The Ministry of Health and Family Welfare (MoHFW) set up the National Telemedicine Portal, which operates along with the National Medical College Network and the National Rural Telemedicine Network, which interlink e-Education and e-Healthcare delivery in rural areas. The establishment of the National e-Health Authority (NeHA, under the National Health Portal) aimed at implementing Information and Communication Technology in Health and allied sectors [21]. AROGYASREE (by the Indian Council of Medical Research and the University of Karlsruhe, Germany) is an internet-based mobile telemedicine platform which aims to bring the expertise of doctors in urban areas closer to rural areas, and they have designed an ECG Jacket, which can monitor the ECG of a person without hospitalized testing [22].

8 Telemedicine During the COVID-19 Pandemic

In December 2019, Wuhan, which is a city in China's Hubei Province, saw an outbreak of the severe acute respiratory syndrome virus, SARS-CoV2, now being called the COVID-19 (coronavirus disease 2019). This outbreak then led to a global pandemic, as officially declared by the World Health Organization [23]. As of July 21, 2020, 14.7 million people have been affected worldwide by COVID-19. With the virus spreading to over 200 countries and territories [24], many governments decided to impose a mandatory lockdown (isolation of citizens at home to prevent public gatherings and hence spread of the virus). With government-mandated rules in place, many services came to a standstill, including non-essential (non-COVID-19 related) hospital/clinic and nursing home visits, as the focus of all healthcare providers was shifted to caring for those affected by the coronavirus disease.

Many countries also decided that patients who are asymptomatic to the disease (still effectively acting as carriers) or patients with mild symptoms should continue home isolation and avoid hospital admission [25, 26].

During turbulent times like these, telehealth and telemedicine services are proving to be a sustainable and effective alternative to physical visits and helping prevent the spread of the virus. A study conducted in the Shandong Province in China in March 2020 showed very clearly the advantages of implementing a successful telemedicine system in compartmentalizing and treating community residents, medical staff, and COVID-19 positive patients [27]. The Shandong Provincial Government and the Shandong Health Committee ensured that there was a preventive telemedicine platform, which included experts conducting remote consultations and preliminary screenings. This led to early detection and also helped to spread awareness and prevention. For treating COVID-19 positive patients as well, the Shandong Health Committee followed a detailed procedure starting from admission in the hospital to discharge, all implemented through telemedicine. This proved to save time and cost and reduce the risk of infection among all involved in close contact. They also created video conferencing platforms and "cloud ICUs" to aid the healthcare workers, which enabled them to exchange crucial information, new findings, case discussions, diagnostic reports, etc.

Patients with non-COVID-19-related medical ailments are especially being benefitted by telemedicine services, offered by companies like TytoCare and MaNaDr in the United States. This helps patients acquire the required medical attention, as well as avoid the risk of infection by entering medical facilities. It was noted that telemedicine offered greater individual attention to the patient and acts as a 24/7 source of comfort as they can be connected to their healthcare providers digitally [28].

Mainly, three huge advantages are seen through the usage of telemedicine during the COVID-19 pandemic:

1. The patients don't have to visit the hospital/clinic and can remotely access their healthcare provider, lowering their chances of infection. This is the most obvious role of using telehealth services in the current situation.

2. Telemedicine services can be used to provide routine care for patients with pre-existing chronic diseases (comorbidities like diabetes, hypertension, lung diseases) who are at greater risk if exposed to the virus.
3. Telemedicine services can greatly lessen the exposure of frontline healthcare provides, thus making their workplace comparatively safer. Healthcare workers are not immune to the virus, and controlling their exposure to the virus will help the patients treated by them as well.

In India as well, a huge number of patients were opting for telemedicine consultations, one example being the LV Prasad Eye Institute, Hyderabad. They used a self-built app for ophthalmologic queries that were of non-emergency in nature. The LVPEI ConnectCare implements Tele Connect 2.0 software, EMRs, payment gateways, and information sharing options [29]. Several Indian healthcare companies like 1MG, Practo, and Portea Medical saw huge boosts in telemedical consultations [30] after the government issued specific guidelines for implementing telemedicine technology in India during the COVID-19 pandemic [31].

However, the majority of the rural population in India still does not have access to smartphones or computers to avail these opportunities worldwide, and it is seen that many hospitals and clinics are not well equipped when it comes to digitalization of health records or secure information exchange. They also lack the necessary hardware and software systems. These are some of the challenges that need to be overcome for hassle-free implementation of telemedical services. Overall, there is a large increase in telehealth and telemedicine services during the COVID-19 pandemic, and it has also contributed to a decrease in the spread of this deadly virus.

9   Conclusion

Undoubtedly, telemedicine is a promising technology that will help in the transformation of the healthcare industry. In the future, telemedicine can ease access to healthcare and enhance the quality and efficiency of healthcare. The well-developed architecture and the different modalities of telemedicine is the solution for the majority of the problems in the healthcare sector. Telemedicine has been successfully implemented in various departments of healthcare such as teleradiology, telesurgery, teleneurology, and so on. Application of telemedicine services in the COVID-19 pandemic emerged as a potential idea by obviating the need to travel and save time. Despite the obvious advantages and the potential of telemedicine, it is not being explored to the maximum due to the risks carried with these telemedicine services. Widespread awareness, technological advancements, major structural changes, training, and funding are some strategies to push telemedicine to its highest potential in the coming years.

References

1. Telehealth. The Health Resources and Services Administration. 2017-04-28.
2. Shaw DK. Overview of telehealth and its application to cardiopulmonary physical therapy. Cardiopulmonary physical therapy journal. 2009 Jun;20(2):13.
3. Masson, M (December 2014). Benefits of TED Talks. Canadian Family Physician. **60** (12): 1080. PMC 4264800. PMID 25500595.
4. Maheu M, Whitten P, Allen A. E-Health, Telehealth, and Telemedicine: a guide to startup and success. John Wiley & Sons; 2002 Feb 28.
5. Zundel KM. Telemedicine: history, applications, and impact on librarianship. Bulletin of the Medical Library Association. 1996 Jan;84(1):71.
6. Health Information Privacy. HHS.gov. Available at: https://www.hhs.gov/hipaa/for-professionals/security/laws-regulations/index.html
7. Chellaiyan VG, Nirupama AY, Taneja N. Telemedicine in India: Where do we stand? Journal of family medicine and primary care. 2019 Jun;8(6):1872.
8. Limor Wainstein (2018). Telemedicine Trends to Watch in 2018. Arizona Telemedicine Program. Telemedicine.arizona.edu. Available at: https://telemedicine.arizona.edu/blog/telemedicine-trends-watch-2018. (Accessed: 19 July 2020).
9. Gupta A, Dogar ME, Zhai ES, Singla P, Shahid T, Yildirim HN, Singh S. Innovative Telemedicine Approaches in Different Countries: Opportunity for Adoption, Leveraging, and Scaling-Up. Telehealth and Medicine Today. 2019;4:10–30953.
10. Pramanik PK, Pareek G, Nayyar A. Security and Privacy in Remote Healthcare: Issues, Solutions, and Standards. InTelemedicine Technologies 2019 Jan 1 (pp. 201-225). Academic Press.
11. Space TH. Enabling Specialty Health Care to the Rural and Remote Population of India. Indian Space Research Organisation, Publications and Public Relations Unit, ISRO Headquarters, Bangalore-560094.:3–5.
12. J. Bell (2016). 4 Types of Telemedicine. Available at: https://keystonetechnologies.com/blog/4- types-of-Telemedicine/.
13. Alvandi, M., 2017. Telemedicine and its role in revolutionizing healthcare delivery. The American Journal of Accountable Care, 5(1), pp. e1-e5.
14. Kontaxakis, G., Visvikis, D., Ohl, R., Sachpazidis, I., Suarez, J.P., Selby, P., Rest, C.L., Santos, A., Ortega, F., Diaz, J. and Pan, L., 2006. Integrated telemedicine applications and services for oncological positron emission tomography. Oncology reports, 15(4), pp. 1091–1100.
15. Weinstein, R.S., Graham, A.R., Richter, L.C., Barker, G.P., Krupinski, E.A., Lopez, A.M., Erps, K.A., Bhattacharyya, A.K., Yagi, Y. and Gilbertson, J.R., 2009. Overview of telepathology, virtual microscopy, and whole slide imaging: prospects for the future. Human pathology, 40(8), pp. 1057–1069.
16. Beck, C.A., Beran, D.B., Biglan, K.M., Boyd, C.M., Dorsey, E.R., Schmidt, P.N., Simone, R., Willis, A.W., Galifianakis, N.B., Katz, M. and Tanner, C.M., 2017. National randomized controlled trial of virtual house calls for Parkinson disease. Neurology, 89(11), pp. 1152–1161.
17. Hall, J.L. and McGraw, D., 2014. For telehealth to succeed, privacy and security risks must be identified and addressed. Health Affairs, 33(2), pp. 216–221.
18. Russell, D., Boisvert, S., Borg, D., Burke, M., McCord, D., Heathcote, S. and Shostek, K., 2018. Telemedicine Risk Management Considerations. Available at: https://forum.ashrm.org/2018/08/21/ashrm-whitepaper-telemedicine-risk-management-considerations/.
19. Pilot Project on telemedicine (2000). Archive of updates from ISRO. Available at : https://www.isro.gov.in/update/16-nov-2000/pilot-project-telemedicine (Accessed 19 July 2020).
20. Dasgupta A, Deb S. Telemedicine: A new horizon in public health in India. Indian journal of community medicine: official publication of Indian Association of Preventive & Social Medicine. 2008 Jan;33(1):3.

21. NeHA. National eHealth Authority (NeHA)|National Health Portal of India [Internet]. Nhp.gov.in. Available from: https://www.nhp.gov.in/national_eHealth_authority_neha_mtl (Accessed: 19 July 2020).
22. Arogyasree – An Internet Based Mobile Telemedicine System. Available at: http://dos.iitm.ac.in/projects/icmr/ (Accessed: 19 July 2020).
23. World Health Organization. WHO Director-General's opening remarks at the media briefing on COVID-19-11 March 2020.
24. Countries where COVID-19 has spread. Worldometer. Available at: https://www.worldometers.info/coronavirus/countries-where-coronavirus-has-spread/ (Accessed: 19 July 2020).
25. India's guidelines (MoHFW) for asymptomatic patients. Available at: https://www.mohfw.gov.in/pdf/RevisedHomeIsolationGuidelines.pdf (Accessed: 19 July 2020).
26. Prevention EC. for D. Guidance for discharge and ending isolation in the context of widespread community transmission of COVID-19-first update Scope of this document. Eur Cent Dis Prev [Internet]. 2020;(April): 1–8.
27. Song X, Liu X, Wang C. The role of telemedicine during the COVID-19 epidemic in China—experience from Shandong province.
28. Siwicki B. Telemedicine during COVID-19: Benefits, limitations, burdens, adaptation. Healthcare IT News. 2020.
29. Success of telemedicine during COVID-19 in India. Euro Times. Available at: https://www.eurotimes.org/success-of-telemedicine-in-india/ (Accessed: 19 July 2020).
30. Megha Mandavia (2020). Indian healthcare companies see big boost with govt move on telemedicine. The Economic Times. Available at: https://economictimes.indiatimes.com/small-biz/startups/newsbuzz/indian-healthcare-companies-see-big-boost-with-govt-move-on-telemedicine/articleshow/74885564.cms?utm_source=contentofinterest&utm_medium=text&utm_campaign=cppst (Accessed: 19 July 2020).
31. Telemedicine Practice Guidelines. MoHFW. Available at: https://www.mohfw.gov.in/pdf/Telemedicine.pdf (Accessed: 19 July 2020).

Advancements in Healthcare Using Wearable Technology

Sindhu Rajendran, Surabhi Chaudhari, and Swathi Giridhar

Abstract In the era of digitization tracking information on a real-time basis was one of the eminent tasks. Wearable technology involves electronics incorporated into items which can be comfortably worn on a body mainly used to detect, analyze, and transmit contemporaneous information. Wearable technology has applications in many fields such as health and medicine, fitness, education, gaming, finance, music, transportation, etc. Wearable devices have become quite inevitable as technology in the medical electronics field advances. These devices are highly cost-effective and portable making it easy to use. Due to the wearable computing devices, tracking the emergency and rescue team becomes easy thus making the workplace more efficient and safer. Development in this scope is being given importance to improvise and add many wearables on the list. Not only is it readily accessible, but it is also extremely useful when it comes to monitoring a patient from a farther distance. Such devices can be made capable of storing reading values for a certain period of time making the data accessible to the doctors without personalized monitoring. Devices such as smartwatch and glasses enhance the efficiency of researchers, engineers, and technicians at their work by storing important data and information. This chapter provides insight into three aims of wearable technology and also the challenges faced by wearable devices. The first aim discusses broadly about how wearable technology has evolved over the years which also includes how wearable devices are popular in different sectors of the industry particularly the healthcare sector. The second aim of this study is to discuss the applications or recent developments along with the possibilities of future development. The third aim is the integration of the Internet of things with wearable devices for the advancements in healthcare monitoring.

Keywords Wearable technology · Wearable device · Internet of things · Healthcare

S. Rajendran (✉)
Department of Electronics and Communication, R.V. College of Engineering,
Bangalore, India
e-mail: sindhur@rvce.edu.in

S. Chaudhari · S. Giridhar
Department of Biotechnology, R.V. College of Engineering, Bangalore, India

© The Author(s), under exclusive license to Springer
Nature Switzerland AG 2021
A. K. Manocha et al. (eds.), *Computational Intelligence in Healthcare*, Health
Information Science, https://doi.org/10.1007/978-3-030-68723-6_5

1   Introduction

In this era of digitalization where people are progressing toward performing their daily activities right from wireless communication to e-shopping, wearable technology has proved its potential with immense applications in almost every sector. Wearable technology can be defined as networked systems capable of gathering information, monitor events, and adapt services to the needs and wishes of user groups. They are also known as "smart devices" which include many components like sensors, microchips, and wireless communication channels [1].

They are usually small in size and are mainly preferred by a majority of people due to their portability. As the name "wearables" implies, it is a device that is literally worn on the body of the user. Wearable devices allow the continuous tracking of human physical activities and habits, as well as physiological and biochemical parameters throughout the daily routine. The most commonly measured data include vital signs such as heart rate, blood pressure, and body temperature, as well as the saturation of blood oxygen, posture, and physical activity using an electrocardiogram (ECG), ballistocardiogram (BCG), and other devices. Wearable cameras or video devices may possibly include valuable clinical knowledge. Shoes, eyeglasses, earrings, gloves, and watches may be added to wearable devices. Wearable devices can also grow to be products that are skin attachable. Usually, a smartphone is connected to these devices to receive the information being collected. There are various ways in which wearable devices can be classified which is discussed in this paper.

2   Classification of Human Wearable Devices

Human wearable devices can be broadly classified into three categories: portable devices, attachable devices, and implantable devices [2].

1. Portable Devices: Customized medical facilities and advanced stages of customized health apps and sensors are introduced by wearable devices. Portable devices can generally be categorized into wrists (smartwatches, bracelets, and gloves), head (smart glasses and helmets), body garments (coats, undergarments, and pants), feet, and sensory function (modulators for the body sugar). Due to the small size of these devices and wireless communication-enabled systems, these devices are easy to carry around and are, hence, known as portable devices.

   (a) Wrist-mounted devices: Smartwatches and fitness trackers are the most popular wrist-mounted devices. Smartwatches are computerized or smaller devices designed to be mounted on the wrist and have improved communication-related functionality. Many of the latest smartwatch models are mobile-based. Several of them function as smartphone-paired apps, offering an external screen to notify the consumer about new notifications, such as incoming texts, calls, or calendar reminders. Features such as waterproof containers, global positioning system (GPS) navigational systems, and health tracking applications are continued by manufacturers. Smartwatches also have the ability to capture hand gestures such as smoking or other activities. Fitness trackers are usually placed on the wrist, chest, or ears and are designed to record and map physical movements and to calculate fitness-related steps, such as pace and distance of running, exhalation, heart rate, and sleeping habits. Fitness trackers are often called activity trackers. In several studies, the accuracy and reliability of several activity trackers were assessed during the counting step. The conclusion was that some trackers perform well indoors and offer valid results, while others are more appropriate for outdoor operations [3].

(b) Head-mounted devices: They usually include smart glasses. New adaptive devices, smart glasses or smart goggle systems, are used with a wide variety of optical head-mounted displays (OHMDs), head-up displays (HUDs), virtual reality (VR), augmented reality (AR), mixed reality (MR), and smart lenses. All smart glasses may be classified in two categories, given variations in functionality and design: devices that need to be displayed on a mobile screen or individual ones, that need a wire linked to their source. Smart glasses may be monocular if the picture is displayed for one eye or binocular if the image is shown for both.

(c) E-textiles: While certain forms of wearable equipment which track the wearer's physical condition can also be included in the smart clothes categories, these include a broad range of sportswear and consumer sports equipment (smart T-shirts and bodysuits), chest belts, medical apparel, work wear monitoring devices, military apparel, and e-textiles. Smart clothing comprises of a variety of products, usually molded in shirts, socks, yoga pants, shoes, bow ties, helmets, and caps with a wide selection of sensors. Wearable smart biometric apps have now called to the attention of professionals in soccer, rugby, cycling, swimming, basketball, and baseball where wearables are used to track players' movements during exercising, minimize injury in the number of athletes, and increase the efficiency of teams. Smart clothing is likely to benefit paramedics, construction sites, and transportation.

(d) Smart jewelry: Smart jewelry is a portable, real-time monitoring system built to warn customers through smartphone notifications, although at the moment they pay or conduct ambient sensing, measuring smart biomedical signaling and biomechanics. Moreover, these wearable devices can monitor human activity, including calorie consumption and distance travel, and calculate sleep quality and duration.

2. Attachable Devices: Smart attachable sensing devices are an important component in real-time health monitoring systems for physiological signals that are closely associated with physical conditions such as blood pressure, heart rate, electrophysiology, body temperature, and various sweating biomarkers.

(a) Wearable skin patches: Wearable skin patches are increasingly prevalent in the market for wearables. Soft, flexible, and stretchable electronic devices are connected to soft tissue and are supplied with a new platform for robotic feedback, regenerative medicine, and continuous medicine. Skin patches are an ideal wearable, as clothes can hide them and more accurate information can be recorded without movement disturbances. Cardiovascular, sweat, strain, and temperature sensors have been used for wearable patches on the human skin.

(b) Contact lens: Smart contact lenses can noninvasively track the physiological information of the eyes and tears. Many forms of contact lenses were produced utilizing optical and electrical methods to track chemical compounds (lactate and glucose) and electrical conductivity of the mucous membrane of the eye.

3. Implantable Devices: Pacemaker is the most popular implanted heart patient medical device; it is used for the diagnosis of irregular heartbeats or arrhythmia which delivers energy-saving electrical stimulation to maintain proper rhythm when irregular heartbeats have been identified. Tattoos are fascinating emotions and vital symptoms monitoring platforms. Electronic tattoos can be adjusted to different skin textures, allowing noninvasive and best methods of attachment to the skin. The texture of the tattoo adhesive layer is completely flexible, allowing the patient to move in any skin movements and providing the physician with natural wearability and exact data. At present, electronic tattoos work for primary care professionals who want optimal treatment options as a way of diagnosis and surveillance.

4. Ingestible Pills: The usage of an ingestible sensor is a secure, noninvasive way to reach the fluid you wish to identify. This sensor is capable of passing lumen and entering organs across the gastrointestinal region via the digestive tract. Therefore, the ingested sensor tracks the genital contents and lumen fluids intrinsic to the organ, as well as enzymes, hormones, electrolytes, microbial communities, and metabolites, and delivers the data.

3 Quality Parameters of Wearable Devices

Wearable devices have the quality features to satisfy specific and implied specifications. While quality characteristics may be used as a criterion for assessment, not all product design, development, distribution, and other similar characteristics are quality characteristics. We know that quality is an inherent property of products according to the definition of quality.

A few of the quality parameters are shown below [4]:

1. Portability: It is the ability of a component to be transferred or carried easily. The component can be a hardware or software. Human wearable devices are expected to be smaller in size and in turn be portable for ease of access.

2. Usability: It is the capacity of the device to carry out a task given to it in the most effective, efficient, and time-saving manner.

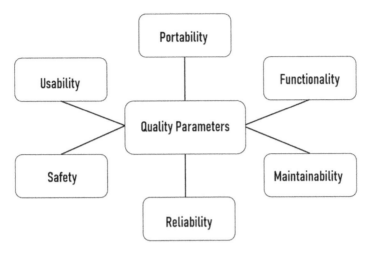

Fig. 1 Quality parameters of wearable technology [4]

3. Safety: It is the ability to protect the health or medical data that is being produced by the wearable devices such that no unauthorized personnel can access, modify, or leak the data.
4. Functionality: It is the ability of a device to be suitable for a specified purpose and deliver the expected results.
5. Maintainability: It is the ease with which a device can be maintained and can be repaired if required.
6. Reliability: The capacity to sustain a given standard of output during usage under the conditions stated. The reliability of the limitations is due to the requirements, design, and implementation failures (Fig. 1).

4 Applications of Wearable Technology in Different Sectors

4.1 In the Mining Sector

Miners are often exposed to life-threatening injuries which may even lead to death. A major contributor to this is the lack of safety and a communication barrier between mine workers. Safety interventions in this sector proved to be a major challenge due to the unpredictable conditions within the mines. Mine workers are exposed to a wide array of hazards which include inhalation of coal dust which leads to severe respiratory problems; the noise from heavy machinery and constant drilling which puts mine workers at risk of hearing damage; exposure to UV for those working in open-pit mines which increases their risk of skin cancer; and the hot and humid environment in mines which exposes miners to the risk of heat strokes. The deployment of wearable devices in this sector could help minimize the major hazards and could potentially lead to a healthier and safer workplace for miners. A healthier and safer workplace could lead to higher productivity and higher efficiency.

The diagram below shows the components of a wearable system used in the mining industry (Fig. 2).

The above figure illustrates the four main components in an Arduino-based wearable technology. The sensor system is used for measuring various parameters. The sensors could be environmental or biosensors. They have the ability to measure parameters such as gas concentration, temperature, oxygen concentration, atmospheric pressure, humidity, and other human characteristic parameters such as heart rate and pulse rate. The microcontroller platform serves to receive the information from the sensor system and transmits this to an actuator module through a communication system that is wireless. The microcontroller is designed using the Arduino, which is a low-cost, easy-to-use, and an open-source platform. The wireless communication system consists of various technologies such as Wi-Fi, ZigBee, and Bluetooth. An actuator is usually an electric device that causes a mechanical device to switch in some fashion [5]. It can be in the form of alarms, buzzers, text messages, etc (Fig. 3 and Table 1).

The successful utilization of such technology can lead to safer workplaces for mine workers. Such solutions increase efficiency and productivity.

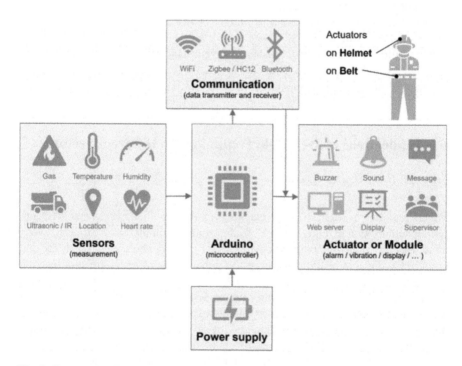

Fig. 2 Components of wearable technology used in the mining industry [5]

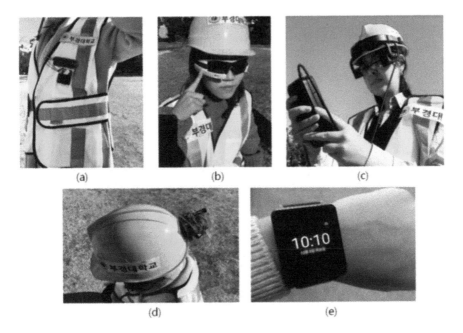

Fig. 3 Different wearables used in the mining industry. (**a**) Safety vest equipped with sensor, (**b**) and (**c**) smart eyewear, (**d**) smart helmet, (**e**) smartwatch [3]

4.2   In Sports and Fitness

Performance tracking and estimation of health and fitness parameters can be done seamlessly with the use of wearable technology. These lifestyle devices are in great demand in recent years, due to people becoming more mindful and inching toward a healthier lifestyle (Fig. 4).

From the figure, we observe that the activities of a user such as daily activity, food consumption, fitness activities, and sleep pattern are monitored by a wearable such as a smartwatch. Through a communication channel such as Wi-Fi, the monitored data is interpreted.

Some of the most commonly used sensors include the microcontroller, the accelerometer, the gyroscope, magnetometer, Global Positioning System (GPS), Heart Rate Sensors, Pedometers, Pressure Sensors [15].

The microcontroller enables the integration of Internet Of Things in this technology. The accelerometer has the capacity to sense different types of acceleration such as linear and gravity. They are commonly used by runners as they can output both speed and acceleration. It is also used to monitor sleep patterns which can in turn help in the diagnosis of seizures. Gyroscopes differ from accelerometers by measuring only angular acceleration. Magnetometers are combined with accelerometers and gyroscopes to form what is known as an inertial measuring unit (IMU). GPS tracks location and time data precisely. It is widely used as a tool for navigation. In

Table 1 Wearable technology in the mining industry

Author	Type of wearable	Specification	Application
Majee [6]	Safety helmet	Microcontroller – Arduino Wireless communication – ZigBee Sensor – Gas, Air Density, Humidity, Temperature Actuator – Alarm system, web server	Environmental condition monitoring and air quality assessment
Harshitha et al. [7]	Safety helmet	Microcontroller – Arduino Wireless communication – ZigBee Sensor – temperature, humidity, smoke Actuator – buzzer, web server	Air quality monitoring, temperature and humidity sensing
Roja et al. [8]	Safety helmet	Microcontroller – Arduino Wireless communication – GSM Sensor – gas/smoke Actuator – buzzer, LCD (liquid crystal display)	Air quality monitoring
Bhuttoa et al. [9]	Leather belt	Microcontroller – Arduino Sensor – gas/smoke, temperature, humidity, ultrasonic Actuator - buzzer	Air quality monitoring, collision detection
Noorin et al. [10]	Safety helmet	Microcontroller – Arduino Sensor – gas/smoke, temperature, humidity, vibration Wireless communication – Wi-Fi Actuator – buzzer/OLED	Air quality monitoring, collision detection
Oliveira et al. [11]	Vibrotactile belt	Microcontroller – Arduino Sensor – heart beat rate Actuator – vibrotactile belt	Navigation heart rate monitoring
Alam et al. [12]	Safety helmet	Microcontroller – Arduino Sensor – gas/smoke, temperature, humidity, heart beat rate Wireless communication – ZigBee Actuator – buzzer, LCD (liquid crystal display)	Air quality monitoring, heart rate monitoring
Dewarkar et al. [13]	Safety helmet	Microcontroller – Arduino Sensor – gas/smoke, temperature, humidity, pulse rate Wireless communication – RF Actuator – buzzer	Air quality monitoring, position monitoring, and pulse rate monitoring

(continued)

Table 1 (continued)

Author	Type of wearable	Specification	Application
Sanjay et al. [14]	Safety helmet	Microcontroller – Arduino Sensor – gas/smoke, temperature, humidity, pulse rate, atmospheric sensor Wireless communication – ZigBee Actuator – buzzer	Air quality monitoring, destructive event detection, and pulse rate monitoring

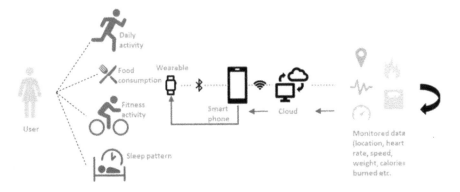

Fig. 4 Block diagram illustrating a fitness wearable technology [15]

professional sport, it eliminates issues related to time-motion analysis and helps coaches track player movements. Measurement of heart rate is carried out through the various heart rate sensors. These sensors can be capacitive sensors which have two distinct components, that is, the electrode and the human skin; the other type of sensor is based on the Photoplethysmography phenomenon, wherein blood flow is measured using light. Pedometers are frequently used in lifestyle wearables and they measure the user's footsteps when the user walks or runs [15] (Table 2).

A majority of the sports wearables rely heavily on accelerometers and gyroscopes. Some of these devices include Fitbit used on the wrist, Lumo Run a wearable used in the lower back, and OptimEye which is used in the lower back as a vest. These examples along with a wide array of other devices rely heavily on the use of accelerometers and gyroscopes as well as pedometers [15].

Inertial measuring units (IMUs) play an important role in the sports wearables industry. They sense measures such as the number of sprints, top speed, distance, hand speed, hip rotation, trajectory vertical and horizontal jump, forward swing and back swing, etc.

An important question that arises is how can the data measured by sensors be understood in terms of performance statistics. The use of filters helps us address such problems. Filters are tools of data processing and have the ability to convert sensor data into performance statistics. This, in turn, can help sports coaches and

Table 2 Different wearable technologies used in lifestyle and fitness [15]

Wearable	Smart category	Application	Body place
Apple Watch 2	Watch	Lifestyle	Wrist
Fitbit	Watch	Fitness	Wrist
Hexoskin	Clothing	Fitness	Upper body
Samsung Gear S3	Watch	Lifestyle	Wrist

teams as a whole to assess their performance and come up with new, better, and winning strategies. Though its advantages are many, the major drawback is in the accuracy of converted sensor data. Data scientists would be required to continuously work in gathering and analyzing sensory data and correlating them with key performance indicators. This would require a lot of time and effort, and multiple sensors need to be working together [16]. Accuracy is higher when doing exercises of low to moderate intensities or when doing consistent movements, such as jogging [15]. The accuracy differs more when doing sports-related activities where players not only experience high intensity, but they also are constantly changing agility, which leads to sensors not producing accurate readings [15].

Apart from playing a major role in performance statistics, wearable technology has a pivotal role in injury tracking as well. The following examples cite the role of wearable technology in injury tracking: American football embeds sensor in the helmets of the players to monitor head injuries. The detection of arm movement and techniques has been achieved with compression shirts [17]. Sleep pattern monitoring trackers can be used to analyze decision-making as irregular sleep patterns can lead to fatigue which in turn can lead to bad decision-making [18]. GPS trackers can measure load variables which in turn can predict if a player is more prone to injury or not [15].

4.3   Emergency Services: Firefighters, Police Officers, and Paramedics

In emergency services which involve police officers, firefighters, and paramedic personnel, time is crucial. The advent of wearable technology has helped emergency services keep up with time in a major way. Currently, wearables are being tested to provide communication and feedback remotely, increased safety, and more reliable audio and visual tools. Wearable devices can largely assist in field communication and give a clear picture of the situation. Improved situational awareness helps in making better decisions. Presently the most commonly used wearable technology in emergency services include smartwatches and wearable cameras.

Smartwatches can assist emergency personnel by improving field communication. Health parameters can be monitored using technology embedded with heart rate sensors, pulse rate sensors, oxygen levels, etc. Wearable cameras have the capacity to get the video footage of what is happening in the field. This in turn can be used as proof against a particular crime in the court of law. It helps protect the public from police violence and other heinous crimes. The wearable cameras can also be used for training purposes, to train and educate the next set of emergency personnel.

Some of the noteworthy examples of wearable technology used in the emergency services sector include MedEx Ambulance Service which uses smart glasses, such that paramedics can show real-time visual footage to the doctors in the hospital, who can make critical diagnosis even before the patient arrives in the hospital. ProTransport-1 also works on a similar principle that uses smart glasses to enable diagnosis before the arrival of the patient to the hospital.

The major challenges include cost and funding, the emergency departments in certain countries do not get enough funding to deploy such technology. The use of such devices gives rise to a plethora of ethical and legal issues related to privacy and confidentiality. The robustness of the device is often questioned, as such devices need to be used in extreme conditions such as fires [19].

4.4   In Wholesale and Retail

Wearable technology in the wholesale and retail industry can aid in a range of activities which include but are not limited to restocking inventory, receiving inbound deliveries, seamless operations in the backend, and smooth customer service and delivery in the customer front.

Some of the proposed applications involve the consumer owning their own wearable device; through this the retailer can create wearable apps and then send personalized offers and promotions to the customers. Apart from this, sales personnel can be equipped with wearable devices like wearable headsets, digital lanyards, smartwatches, smart glasses, etc. This eliminates the need for searching customer records on the computer and allows the sales personnel by the side of the customer throughout the sales cycle.

Total Wine and More makes use of Theatro's wearable computer, which can track sales staff, improve in-store and warehouse communication, and provide key performance indicators. The device is voice-driven and hands-free.

The major challenges include the cost of scaling up to a new technology and the battery life and robustness of the product [19].

4.5   In Travel and Hospitality

In the travel, tourism, and hospitality industry, wearable technology serves two main purposes: to accelerate customer experience and brand promotion. Employees can rely on wearable technology to provide a seamless customer experience, while big brands can make apps which are interconnected with a particular wearable to provide personalized ads, coupons, offers, and other promotional information.

Some of the noteworthy use cases include the Virgin Atlantic staff greeting their first-class passengers with Google Glass and Sony SmartWatch. These devices provided personal information about the passengers which enabled the staff to provide a personalized and comfortable journey. This project piloted at the Heathrow Airport. Walt Disney World Resorts offered to its guests a wearable band with which guests could enter parks and hotel rooms and make purchases. Walt Disney uses this data to provide better experiences to its guests. Westin Hotel deployed sleep sensing and monitoring wrist bands for the well-being of their guests. Starwood developed apps for Google Glass and Apple Watch which allowed guests to perform all activities such as booking a room and entering one without a key. Schiphol Airport gave its airport authorities Google Glass which enabled them to look up gate numbers and flight information instantly. Vueling partnered with Sony SmartWatch to provide a wearable boarding pass. British Airways came up with an innovative blanket which tracked the emotions and mood of the passenger by subtly changing colors to provide better service and better customer experience [19].

4.6 In Logistics

Logistics is important in warehousing. Companies are at a constant outlook of reducing costs and boost performance. This can be achieved using wearable technology. The most popular wearable devices used in logistics include smart glasses with augmented reality, wearable computers such as the HC1 Headset Computer and the RS419 Ring Scanner, and voice-directed wearable solutions.

A few noteworthy use cases of wearables in logistics include DHL which made use of Smart Glasses along with augmented reality software to improve its warehousing operations. The technology-enabled barcode scanning and real-time object recognition allowed for the integration of information with the warehouse management system. DHL reportedly had a 25% increase in its efficiency with the deployment of this technology. FedEx deployed wearable ring devices for its parcel handlers, during the loading of goods/parcels in a van. Wynsors World of Shoes also deployed a similar wearable ring. UPS along with HP created a wearable scanner and printer which accelerated the loading of packages and enabled employees to store barcode images at a much faster rate than they would with a mobile scanner [19].

The major challenges in the widespread use of this technology are the cost to scale up, battery life, and robustness.

4.7 In Healthcare and Medicine

The healthcare and medicine industry are the major team players in the wearable technology space. Wearable devices are used in three unique ways in this industry – it is used by physicians and other healthcare providers, it is used on patients with chronic conditions to monitor their vitals, and it is used for health-related applications such as lifestyle, nutrition, sports, and fitness [19] (Table 3).

4.8 In the Oil and Gas Industry

The energy industry is facing a plethora of challenges in the current scenario. The major hurdle lies in the high production cost but low production rate. The introduction of wearable technology in this industry could increase efficiency by cutting costs. The wearable devices such as Smart Glasses, Virtual Reality Devices, Smart Watches, Smart Helmets, Wrist bands, Clothing embedded with sensors which serves the purpose of both collecting and transmitting data.

Schlumberger used smart glasses to generate data needed to improve the safety and efficiency of workers. Baker Hughes came up with an innovative idea of generating "Man Down" alerts, which notified the company when one of their employees was unwell; they used a wearable that monitors workers' vitals. Marathon Petroleum used a wearable monitoring system with the capability to detect multiple types of potentially harmful gases. They termed this as a "Life Safety Solution," and it also encompasses GPS, panic button, and motion sensors [19].

Table 3 Representing the application of wearable technology used in certain hospital settings [19]

Hospital	Type of wearable	Application
UC Irvine Health	Smart glasses	Monitor resident procedures
Yale New Haven Health System	Smart glasses	Evaluation of patient experience
Rhode Island Hospital	Smart glasses	To live stream patient condition in the emergency department, to a remote doctor
Seattle Children's Hospital	Wearable device	Attached directly to the patient's body, to measure body vitals such as blood pressure, blood sugar, heart rate, etc.
Desert Valley Medical Center	Wearable leaf monitoring system	Monitoring patients with higher efficiency
Beth Israel Deaconess Medical Center	Smart glasses	Accession of patient records with QR codes

5 Wearable Devices with Internet of Things Technology for Healthcare Monitoring

Internet of things abbreviated as IoT is an amalgamation of hardware and software technology, which is capable of producing vast volumes of data by connecting multiple devices and sensors with the cloud. Other intelligent tools aid in analyzing this vast amount of data. The integration of IoT with healthcare and medicine will bring about a revolution in the healthcare industry by curbing costs, increasing efficiency, and saving a larger number of lives [20].

The figure below shows a transformed healthcare system that is integrated with IoT technology (Fig. 5).

From the figure, we observe that the patient has a unique ID card, which is scanned using an RFID reader. Once scanned, the patient records which are stored in a secure cloud can be accessed. The patient records include the EHR (electronic health records), which contain the complete medical history of the patient. The IoT-enabled hospital will also have a virtual biobank with all the clinical trial records. A majority of the data stored in the cloud comes from the parameters tracked by the wearable devices.

A vast amount of patient data are manually collected from hospitals using various medical devices and are often not integrated with the electronic health records.

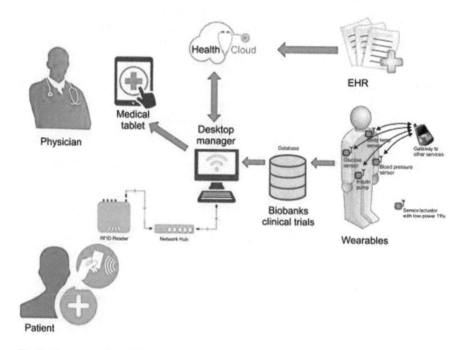

Fig. 5 Illustration of an IoT technology-integrated hospital [20]

Hence, it becomes difficult for healthcare providers to combine the vast amount of data and analyze it. IoT provides a solution to overcome these hurdles [21].

The IoT in the healthcare sector has a unique architecture which is depicted in the following figure (Fig. 6):

The four distinct layers, acquisition [21], storage, processing, and presentation, make up the architecture of IoT in a healthcare setting.

Acquisition: Collection of data using various tools known as "smart health objects," and these include all the wearable technology.

Storage: The vast amount of data collected is stored in personal health records. The data is stored in a highly interoperable and highly scalable form. Cloud computing technology is used for this purpose.

Processing: Processing involves the use of artificial intelligence (AI) and machine learning (ML) algorithms instead of traditional heuristic approaches.

Presentation: It involves presenting the analyzed data in the form of pictorial representations such as graphs, pie charts, scatter plots, box plots, etc.

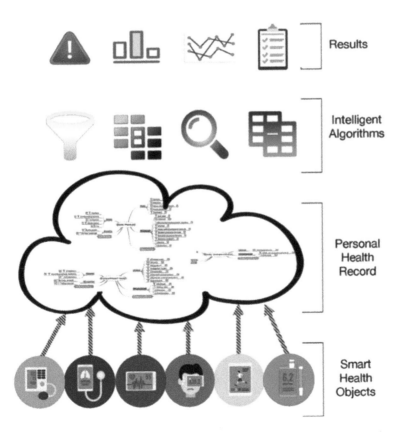

Fig. 6 Architecture of Internet of things, with four Layers: acquisition, storage, processing, and presentation [21]

5.1 IoT in Vital Signs Monitoring

There are eight typical vital signs which are used to monitor patients in hospitals. These include blood pressure, body temperature, heart rate, respiration rate, oxygen saturation, level of pain, level of consciousness, and urine output [21].

5.1.1 Pulse Rate and Heart Rate

Pulse rate is an important vital sign, which can determine the severity of critical emergencies such as cardiac arrest, pulmonary embolism, etc. Therefore, pulse sensors are of great importance and are being researched to a great extent. Apart from its applications in the emergency department, they are also widely used in fitness trackers. Pulse is most commonly read from the chest, wrist, and neck, but pulse reading from the earlobe or fingertip provides higher accuracy.

Similar to pulse rate, heart rate is also an important parameter in the measurement of the patient's total well-being. The table below summarizes the various IoT-based wearables for the measurement of heart and pulse rate (Table 4).

From the table, we see various studies that integrate wearable technology with IoT technology. The specifications vary from study to study. There are a variety of sensors that are used; in studies like that done by Reshma et al. [24], IR-based sensors are used, whereas in studies done by Brezulianu et al. [25], inductive sensors are used. The wearable devices in this space are usually specific to the parts of the body where strong pulse reading can be obtained. Other studies that measure similar parameters are done by Kumar et al. [27], Chao et al. [28], and Arnob et al. [29].

5.2 IoT in ECG Monitoring

ECG, known as electrocardiogram, is a graph of voltage versus time of the electrical activity of the heart measured using electrodes placed on the skin [30]. Small electrical changes that occur due to the depolarization followed by repolarization of the cardiac muscle during the cardiac cycle are measured by these electrodes. Anomalies in the normal cardiac cycle occur due to a variety of cardiac abnormalities such as cardiac arrhythmias, atrial fibrillation, ventricular tachycardia, etc.

There are three main components to an ECG: the P wave, which represents the depolarization of the atria; the QRS complex, which represents the depolarization of the ventricles; and the T wave, which represents the repolarization of the ventricles. The figure below shows the P wave, QRS complex, and T wave during a normal sinus rhythm (Fig. 7).

ECG is traditionally detected through medical stationary devices present in hospitals. There are 12 electrodes that measure ECG in a short span of time. The electrodes are placed on the patient's limbs and the surface of the chest. The magnitude

Table 4 Studies highlighting wearable technology in heart and pulse rate monitoring

Author	Application	Methodology	Type of wearable	Specification
Jayant et al. [22]	Reminder alert for timely medication	Wearable device monitors heart rate and generates an alert in case of any abnormality	Wearable on the hand	Heart beat sensor – SFH7051; Wi-fi module, CMOS battery
Abba et al. [23]	Heart rate monitoring using a heart pulse sensor	The pulse rate sensor gets data from the fingertip of the user, data is converted to a digital signal, the digital signal is processed by the microcontroller, and the results are displayed on an LCD screen	Wearable at the fingertip of the user	Fingertips capturing unit, heart pulse sensor unit, microcontroller (ATmega32p), LCD screen
Reshma et al. [24]	Heart rate monitoring	The system allows its users to measure their mean blood vessel weight (MAP) and measure the body temperature to be displayed on the Android screen for viewing	Wearable to measure pulse	IR-based heart beat sensor, Arduino UNO
Brezulianu et al. [25]	Mechanical activity of the heart	A sensor placed inside the clothing detects the cardiorespiratory activity	Clothing fabric	Inductive sensors to monitor the mechanical activity of the heart
Mehmet et al. [26]	Heart rate, heart rate variability, body temperature	The wearable sensors continuously measure the patient's cardiovascular signs by a wearable wireless connectivity. The system then transmits the sensed signals to an Android interface through wireless connectivity.	Wearable pulse sensor and body temperature sensor	Arduino Pro Mini, body temperature sensor, pulse sensor, Blynk application, Bluetooth module

of the heart's electric potential is measured at 12 different angles which are known as leads over a period of 10 seconds.

The ECG machines are limited to monitoring the patient only while they are present in the hospital, and hence remote monitoring of the patient is a challenge. IoT technology enmeshed with wearable technology can provide a potential solution for this problem. Wearable ECG monitoring systems have been deployed which can detect ECG signals and send alerts to physicians if any abnormality arises, saving time which is crucial in saving the life of an ailing patient.

The wearable sensors are usually embedded in clothing; wearable nodes are also used for this purpose. In the work done by Yang et al. [31], the wearable ECG sensor adopted has little impact on the daily life of the user, and the sensor collects physiological data from the body. The ECG data is then transmitted to the IoT cloud via wireless communication modules, like Wi-Fi, Bluetooth, and ZigBee. The graphical

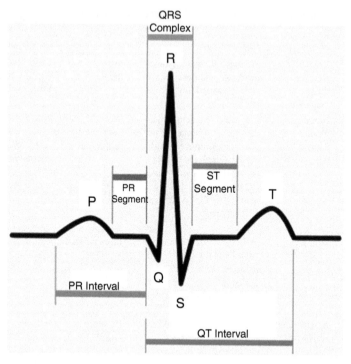

Fig. 7 ECG during normal sinus rhythm [30]

user interface enables physicians and patients to take the next steps, hence aiding in rapid diagnosis. In their study, Miao et al. [32] deployed an ECG monitoring sensor, which uses wearable technology and is placed on the user's chest. This sensor is integrated with a smartphone that already has built-in kinetics sensors. The ECG signals are transmitted to the smartphone, and real-time results are displayed. Zhe et al. [33] showed that the wearable ECG monitor collects data from the body and transmits it to the IoT cloud via Wi-Fi.

5.3 *IoT in EEG Monitoring*

Electroencephalography is the electrophysiological method to measure brain activity. EEG measures voltage fluctuations resulting from ionic current within the neurons of the brain [34]. Patient follow-up is a major problem for neurologists, hence the need for EEG emerged (Fig. 8).

The common wearable EEG is the ear EEG. In the work done by Goverdovsky et al. [36], the ear EEG was a sensor based on viscoelastic substrate and conductive fabric electrodes which show highly desirable mechanical and electrical properties. The viscoelastic property enables good conformance of the earpiece. The in-ear

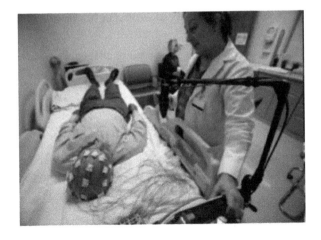

sensor can potentially produce high-quality EEG signals. They also showed that the device is immune to pulsatile ear canal movements [35] and also addresses in-ear EEG wearables. In the work done by Kannan et al. [35], the EEG acquisition system consists of three electrodes, one of which obtains EEG signals from the ear while the other two are placed behind the ear and act as reference electrodes. There is an amplification unit and a signaling unit and an Arduino microcontroller. The microcontroller analyzes the analog signal and produces the desired output which can be viewed on the screen. Wild et al. [37] demonstrated a Bluetooth-brain computer interface for the detection of the EEG signal. Billeci et al. [38], in their research study, included five children with autism spectrum disorder. The architecture of the system included a biosignal sensor unit, a video mobile unit, and a central unit. The biosignal sensor unit was composed of wearable EEG and ECG monitors. The EEG monitor was a wireless device, Enibo, while the ECG monitor was a wireless chest belt. The EEG and ECG data obtained were further analyzed using the video mobile unit and the central unit.

5.4   IoT in Clinical Trials

A study done by [39] revealed that, as of the year 2015, 299 clinical trials reportedly used wearable technology. A noteworthy example of IoT in clinical trials was AstraZeneca's human factors study, which evaluated six different body sensors and wearables over the period of 1 month [40]. The same study also stated that a major reason pharmaceutical companies are turning to IoT devices and wearables in their clinical trials is to increase accuracy while reducing the overall cost to conduct the trial [40]. The use of IoT in this sector makes it easier for researchers to follow-up with patients in timely intervals.

6 Challenges in Wearable Technology

The following are some of the major challenges associated with the wearable technology [41]:

1. Battery life: It is a critical issue when it comes to the battery life of wearable devices. One of the major drawbacks of wearable devices is that the battery does not last long. It needs to be charged every now and then which can be quite frustrating. This can be overcome by using other potential energy sources like using solar, kinetic, or electromagnetic emission technology.
2. User acceptance: Wearable devices will be of no use if the users are not familiar with the technical skills to use them. For this, the interface, design, and language should be user-friendly, and they should be able to use these devices without any interruption.
3. Price: Many studies have shown that the majority of people find wearables expensive for what they offer. Modifications need to be made in the future to reduce the cost of these devices.
4. Weight: Few of the wearable devices are heavy and can make the user uncomfortable carrying it around. Therefore, it is important that the appropriate choice of materials is made which can make the device as light as possible.
5. Security: Privacy and security issues in wearable technology have always been a critical issue. These devices collect a lot of sensitive information that needs to be protected from third-party attackers. The sensors in these devices are able to detect some extremely personal information like religious or spousal activity or can indicate when no one is home. Such data needs to be encrypted, and various algorithms need to be developed to prevent any sort of threat to personal data.
6. Design: Many users often expect these devices to have an aesthetic touch and preferably obscured. These devices often disturb the user's daily activities and frequent wearing of these devices becomes difficult.
7. Big data handling: Wearable sensors gather a significant amount of data due to their ability to continuously track data for a very long time. Efficient algorithms need to be used to train these devices to handle a large amount of data.

References

1. Thierer AD. The internet of things and wearable technology: Addressing privacy and security concerns without derailing innovation. Adam Thierer, The Internet of Things and Wearable Technology: Addressing Privacy and Security Concerns without Derailing Innovation. 2015 Feb 18;21.
2. Guk K, Han G, Lim J, Jeong K, Kang T, Lim EK, Jung J. Evolution of wearable devices with real-time disease monitoring for personalized healthcare. Nanomaterials 2019 Jun;9(6):813.
3. Mardonova M, Choi Y. Review of wearable device technology and its applications to the mining industry. Energies 2018 Mar;11(3):547.
4. Li Y, Zhang F, Yang C, Yang D The Wearable Level for Wearable Devices. 2015.

5. Kim SM, Choi Y, Suh J. Applications of the Open-Source Hardware Arduino Platform in the Mining Industry: A Review. Applied Sciences. 2020 Jan;10(14):5018.
6. Majee, A. IoT Based Automation of Safety and Monitoring System Operations of Mines. Int. J. Elect. Electron. Eng. 2016, 3, 17–21.
7. Harshitha K, Sreeja K, Manusha N, Harika E, Rao PK. Zigbee based intelligent helmet for coal miners safety purpose.
8. Roja P, Srihari D. IoT based smart helmet for air quality used for the mining industry. Int. J. Res. Sci. Eng. Tech. 2018;4(8):514–21.
9. Bhuttoa GM, Daudpotoa J, Jiskanib IM. Development of a wearable safety device for coal miners. International Journal. 2016 Dec;7(4).
10. Noorin M, Suma KV. IoT based wearable device using WSN technology for miners. In2018 3rd IEEE International Conference on Recent Trends in Electronics, Information & Communication Technology (RTEICT) 2018 May 18 (pp. 992-996). IEEE.
11. Oliveira, V.A.D.J.; Marques, E.; de Lemos Peroni, R.; Maciel, A. Tactile interface for navigation in underground mines. In Proceedings of the 2014 XVI Symposium on Virtual and Augmented Reality, Piata Salvador, Brazil, 12–15 May 2014; pp. 230–237.
12. Alam, M.M.; Chakraborty, P.P.; Biswas, S.; Islam, A.J. Design of an intelligent helmet for mine workers. In Proceedings of the International Conference on Mechanical Engineering and Renewable Energy 2015, Chittagong, Bangladesh, 26–29 November 2015; pp. 1–5.
13. Dewarkar, A.; Lengure, R.; Thool, S.; Borakhade, S. Smart Device for Security of Coal Mine Workers. Int. J. Innov. Res. Technol. 2019, 5, 351–353.
14. Sanjay BS, Dilip KA, Balasaheb TA, KinnuKumar S, Chandrabhushan P, Saware NP. Smart Helmet Using Zigbee.
15. Aroganam G, Manivannan N, Harrison D. Review on wearable technology sensors used in consumer sport applications. Sensors 2019 Jan;19(9):1983.
16. Wundersitz DW, Josman C, Gupta R, Netto KJ, Gastin PB, Robertson S. Classification of team sport activities using a single wearable tracking device. Journal of biomechanics. 2015 Nov 26;48(15):3975–81.
17. Awolusi I, Marks E, Hallowell M. Wearable technology for personalized construction safety monitoring and trending: Review of applicable devices. Automation in construction. 2018 Jan 1;85:96–106.
18. Arriba-Pérez D, Caeiro-Rodríguez M, Santos-Gago JM. Collection and processing of data from wrist wearable devices in heterogeneous and multiple-user scenarios. Sensors 2016 Sep;16(9):1538.
19. https://uploadsssl.webflow.com/5c1002a3f554acc315019809/5e1e0b6e9d2a918110c4712b_ Wearable%20Technology%20By%20Industry.pdf
20. Dimitrov DV. Medical Internet of Things and Big Data in Healthcare. Healthc Inform Res. 2016 Jul;22(3):156–63. doi: https://doi.org/10.4258/hir.2016.22.3.156. Epub 2016 Jul 31. PMID: 27525156; PMCID: PMC4981575.
21. da Costa CA, Pasluosta CF, Eskofier B, da Silva DB, da Rosa Righi R. Internet of Health Things: Toward intelligent vital signs monitoring in hospital wards. Artificial intelligence in medicine. 2018 Jul 1;89:61–9.
22. S. Jayanth, M. B. Poorvi, R. Shreyas, B. Padmaja and M. P. Sunil, "Wearable device to measure heart beat using IoT," 2017 International Conference on Inventive Systems and Control (ICISC), Coimbatore, 2017, pp. 1–5, doi: https://doi.org/10.1109/ICISC.2017.8068704.
23. Abba S, Garba AM. An IoT-Based Smart Framework for a Human Heartbeat Rate Monitoring and Control System. In Multidisciplinary Digital Publishing Institute Proceedings 2019 (Vol. 42, No. 1, p. 36).
24. Reshma, S.P.T.; JaiSurya, Y.; Sri, L.M.; Heart Rate Monitoring System using Heart Rate Sensor and Arduino Uno with Web Application. Int. J. Eng. Adv. Technol. (IJEAT) 2019, 8, 350–352.
25. Brezulianu, A.; Geman, O.; Zbancioc, M.D.; Hagan, M.; Aghion, C.; Hemanth, D.J.; Son, L.H. IoT Based Heart Activity Monitoring Using Inductive Sensors. Sensors 2019, 19, 3284, doi:https://doi.org/10.3390/s19153284.

26. Mehmet, T. IoT Based Wearable Smart Health Monitoring System. Celal Bayar Univ. J. Sci. 2018, 14, 343–350.
27. Kumar, A.; Balamurugan, R.; Deepak, K.C.; Sathish, K. Heartbeat sensing and Heart Attack detection using internet of things (IoT). Int. J. Eng. Sci. Comput. (IJESC) 2017, 7, 6662–6666.
28. Chao, L.; Xiangpei, H.; Lili, Z. The IoT-Based Heart Disease Monitoring System for Pervasive Healthcare Service. In Proceedings of the International Conference on Knowledge Based and Intelligent Information.
29. Arnob, S.; Akash, M.; Nilay, S.; Abhishek, K.K.; Binanda, K.M.; Souvik, C. An IOT based Portable Health Monitoring Kit. Int. J. Res. Appl. Sci. Eng. Tech. (IJRASET) 2018, 6, 701–708.
30. Lilly, Leonard S, ed. (2016). Pathophysiology of Heart Disease: A Collaborative Project of Medical Students and Faculty (sixth ed.). Lippincott Williams & Wilkins.
31. Yang Z, Zhou Q, Lei L, Zheng K, Xiang W. An IoT-cloud based wearable ECG monitoring system for smart healthcare. Journal of medical systems. 2016 Dec 1;40(12):286.
32. Miao, F., Cheng, Y., He, Y., et al., A wearable context-aware ECG monitoring system integrated with built-in kinematic sensors of the smartphone. Sensors 15:11465–11484, 2015. doi:https://doi.org/10.3390/s150511465.
33. Zhe, Y.; Qihao, Z.; Lei, L.; Kan, Z.; Wei, X. An IoT-cloud Based Wearable ECG Monitoring System for Smart Healthcare. J. Med. Syst. 2016, 40, 286, doi:https://doi.org/10.1007/s10916-016-0644-9.
34. Niedermeyer E.; da Silva F.L. (2004). Electroencephalography: Basic Principles, Clinical Applications, and Related Fields. Lippincott Williams & Wilkins.
35. Kannan R, Ali SS, Farah A, Adil SH, Khan A. Smart wearable EEG sensor. Procedia Computer Science. 2017 Dec;105(C):138–43.
36. Goverdovsky V, Looney D, Kidmose P, Mandic DP. In-ear EEG from viscoelastic generic earpieces: Robust and unobtrusive 24/7 monitoring. IEEE Sensors Journal. 2015 Aug 21;16(1):271–7.
37. Wild, M., Pegan, R., & Lera, M. Wearable Bluetooth Brain-Computer Interface for Detection and Analysis of Ear-EEG Signals.
38. Billeci L., Tonacci A., Tartarisco G., Narzisi A., Di Palma S., Corda D., Baldus G., Cruciani F., Anzalone S.M., Calderoni S. et al. (2016) An integrated approach for the monitoring of brain and autonomic response of children with autism spectrum disorders during treatment by wearable technologies. Front. Neurosci., 10, 276.
39. A, E. and C, C. (2015) Big pharma hands out fitbits to collect better personal data. First Published on September 14 2015.
40. Hale C. (2018) Sensors and wearables transform clinical trials but challenges remain, experts say. First Published on February 19th 2018.
41. Al-Eidan RM, Al-Khalifa H, Al-Salman AM. A review of wrist-worn wearable: Sensors, models, and challenges. Journal of Sensors. 2018 Dec;2018.

Machine and Deep Learning Algorithms for Wearable Health Monitoring

Chengwei Fei, Rong Liu, Zihao Li, Tianmin Wang, and Faisal N. Baig

Abstract Because people desire a high quality of life, health is a vital standard of living factor that is attracting considerable attention. Thus, the development of methods that enable rapid and real-time evaluation and monitoring of the human health status has been crucial. In this study, we systematically reviewed the techniques of data mining and machine learning (ML) for wearable health monitoring (WHM) and their applications, including conventional ML methods (artificial neural networks, the Kriging model, support vector machines, and principal component analysis) and the latest advance in deep learning (DL) algorithms for WHM; specifically, the advantages of the DL-based approaches over the traditional ML methods were analyzed in line with metrics associated with data feature extraction and identification performances. Moreover, to attain an intuitive insight, this study further reviewed the developments on the classifier performance with regard to detection, monitoring, identification, and accuracy. Finally, with regard to the characteristics of time series data acquired using health condition monitoring through sensors, recommendations and advices are provided to apply DL methods to human body evaluation in specific fields. Moreover, future research trends required to improve the capability of DL algorithms further are offered.

Keywords Machine learning · Deep learning · Wearable health monitoring · Data mining

C. Fei · Z. Li · T. Wang
Department of Aeronautics and Astronautics, Fudan University,
Shanghai, People's Republic of China
e-mail: cwfei@fudan.edu; 17300290038@fudan.edu.cn; 17300290018@fudan.edu.cn

R. Liu (✉)
Institute of Textiles and Clothing, the Hong Kong Polytechnic University,
Hong Kong, SAR, China
e-mail: rong.liu@polyu.edu.hk

F. N. Baig
Department of Health Technology and Informatics, Institute of Textiles and Clothing,
the Hong Kong Polytechnic University, Hong Kong, SAR, China
e-mail: faisal.n.baig@polyu.edu.hk

© The Author(s), under exclusive license to Springer
Nature Switzerland AG 2021
A. K. Manocha et al. (eds.), *Computational Intelligence in Healthcare*, Health
Information Science, https://doi.org/10.1007/978-3-030-68723-6_6

1 Introduction

With improvement in the living standard and increase in the aging population, people are becoming increasingly aware by the significance of healthcare in their daily lives. Wearable health monitoring (WHM) is a rising technology that enables steady ambulatory monitoring of humans to record vital information related to their health and body without much discomfort and interference with their routine activities when they are staying at home, workplace, or other exercise-focused places, or clinical environment [124, 131, 164]. The four major areas of focus of the technical designs of WHM devices are reliable and safe, low power consumption, ergonomic, and comfortable [179, 220]. Considerable attention is concentrated on smart WHM systems, which are fabricated using actuators, sensors, and smart fabrics and involve the technologies such as electronic surveillance, wireless sensor networks, and so on. The reason for the considerable attention is that smart WHM systems enable synchronization to domestic patients and allow real-time consultation with the healthcare providers without incurring any traveling cost [136, 141, 189]. Smart WHM systems are provided in various forms—skin-contact devices, implantable devices, smart clothes, and other wearable small things [76, 158]—and have been applied for monitoring vital signals related to health and body, body movement, fall prevention, and location [18, 60, 114, 168]. However, the acceptance level of WHM devices by end users is low [4, 117, 153], because the data processing technologies used in WHM systems or devices cannot efficiently manage the data collected by the varieties of sensors installed in the system during the stages of data preprocessing, extraction of discriminative and salient features, and data recognition [33] in body activity recognition. To overcome the aforementioned problem in body activity recognition, machine learning (ML) techniques serve crucial roles in interpreting the activity details. The ML methods include the support vector machine (SVM) [8, 55, 56, 104], hidden Markov model [172], decision tree [96, 98], K-nearest neighbor (K-NN) [182], and Gaussian mixture model [165]. These techniques provide WHM with efficient solutions for processing human activity recognition through wearable sensor. Moreover, deep learning (DL), a new ML branch, models high-level features present in data through automatic feature extraction with less human efforts. Thus, the technology has been highly applied in machine fault diagnosis and system health monitoring [102, 166, 167, 173, 186, 230]. However, up to date, few researches have systematically focused on the use of ML and DL algorithms in WHM system and technologies.

This review study aims to explore the processes involved in developing wearable health monitoring devices through ML and DL and offers a deep review of the related technologies and the process of implementation and feature learning. The rest of the paper is organized that Sect. 2 presents the existing problems of WHM, an analysis of traditional ML-based approaches and their subdivisions is presented in Sect. 3, in Sect. 4 the investigations of DL-based advanced approaches and its subdivisions are proposed, Section 5 provides the discussion of various ML algorithms used for WHM, Section 6 presents the limitations and challenges for future works on WHM based on ML and DL methods, and Sect. 7 finally concludes this investigation as well.

2 Key Technologies of WHM

Since the beginning of the twenty-first century, the population in the developed countries is aging at an extraordinary rate. Currently, approximately 600 million people who are above 60 years old and approximately 860 million people have chronic heart disease around the world [85]. For instance, in Japan, aging is sharply rising. More than 23% of the population in Japan was above 65 years old in 2010, and this value is expected to exceed 30% in 2025 [85]. Both medical expenditure and lifestyle disease risks are being increased by increasing aging population. Therefore, it is urgent to implement preventive medicine and health management to improve the quality of life of individuals and reducing their medical expenses, rather than passive medical care.

Health or healthcare monitoring is a preventive medicine and health management technique that can be used in the daily lives of human beings. Healthcare monitoring is applied due to the following reasons: to ensure a better support in medical diagnosis, provide faster recovery after medical treatment or injury, monitor athletes' performance in sport or fitness activities, and guide professional personnel for evaluating and monitoring their physical response under different dangerous conditions to manage the tasks assigned to them and their occupational health better [167].

Information and communication technology (ICT) are a crucial aspect of health monitoring because the use of ICT enables several applications, such as telesurgery and teleconsultations, to support independent living and wellness. Moreover, environment sensors installed in a patient's body surroundings can make the health information of the patient accessible from any part of the world by continuously supervising and evaluating the patient's domestic activity. However, the use of the pervasive ICT system is still constrained to the environment which is closed. Lastly, the advanced wireless communication systems like Bluetooth, WiFi, near-field communication, ANT+, and Zigbee are adopted in healthcare devices, mobile phones, and smartphones [31, 44]. Furthermore, the development of micromechatronics such as micromachine and large-scale integrated circuits has enabled the development of miniature and lightweight wearable sensors. Nonintrusive wearable sensors equipped with wireless ICT address the restrictions of emergency and hospitalization care and thus allow WHM for individuals. A comparison between the medical service evolution of different micromechatronic system is shown in Table 1.

As indicated in Table 1, unlike hospitalization (or emergency care) and home care, WHM is a promising method which can monitor patient's health anytime and anywhere in real time at a low cost through miniature, lightweight, and portable sensors. Obviously, the WHM devices are key systems for performing healthcare. The following subsections offer a review of the general system architecture of

Table 1 Medical service evolution with different micromechatronics

Medical service	Hospitalization and emergency care	Home care	Wearable healthcare monitoring
Cost/ performance	Low (treatment medicine)	Medium (regular monitoring)	High Anywhere, anytime, (preventive medicine)
Care place	Medical facilities	Any individual's home	
Medical devices (sizes)	Any (big)	Designed for use in house (portable)	Wearable sensors (tiny and light)

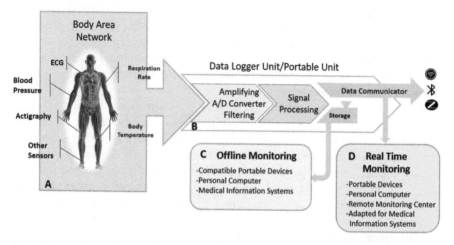

Fig. 1 Commonly used framework of wearable health system comprising devices [47, 101]

WHM and elaborate on the system or devices used, vital signals obtained, and data and signals analyses conducted in WHM.

2.1 Generic System Architecture of WHM

An increase in aging population and chronic heart diseases has led to increasing concern about the development of cost-effective wearable physiological measurement devices for nondomestic consumer with data storage facility [220]. An abstract generic WHM architecture was designed in this study by conducting a thorough literature investigation (Fig. 1). The architecture is decomposed into four parts (or modules)—(i) a body area network (BAN) module that can employ different techniques, (ii) a data logger or portable unit (PU), (iii) data analysis module, and (iv) real-time monitoring module that enables the visualization of health-related data [47, 101].

The *BAN* can be applied to many types of wearable devices due to its structure. A network of sensors, known as the BAN, can be created by placing an interconnection of these sensors around the human body. The signals of this network are transmitted to the portable processing module (or unit). Data centralization to a single PU is possible by connecting all sensors through a network. Thus, information can be gathered from numerous sensors and then sent to external networks from body for teleprocessing. Moreover, the BAN intensifies the synchronization, control, programming, and scheduling of the entire system. The system enables the WHM system to readjust according to the current physical condition and external situations. These merits optimize the resource usage [151]. Wireless connection is a crucial asset and enables systems to become mobile and ubiquitous.

The *PU*, a data logger unit or user interface box, is a unit in which all the information is gathered and contains output and input ports of the WHM devices. The primary input information are the decisive signals obtained from sensors and other portable devices connected. The exchange between sensors and the PU is generally conducted using wires. Such a communication provides easier and more economical WHM device. Currently, some alterations have been emerging in this communication technique due to the development of technologies, such as smart clothes. Smart clothes contain various interconnections (wires) that are woven and embedded into the fabricable clothes that are worn by patients. This is a much more favorable WHM technology, because it can avoid the inconvenience of loose wires around the body. The absence of wires leads to higher degrees of comfort and freedom. An inventive approach was proposed in which communication is made using biological channels [220]. In this method, the human body serves as a transmitter through electrostatic engineering fields. After getting the analog vital signals, the PU amplifies and/or filters the obtained signals and then converts them into the digital signals. *Signal processing* is conducted in the PU or in the other device after transmitting the data. The signal features are extracted through signal processing to evaluate a subject's health condition through anomaly detection and disease prediction. The original data received from the PU may be wirelessly transmitted or saved in a memory card. The PU receives data from real-time monitoring equipment and stores it in a local memory unit (Fig. 1). This bidirectional communication allows other devices to establish a wireless contact with a primary device and facilitates the storage of data collected from several storage sensors or devices. This system is beneficial to tracking the time of incidence and maintaining records [47, 151, 220]. The popular WHM-based wireless controls include WiFi, Bluetooth, Zigbee, and LoRa (more advanced technology). The features of these technologies are listed in Table 2.

Mobile telecommunication technologies are also employed to transmit data via general packet radio service (GPRS) in real time. The GPRS is a standard mobile data service for global mobile communication. The communication protocol is a fundamental aspect of a wearable device and aids in minimizing the energy consumption of the device [11]. The battery half-life can be improved by lessening the

Table 2 Comparison between primary features of wireless protocols [46, 128]

Protocol types of wireless	Max range (m)	Max data rate (Mbps)	Power consumption (mW)
Bluetooth low-energy (BLE)	100	1	10
Bluetooth (before version 4.0)	100	1–3	2.5–100
LoRa	50,000	0.0007	(customizable)
Zigbee	100	0.25	35
Wi-Fi	150–200	54	1,000,000

amount of data transfer. Data can be conveyed merely when the data are saved in the internal memory for offline data analysis. Data is able to be saved in a micro secure digital card or an internal digital memory and can be transmitted through a USB link between a WHM device and another device. The energy consumption of a WHM device can also be minimized through integrating compression techniques and transmission protocol [11]. Moreover, this method is helpful when network bandwidth limitations occur, the data storage capacity is limited, or data compression is required [23].

Real-Time Monitoring Distant monitoring through WHM allows prompt actions to be taken for of hospitalized patients in a timely manner by alerting the medical staff and the patient in case of any clinical emergency. Moreover, daily vital signals can also be monitored [151]. Patients inside a specific area like hospital can be monitored using WHM. The patients can freely move in the specific area, while their fundamental information like patient location is being sent to a distant monitoring center wirelessly. These real-time monitoring systems can be equipped with a set of alarms [47, 103], to alert the medical staff and patient during an emergency so that the patient can have a healthy life and freely move while their vital signals are being continuously or intermittently transmitted to a remote monitoring center. The data collected from patients can also be useful to reveal their ambient temperature (excessive cold or heat) [35, 47]. Finally, the key signals can be sent via Bluetooth to personal computers or portable devices, to visualize and analyze the health conditions of a person. Mobile technologies, such as GPRS, can be used in this real-time monitoring method to analyze athletes' vital signals during their exercises, sports activities, and daily workouts and to analyze the health information of combatants and firefighters [46, 47].

Offline Monitoring The data of the key signals may be saved in a PU such as tiny SD card, for the applications in medical diagnosis and analysis or only for individual record. The data storage and real-time monitoring are conducted simultaneously to keep a record of vital data for the diagnosis and prediction in hospital [46, 114].

2.2 Device or System of WHM

Many WHM devices have been developed to conduct one or several physiological parameter measurements. Figure 2 illustrates the various WHM devices attached to end users' bodies.

A smartwatch is a typical WHM device and can monitor the blood oxygen saturation, heart rate, and the temperature on the skin through a data communication module that is wireless [123]. Recently, novel smartwatches provide high wearing comfort due to their design, enable mobile and wireless connection, and provide a long-time vital monitoring (more than 24 h) proposed in [28]. These novel smartwatches monitor physical activity parameters, such as calories burned, distance traveled, and heart rate. More recently, PEAKTM shown in Fig. 2-(4) was proposed and is the first smartwatch that could track the cycles of sleep [20, 211]. The Moov shown in Fig. 2-(7) is a new wearable bracelet, monitoring the movement and being worn in any positions of the body based on the sports type. For example, the bracelet can be worn in the wrist while swimming or the leg while conducting running activities.

Google Contact Lens illustrated in Fig. 2-(2) is a type of WHM device that indicates the development direction of wearables. In the future, such wearables will reduce in size from the macroscale to the microscale and then will be available in

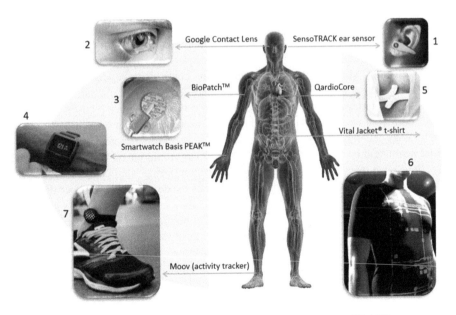

Fig. 2 Several wearable health monitoring devices, including (1) SensoTRACK ear sensor, (2) Google Contact Lens, (3) BioPatch™, (4) Smartwatch Basis PEAK™, (5) QardioCore, (6) Vital Jacket® t-shirt, and (7) Moov

the nanoscale so that they can be introduced into the body [112]. The ear accessory device is another class of wearable device. The device is emerging and can obtain many physiological feature parameters like heart rate and oxygen saturation level. These types of devices demonstrated in Fig. 2-(1) are connected to the ear as reasonable sensors, because muscle interference can be eliminated due to the composition of the central cartilage and the existence of arteries near the surface of the ear. Valencell which supplies major sensing technology revealed that the signals obtained through devices connected the ear were 100 times clearer than those obtained through devices connected to the wrist. Thus, the use of ear-based WHM devices is trending [61].

Most of the wearable devices are connected with heart activity. These WHM devices are divided into three main types: chest straps shown in Fig. 2-(5), adhesive patches displayed in Fig. 2-(3), and t-shirt revealed in Fig. 2-(6) with the sensors that are embedded. The former two types of devices efficiently acquire signals pertaining to several vital parameters of the user's body and heath. However, these wearable devices are not as comfortable and convenient as the t-shirt with the embedded sensors. E-textiles are prepared using electronic technologies and cloth materials and can obtain a larger number of physiological signals because they cover a larger body area than other WHM. To appropriately analyze the three types of WHM devices (electronic chest straps, t-shirts, and adhesive patches), the quality of heart-activity-signal monitoring was analyzed.

The concept of e-textiles is employed to many fields from fashion (e.g., light dresses) to medical science (e.g., monitoring of vital health and body parameters). Studies are being conducted to develop the smart (intelligent) fabrics into textiles that contain the unique properties of electronic systems. These smart fabrics can be classified into two categories, i.e., metal yarns comprising conductive fibers and electroconductive yarns containing carbon-coated or polymeric threads. The development of smart textiles for realization in WHM devices mainly focuses on textile electrodes (known as tetrodes) to obtain the signals from the human body. This technology has already been involved in some acquisition methods pertaining to vital health and body parameters. Currently, smart textile-based WHM devices can be developed for many lifestyle and sport monitoring applications. However, detailed materials are required chiefly in clinic as the demand of device certification and signal quality.

Wet electrodes are the gold standard in field of medicine for acquiring electrocardiograms (ECGs). However, these electrodes cause skin discomfort and irritation. Thus, textile-based electrodes are the other solution to wet electrodes but with a slight compromise in terms of signal quality. When wet electrodes are used, the total contact conductivity of electrodes may increase because the adhesion between the electrode and the skin reduces due to sweat. The quality of heart activity WHM devices can undergo from measuring a pure heart rate to measuring an ECG waveform quality signal based on the touch between the sensor and the skin as well as the influence of the hardware acquisition device on the accuracy level of the extracted signal [6]. In this study, the WHM devices include three kinds of heart-activity-monitoring devices: (1) HR devices that is to acquire the R-peaks to evaluate heart rate, (2) R-R interval devices that are adopted to determine the time of gaining each R-peak of an ECG signal, and (3) ECG devices that are used to acquire the ECG waveform and to mine morphologic feature parameters (peaks and valleys of ECG waveform), diagnose cardiovascular diseases, and analyze the rehabilitation of cardiovascular.

One the basis of the brand specifications of proposed devices [1, 10, 29, 67, 77, 78, 145, 185, 203–206, 226, 227], the heart-activity-monitoring wearable devices are assessed using two approaches (Fig. 3): type of wearable device (adhesive patches, chest straps, and t-shirts) and the aim of using the device (fitness, sports, medical, and health). The purpose of using the devices determines the heart-activity measure accuracy required (ECG < R-R interval < HR). Figure 3 presents that higher-accuracy and higher-quality heart-activity signals are required for medical and health-related applications compared with those required for fitness and sports applications.

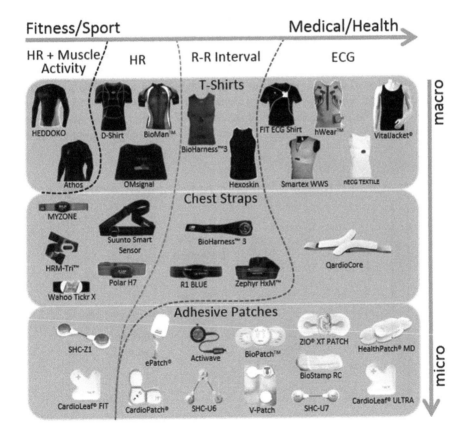

Fig. 3 Heart trackers characterized by different types of WHM devices

2.3   Vital Signals for WHM

Different physiological signals pertaining to the human body may be tested from electrical signals to biochemical signals. Human biosignals can be utilized to appropriately figure out the health condition of the human body and then to respond to external factors. Before understanding how to generate and acquire the signals by adopting wearable devices and sensors, the main biosignals that contribute to an efficient analysis of the human body health should be determined. Currently, technology and wearable scenarios enable the classification of WHM into three categories (Fig. 4): the situations of uses such as in home, remote, or clinical environment, kind of monitoring comprising offline and online, and type of user including healthy and patient as well [19]. In Fig. 4, the solid line indicates that the devices are used for medical purposes, and the dotted line represents that the device is used for activity purposes.

In respect of application, the WHM devices are generally categorized into activity applications involving fitness monitoring and wellness monitoring, nonmedical applications involving self-rehabilitation monitoring, and medical applications as well. The medical applications can be further decomposed into three main subcategories, i.e., prediction, anomaly detection, and diagnosis support. Prediction includes the identification of events to provide medical information for preventing chronic problems further and building a diagnosis [19]. Anomaly detection involves the identification of unusual patterns to distinguish between standard data and outlier data and then provide an alarm as a subtask particularly for anomaly detection [19]. Diagnosis-based support is one of the basic tasks of clinical observations and monitoring and is used for making a clinical decision by incorporating essential

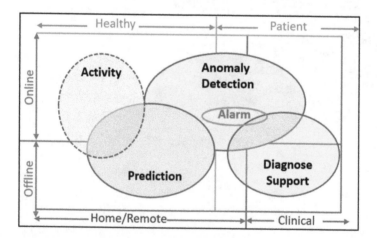

Fig. 4 Illustration of four types of main data comprising prediction, activity, diagnose/ decision support, and anomaly detection concerning different perspectives of wearable sensing in WHM systems and devices

retrieved information of health records, anomaly detection data, and vital signals [19].

From all the possible health-related parameters that are acquired through the human body, it is necessary to discern the most helpful nonmedical and medical parameters (pertaining to activity, exercise, or sports). To appropriately illustrate the advance of scientifically investigating the WHM devices, a survey and investigation in the dataset "Web of Science" with criteria are performed and presented in Table 3. In the survey, the criteria are followed to conduct the search for *Wearable Device* for two different periods (2010–2015 and 2016–2019). For each analyzed period (i.e., each search in Web of Science), we searched for the "pairs" of purpose and vital sign data for all combinations, excluding all others (purpose and vital signals). The following description presents an example of a search: "Topic: (Wearable) AND Topic: (Medical) NOT Topic: (Activity) AND Topic: (Body Temperature) NOT Topic: (Blood Pressure) NOT Topic: (Respiration) NOT Topic: (Glucose) NOT Topic: (Heart Rate) NOT Topic: (oxygen saturation) NOT Topic: (Electrocardiogram); Timespan: 2010–2015." In this search, we selected the revealed vital signals according to the most frequent vital signals observed in the acquired literatures and segregated into the two main fields of activity and medical (Fig. 5).

Overall, five traditional vital signals including HR, BP, RR, SpO2, and BT were identified to be crucial. We generally consider the five signals to recognize human health conditions and to continuously monitor them for patients. Ahrens et al. [3] presented two novel physiological markers, capnography and stroke volume, and suggested that these signals should be immediately measured if patient is in critical medical condition. Similarly, Elliott and Coventry et al. [52] described three vital signals pertaining to human health, i.e., pain, urine output, and level of consciousness. These signals should also be regarded as part of the regular patient monitoring. These researchers indicated that a combination of the three additional signals with the five vital signals could accurately recognize the variation in the physiology of a patient. The electrocardiography method is significant in electrical heart analysis and the prediction and diagnosis of cardiovascular diseases [215]. The monitoring of the blood glucose level is essential in patients with diabetes mellitus, which is an endocrine disorder. Numerous studies have been conducted to develop noninvasive method for blood-glucose-level monitoring [35]. For conducting WHM, vital signals should be analyzed and identified using data mining techniques. The next subsection illustrates data analysis of vital signals used for WHM.

Table 3 WHM devices survey topics and restrictions

Topic	Years	Intention	Vital signals words
Wearable healthcare monitoring (WHM)	2010–2015; 2016–2019	"Medical", "Activity"	"Body temperature," "blood pressure," "respiration," "glucose" "Heart rate," "oxygen saturation," "electrocardiogram"

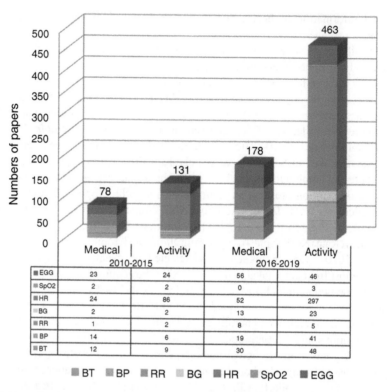

The chart data table:

	Medical 2010-2015	Activity 2010-2015	Medical 2016-2019	Activity 2016-2019
■ EGG	23	24	56	46
■ SpO2	2	2	0	3
■ HR	24	86	52	297
BG	2	2	13	23
■ RR	1	2	8	5
■ BP	14	6	19	41
■ BT	12	9	30	48

■ BT ■ BP ■ RR BG ■ HR SpO2 ■ EGG

Fig. 5 The related scientific papers retrieved to the topics of WHM and monitored physiological signals. *Note:* BP, blood pressure; BT, body temperature; BG, blood glucose; RR, respiration rate; HR, heart rate; ECG, electrocardiogram; SpO2, blood oxygen saturation

2.4   Data Analysis of Vital Signals Used for WHM

Due to the technological advances in healthcare and sensors, numerous data mining approaches have been proposed [13, 18, 22, 35, 138]. Sow et al. [187] categorized the primary procedure of sensor data mining into five stages, i.e., data acquisition, data preprocessing, data transformation, data modelling, and data evaluation. Moreover, in other studies [22, 222], data mining algorithms were subdivided into two types: (1) unsupervised or descriptive learning (i.e., clustering, association, summarization) and (2) supervised or predictive learning (i.e., regression and classification). However, these studies lack an in-depth study into algorithms applicability in handling specific sensor data features in WHM systems and devices.

In recent years, the research area of WHM systems has changed from the simple calculation and measurement of wearable sensor such as computing sleep time or number of steps in single day to a higher level of data and signal processing which are promising to provide more beneficial details to the end users. Thus, healthcare has focused more on in-depth data mining to obtain profound information representation. Three kinds of data mining tasks were identified in this study based on the studies selected for analysis. The three data mining tasks include anomaly detection, prediction, and diagnosis. Herein, the anomaly detection contains raising alarm as occurring an anomaly. The diagnosis is a decision-making process, by which the data is often classified into many categories in respect of the diseases or other conditions. Figure 4 illustrates the three tasks from a three-dimensional (3-D) perspective. The first dimension is the setting where monitoring is conducted. Most monitoring applications that involve the home and remote monitoring settings predominantly pertain to anomaly detection and prediction, while the uses of clinical settings pay general attention to the diagnosis [35, 188]. The fact is because the increasing attention is paid to gain a more preventive technique (prediction) by using wearable sensors, to consider the possibility of promoting independent living in home environment by the increasing sense of security (alarm). Similarly, enough information in clinical settings is available for diagnosis and decision-making [22]. A second dimension displays the important tasks of data mining used for users. For the patients who have known medical records, the WHM devices with the diagnosis capabilities and the possibility of raising alarms are crucial. Individuals who use such devices to maintain good health by monitoring, prediction, and anomaly detection, were reported in the literature [135]. The final dimension pertains to how the data are dealt with. As for all the three tasks, the data were resolved in an offline and online manner. Moreover, a large number of alarm-related tasks are being adopted for continuous monitoring in online method [187].

The central status of data mining in WHM systems is information retrieval such as anomaly detection, diagnosis decision-making, and prediction. According to previous studies [138, 187], most healthcare systems deal with issues related to the following aspects: (1) data acquisition through an enough sensor set, (2) data transmission from a patient to a doctor, (3) data integration with other descriptive data, and (4) data storage as well. The aforementioned tasks were included in all physiological data processing frameworks that is to conduct data mining tasks, i.e., noise removing, data cleaning, data compression, and data filtering. Several data mining techniques are commonly applied such as wavelet analysis for both data compression [49] and artifact reduction [139], rule-based methods for data transmission and summarization [2, 223], and Gaussian processing approach for secure authentication [209], to conduct these tasks. These tasks must be conducted because in real world the WHM systems often handle continuous data and unlabeled data [18].

The role of data analysis in health monitoring system is to acquire data information which are from low-level sensors and to change the information from high-level sensors. Thus, the novel health monitoring system has paid more attention on the phase of data processing to obtain a higher amount of information that is valuable based on requirements of expert user. Data mining techniques were initially used on the data of wearable sensors in the health monitoring system. In the subsection, we summarize the approaches that are frequently applied to process the data of wearable sensor for providing the valuable information. Apart from the data mining technique, the most extensively applied and standard method to mine information from the wearable sensor is presented in Fig. 6.

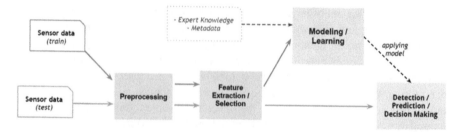

Fig. 6 The generic architecture for the data of wearable sensors of the advanced data mining method

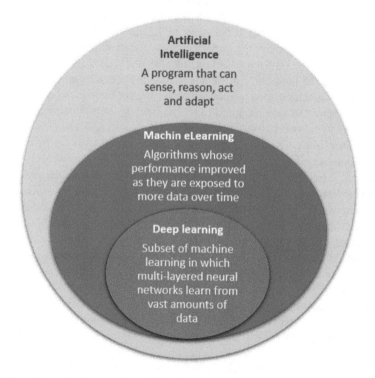

Fig. 7 The relationship between the artificial intelligence (AI), the machine learning (ML), and the deep learning (DL)

Raw data from the sensor are applied as the origin of the data mining method typically (Fig. 7). In this study, the sensor data were used as training data to study from the system and establish models of the feature and applied for testing the data of the model designed to determine the usage in the real world and derive results. This data mining method is deemed as a common flow for not only the supervised but also the unsupervised data mining solutions for obtaining results from any task of data mining. The primary procedures of the data mining method are as follows:

1. *Preprocessing of the data* Preprocessing of the raw data obtained in the health-care domain is necessary because of the appearance of possible motion artifacts, noise, and errors of sensor in any networks of wearable sensors in real-life scenarios. This preprocessing involves the following steps: (1) filtration of unusual data to remove artifacts usually by applying threshold-based methods [129] or statistical measures to insert the missing point of data [86] and (2) removal of high-frequency noise [69, 187]. The major aspects that challenges the preprocessing period of healthcare systems were presented in a previous study [187]. This study included the formatting, normalization, and synchronization of data because the accumulated sensor data are often unreliable and abundant [69].

2. *Extraction and Selection of Features* Commonly, data mining is conducted on extensive and datasets in the real world for retrieving valuable information. The feature extraction is aimed to find the main features of data sets [74]. In particular, feature extraction provides a meaningful representation of the abundant and complex raw data obtained from wearable sensors to formulate a relationship between the expected message and raw data for making decision [24]. Because wearable sensor data pertaining to vital parameters is tending to be in the successive format of time series, the majority of the features that are considered are correlated to the properties of signals in time series [40]. Signals can be analyzed in the domain of time and spectrum [15]. In the domain of time, the acquired features generally contain characteristics of basic waveforms, and statistic parameters are correlated to the apparent nature in the data stream, for instance, variance, mean, and pick counts [9]. The features in time domain are commonly found in physiological data due to that the traditional frameworks of decision-making, which are suitable for vital parameters, are on basis of the remarkable tendencies in the signal [203]. However, to obtain additional information related to the periodic action of data in time series, the researches in the medical aspect focused more on the obtained features from the frequency domain, for instance, the power spectral density, high-pass or low-pass filters, spectrum energy, and signal wavelet factors [68, 69]. For example, even though Bsoul et al. [32] have proposed a great number of characteristics for ECG signals, the major concern of their study was to take R points (each beat's pick point) into account and their performances in ECG pulses, for instance, the R-R interval and the pick count [24, 190].

The feature selection is an available solution to select more distinct characteristics based on the feature size acquired from the raw data and the capability of the learning approach to deal with these data. The method of feature selection often discovers a subset of the obtained high-dimensional data that are unrelated and make contribution to the property of learners [129]. The technique of feature selection used for physiological data can cut down the scale of the input data. The three most prevalent methods in the medical field used for dimension reduction are LDA, ICA, and principal component analysis (PCA) [210]. These approaches select the subset of the features that are most important in statistic [74, 116]. Other implements for the feature selection consist of Fourier transforms [99], analysis of variance (ANOVA) [63], and threshold-based principles [9].

Even though the bulk of the frameworks presented in healthcare include the feature acquisition or selection phase, the capital challenge is remaining to balance between characteristic acquisition (or selection optimum methods) and system expenses. For example, the utilization of the feature selection in the systems of real time is costly because the modeling technologies decrease the accuracy of these results. The aforementioned challenge is interrelated with (1) the health parameters that are selected in the system and (2) data mining missions or the objective of health monitoring system directly. Nevertheless, the solution to challenge is yet to be illustrated.

3. *Modeling and Learning Method* The methods of modeling and learning are crucial in WHM and the core of this study. In general, the methods involve statistical algorithms and ML algorithms. Statistical algorithms include decision tree [121, 152, 219], Gaussian mixture models [43, 209], HMMS [17, 156, 198, 233], rule-based methods [5, 97], statistical tools [87, 190], and wavelet-based analysis approaches in the frequency domain [36, 49, 99, 178]. ML has been progressing rapidly in the recent decades and is studied in the next section.

Other parameters pertaining to ML and data mining approaches are essential, for instance, electronic health records, historical data measurements, expert knowledge, and anthropometric parameters (e.g., sex, age). The metadata supplies the analysis from context and ameliorates the knowledge acquisition process [68, 209]. For example, each healthcare system that uses HR sensor data is required to study effects of metadata, such as medicine, weight, age, and sex, for obtaining a meaningful reasoning (i.e., basic heart rates which are irregular) or to personalize the pulses which are critical on basis of mentioned metadata [82].

3   Traditional Machine Learning-Based Approaches

Extensive data is produced when WHM sensors are deployed for monitoring the health of a person in a home environment. Moreover, this data can be multivariate with possible dependencies when multiple sensors are employed. Thus, suitable data processing methods are indispensable to make the data intelligible [187]. In this section, we sketch the most familiar ML algorithms that are applied with the data of wearable-sensor. The technical details of each algorithm are presented with the most typical instances to understand how to utilize the algorithm in the healthcare services. Moreover, the usability, efficiency, and relevant challenges of every technique in the medical field are instructed. Artificial intelligence (AI) is an emerging technology for the last two decades. ML and DL are the present state-of-the-art techniques used for system health monitoring and machine fault diagnosis [55, 56, 230] and are promising for rapidly and precisely performing WHM for human activities. The relationship between AI, ML, and DL are presented in Fig. 7.

Before ML gets more deep, various classical ML and data mining algorithms have emerged for decades of years, i.e., artificial neural networks (ANN) based on backpropagation (BP-ANN), SVM. The application of classification ML algorithms requires considerable expertise and sophisticated feature engineering because an in-depth exploratory data analysis has to be often conducted on the dataset firstly. Subsequently, a dimension reduction step can be performed using techniques, such as PCA, for enabling easier handling. Ultimately, the best characteristics have to be selected attentively to transfer these characteristics to ML algorithms. Knowledge pertaining to typical ML for distinct fields and utilizations is very distinct and often needs massive professional expertise within every domain. Because the major focus of the retrospect study concerns the DL-based methods, a concise sum up of every classical ML method is introduced in the part with a complete reference list.

3.1 ANN

Neural network (NN) is one of the AI approach, which is extensively utilized for classifying and forecasting [150], and its structure is displayed in Fig. 8. NNs are used to model the training data through studying the classification which is known of records and make a comparison with given categories with the forecasted categories of the records to alter the weights of network for the next iterations of learning. The use of NNs is currently the most prevalent method for data modeling used in the medical field due to the acceptable predictive performance of NNs [21, 22]. NNs can model nonlinear systems, for instance, physiological records in which the relationship between the import parameters is difficult to detect.

A broad scale of decision-making and diagnosis missions has been performed by NNs in the medical field. NNs have been used to multisensor networks and to conduct sophisticated multivariate data analysis. The multilayer perceptron (MLP) NN has been utilized in a previous study [115] to evaluate the pulse quality in PPG. In the NN, several quality metrics of individual signal are utilized as the import. Then,

Fig. 8 ANN structure

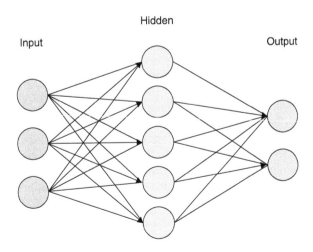

the node number (2–20) of the underground layer invalidation iterations is optimized. The result conducts two categories of signal quality as output. Some standard indices, such as specificity, accuracy, and sensitivity, were employed for evaluating the task. Vu et al. [207] presented a framework for recognizing the variability patterns of heartrate by accelerometer sensors and ECG. This approach utilizes a NN with three layer to learn the obtained patterns incrementally and make the classification. In the output layer, three nodes were utilized for three data classes—activity, location, and heart status. The replicator NN (RNN) [30] is another kind of NN, which is usually applied for outlier and abnormal detections. Recently, Chatterjee et al. [37] proposed an RNN to forecast levels of blood glucose. A network was designed with 11 input variables and 1 output node which is used for providing the predicted level of blood glucose, together with 3 underground layers with 8 neurons for each layer. Another study conducted an online classification of sleeping-awake states [99] through a feedforward NN on ECG and RR characteristics in the domain of frequency. The network was devised utilizing three frameworks (no hidden layers) which is different from the type of input signal applied. To make the estimation, the investigation utilized other clinical parameters (e.g., EEG) for monitoring and labeling collected data. Many other studies have included NNs [69, 147].

In summary, because learning is a complicated task in NNs, the NN method is generally applied for making decision in clinical situations that contain complex and large datasets. However, this model cannot handle the domain knowledge for enriching results. Moreover, because the process of modeling in NN is in the black box, the methods employing NNs must justify each input data. Thus, the methods using NNs are not considered as techniques that can be easily applied to diverse datasets.

3.2 Kriging Model

Kriging surrogate model was proposed by Danie G. Krige in 1951 in the geostatistics field for the first time [48]. The term "Kriging" was forged by Matheron who firstly formulated the Kriging model mathematically in 1963 [64]. In 1973, Matheron utilized the Kriging model in the field of the mineral reserve and corresponding error evaluation [65]. Sacks et al. conducted the utilization of Kriging models firstly in the process of analysis and design of computer tests [91]. In the method, they made the analogy of the input space points to the geographic coordinates. The Kriging models have been widely utilized in many application scenarios in recent decades, for instance, the optimization of design of engineering structures or other systems. Li et al. discussed the use of the Kriging model with the multiobjective genetic algorithm for the engineering optimization of a gear train [125]. In the biomedical engineering field, Li et al. studied the stent design optimization and relevant dilatation balloon by using the Kriging surrogate model with high-accuracy analysis [84]. Simpson et al. applied the Kriging model on an aerospike nozzle for the design optimization in multidisciplinary aspects [193]. Zhao et al. developed a dynamic Kriging modelling method to address the transient problem pertaining to structural design optimization [107]. Liem et al. combined an expert's method with the Kriging model for predicting the aerodynamic property to enable an accurate and efficient analysis procedure of aircraft mission [57, 107, 161, 193]. The Kriging model was also applied in the structural reliability analysis field [57, 84, 91, 107, 125, 161, 193]; meanwhile, it was proved to be fairly efficient and accurate for dealing with the high-dimensional and highly nonlinear problems.

3.3 SVM

SVM is one major statistical learning theory that can itemize unknown information by deriving chosen characteristics and establishing the hyperplane with a high dimension to divide the data points into two categories to develop a decision model [45]. SVMs are extensively used currently for mining physiological data in applications of medical field due to its ability to manage high-dimensional data through using a set of mining training features.

The standard health parameters considered in SVM method include SpO2, HR, and ECG. Hu et al. [86] utilized SVM for diagnosing arrhythmia by ECG signals. They used an SVM classifier version with binary system to separate ECG signals into the categories of regular and arrhythmia. Similarly, another study [111] put forward an SVM method to detect seizure episodes and arrhythmia by ECG signals. The study indicated that the application of the SVM with polynomial kernels performs better than that with other kernels. In another study [25], researchers utilized a one-against-all SVMs method for managing multilabel category to detect the condition of the patient. On basis of the labels of experts on the data of the episodes (level 4 severity), some binary SVMs with distinct kernels, such as sigmoid, polynomial, and RBF, were united with simulated input data obtained from multisensor features. Researchers also discussed the special application of SVM classifiers [197]. The study confirmed the deterioration in the patients' condition with chronic arthritis and gastritis by conducting binary categories of abnormal and normal ECG radial pulses by applying the SVM algorithm. The performance of this approach was estimated in terms of accuracy, specificity, and sensitivity.

General, SVM techniques are usually presented for abnormal inspection and making decision in services of healthcare. Nevertheless, in the SVM method, domain knowledge of using symbolic knowledge or metadata cannot be integrated with the sensors' measurements. Moreover, SVM cannot be used to find out the unexpected information that is acquired from unlabeled data like other classifiers.

3.4 PCA

PCA is the algorithm that interprets the structure inside in the way best explicating the change of the data. In case a dataset, which is multivariable, is visualized as a group of coordinates in the data domain of high dimension (each axis has a variable), PCA can supply a projection of the resulting object in lower dimension with the user when the most informative viewpoint is adopted. Because the different features' sensitivity which are the characteristics of a bearing defect may change remarkably in various operating conditions, it is proven that PCA is a systematic and practical feature selection option which enables the manual partition of the most representative features in the defect categorization.

In a previous study, one of the earliest adoptions of PCA on the bearing fault diagnosis was found [88]. This investigation illustrated that the PCA method can classify bearing faults with the higher precision and less feature inputs. Similarly, the remaining studies based on PCA [214] have utilized this data mining ability of PCA to benefit the selection process of manual feature. Recently, the PCA was also applied to the automated diagnosis of coronary artery disease [69].

3.5 k-NN

The k-NN algorithm is a nonparametric approach for either regression or categorization. In the k-NN categorization, the output is the object's class member, which is classified by the neighbors' majority vote. The application of k-NN in personable health monitoring and ill diagnosis has not been found to date, though k-NN was widely adopted in rotor fault diagnoses [92, 170]. In a study, the early realization of the k-NN classifier in the fault diagnosis of bearings was found [47]. In this investigation, k-NN functions serves as the central leading algorithm of the data mining classifier of ceramic the bearing faults that on basis of acoustic emission signals. Similarly, some other investigations [11, 23, 103] have applied k-NN for conducting distance analysis on every new data sample and determining whether the sample is belonging to a specific fault type.

3.6 Other Traditional ML Algorithms

In addition to the generally applied ML methods mentioned above, a great deal of other algorithms with different features have been used on the WHM, such as decision tree [121, 152, 219], Gaussian mixture models [43, 69], HMMs [17, 156, 198, 233], rule-based methods [5, 97], statistical tools [87], and wavelet-based analysis approaches in frequency domain [36, 178].

Feature acquisition is the most important step in each stage of WHM framework, because the performance of WHM system is closely related to the extraction of distinctive and relevant eigenvectors. Many researches have been performed for improving the WHM recognition system through obtaining expert-driven features [58]. Traditional artificial set feature learning methods are simple and easy to understand and have been universally used in activity recognition. However, the eigenvectors extracted by these methods depend on the application or task and are not suitable for similar activity tasks. In addition, the features cannot represent significant features of complex activities, and time-consuming feature selection techniques are required to select the best features [218]. What's more, there is no general procedures in selecting appropriate features. Therefore, many researches use heuristic methods to study feature engineering knowledge.

In order to solve the above problems, researchers have studied some automatic feature extraction technologies through DL techniques, which require less manpower and material resources [109]. DL is a new branch of ML, which models the high-level data features and has develop into an important technology of human health recognition. DL is composed of multilayers of NNs, which represent features from low to high levels, and has become an important research field in natural language processing, object recognition, imaging analysis, environmental monitoring, and machine translation [73]. In recent year, various DL methods can be utilized in different levels to form DL models, to enhance the robustness, flexibility, and performance of the system, which is promising to eliminate the dependence on traditional manual setting features.

4   Advanced Methods Based on Deep Learning

DL is a part of ML and AI techniques and thus provides considerable power and flexibility for feature extraction through learning to represent the world as a concepts' nested hierarchy. Here, per concept is made up of the simpler concepts, and less abstract ones are applied to compute the more abstract expressions. The framework of the DL network is displayed in Fig. 9.

DL has advanced considerably since its discovery in 2006 [80]. The prevalent research of DL is owing to the ability of DL in acquiring prominent characteristics from raw sensor data without depending on setting features manually. Moreover, in the human activity identification field, for example, complicated human activities are hierarchical and translational invariant. Thus, the same activities can be conducted through different manners by the same participants. Sometimes, the activity can become a preliminary stage for other complicated activities. Jogging and running activities might not be differentiable relying on the health and age conditions for persons who are performing the activities. As an ML technique, DL [26] uses typical learning for automatically conducting feature characterization for the raw data of sensors. DL techniques are different from classical ML techniques (such as SVM, k-NN, and k-mean), which require manually set features to perform optimally [109]. Over the years, DL has been extensively used in speech recognition [80], image recognition [192], natural language processing [191], and medicine and

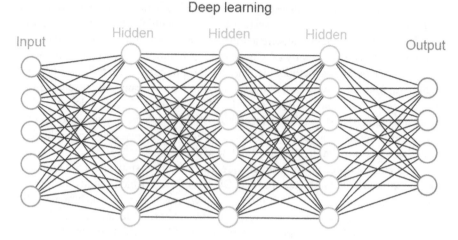

Fig. 9 The framework of deep learning network

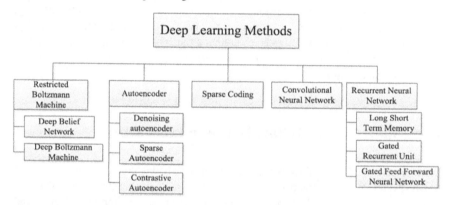

Fig. 10 Different framework of deep learning algorithms

pharmacy [127]. Recently, DL has found applications in human activity recognition [118, 157, 167].

Many DL methods [109, 177] have been put forward in recent years. Some of the methods are listed in Fig. 10, such as deep autoencoder, restricted Boltzmann machine (RBM), recurrent NNs (RNNs) and sparse coding, and convolutional NN (CNN). These methods are commented in the following subsection, and the features, merits, and weaknesses of each method are summarized.

4.1 RBM

RBM [59] is a derived model that functions as the main component in the rapacious layer-by-layer feature training and learning of the deep NNs. The model is trained with contrastive difference for providing unselfish assessment of the maximum likelihood learning. However, RBM is hard to converge to the local minimum point for the data representation of variants. Moreover, information about the automatic adjustment of parameters such as momentum, weight decay, learning rate, sparsity, and mini-batch size is crucial for achieving the optimal result [38, 80]. However, obtaining this information is challenging. RMB comprises a visible unit together with several hidden units, which are restricted for generating two-part graph to execute the algorithm effectively. Accordingly, the weights of neurons that are connected between the hidden and visible units are independent with no hidden-hidden or visible-visible connections under certain conditions. For providing efficient feature acquisition, several RBMs are piled up to produce visible to hidden units; meanwhile, top layers are embedded or connected fully with classical ML to distinguish between eigenvectors [59]. However, problems such as class variation, inactive hidden neuron, and intensity and sensitivity to large dataset make it difficult for training RBM. Recently, the methods such as regularization have employed a noisy rectified linear unit [137] and temperature-controlled RBM [113]. These methods have been proposed to resolve the problems. RBM has been widely investigated in feature acquisition and dimension reduction [79], together with modeling high-dimensional data in the motion and video sensors [195]. The two well-known RBM methods mentioned in literature are deep Boltzmann machine (DBM) and deep belief network (DBN), which are shown in Fig. 11.

DBN [80] is a DL algorithm that is trained with the greedy layer-by-layer way by piling up a few RBMs for acquiring the hierarchical characteristics from the raw data of sensors. There are directed links in the lower layer and undirected connection in the top layer with DBN which make the modeling of detected distribution possible between hidden layers and the vectors space. Similarly, the training is conducted in a layer-by-layer manner with the fine-tuning weight through the contrastive convergence. Next, the data distribution with conditional probability is computed for learning the robust features that are invariant to displacement, noise, and transformation, [80]. The DBF is depicted with the different color boxes in Fig. 12.

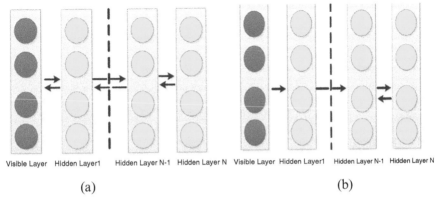

Visible Layer Hidden Layer1   Hidden Layer N-1 Hidden Layer N   Visible Layer Hidden Layer1   Hidden Layer N-1 Hidden Layer N

(a)   (b)

Fig. 11 Representation of restricted Boltzmann machine. (**a**) Deep belief network. (**b**) Deep Boltzmann machine

Fig. 12 The architecture of DBN [80]

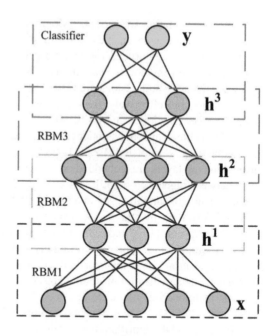

DBM [173] is a generation model. It has several hidden layers, which are located in the indirect connection of the whole network layers. DBM learns features hierarchically from the data, and in the next layer, the characteristics learned in the first layer are applied as potential variables. Similar with DBN, DBM uses Markov random field to pretrain massive unlabeled data layer by layer and uses bottom-up method to provide feedback. Moreover, the algorithm is adjusted by the backpropagation method. Fine-tuning allows for change inference and describes the algorithm to be deployed to identify tasks for a specific category or activity. The RBM training process [173, 174] contains maximizing the likelihood lower bound by the random maximum likelihood algorithm [224]. In this event, the training strategy has to determine the weight initialization and training statistics, to update after every small batch, and replace the random binary values with the determined real probability. The main disadvantages of DBM is that it takes a lot of time when considerable number of understandable optimization parameters are involved. Montavon et al. [134] proposed a central optimization method of stable learning algorithm and proposed a medium-sized DBM for discrimination and generation model.

4.2 Autoencoders

The use of autoencoders was proposed in the 1980s as an unsupervised pretraining approach for ANN [177]. After decades of development, autoencoders have been extensively applied as a greedy pretraining tool for layer-wise NN and a learning tool with no supervision. The training procedure of an autoencoder with single

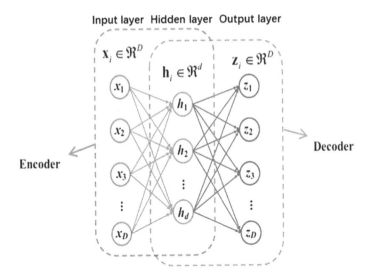

Fig. 13 Training process of a single hidden layer autoencoder [180]

hidden layer is described in Fig. 13. An autoencoder is trained through the use of an ANN. An ANN consists of two portions— encoder and decoder. The encoder's output is sent to decoder as input. The ANN regards the mean square error between the output and original input as loss function, and its main purpose is to imitate the input as the eventual output. After training the ANN, the decoding unit is abandoned, and the part of encoder is retrained alone. Thus, the encoder's output is a feature characterization which can be applied in the classifiers of next stage.

The deep autoencoder approach copies the values of input as output values, as described in Fig. 14. The deep autoencoder method generates the most distinctive characteristics from the sensor data that is unlabeled during WHM, and they are projected into lower-dimensional space in the way of utilizing decoding and encoder units. The encoder transforms the input of sensor data into the hidden characteristics; furthermore, these features are reconfigured by the decoder to approximate values for minimizing error rates [119, 208]. The extraction techniques of data-driven learning feature are provided by the method for avoiding problems that are commonly inherited by manually set features. An autoencoder should be trained in a manner such that the hidden units are smaller than the inputs or outputs, so it can provide lower dimension distinctive characteristics for activity recognition with less computation time [160]. In addition, the deep autoencoder algorithm uses multi-layer encoder units for transforming high-dimensional data into low-dimensional eigenvectors, which make the computation easier. The deep autoencoder algorithm is pretrained using RBM due to its complexity [79], and higher feature characterizations can be obtained by piling up multiple levels of automatic encoder algorithms [208]. In general, different kinds of autoencoder, such as contractive autoencoder, sparse autoencoder, and denoising autoencoder, have been put forward for ensuring robust features characterizations of ML applications.

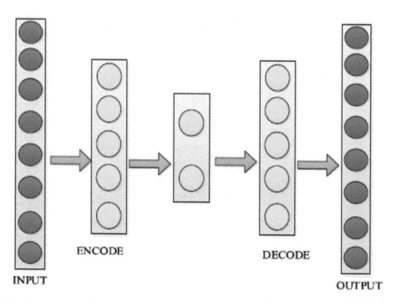

INPUT

ENCODE

DECODE

OUTPUT

Fig. 14 Deep autoencoder encoding and decoding process

Firstly, denoising autoencoders were introduced for learning robust feature characterization stochastically from damaged data (such as sensor values) through destroying original input samples partially [201]. Therefore, we train a denoising autoencoder and assign zero to random sample data values in way of stochastic mapping, to regenerate input data samples from the damaged data. It is similar to other DL models, which are unsupervised; the denoising autoencoder is trained by layer-to-layer initialization. It is trained with every layer for producing the next higher level of input data, which ensures the robust structure of the autoencoder network and observes the statistical dependence and regularity related to the distribution of input data. What's more, a stack denoising autoencoder can train and learn useful damage version of input sample data and with low classification errors [202]. Recently, a stacked denoising autoencoder was used for recognizing complicated activities [148].

Sparse autoencoder [130] is an unsupervised DL model that is proposed for over complete and sparse feature characterization of input data. In this kind of autoencoder, the sparse term is imposed on the model loss function, and some active units are set close to 0. Sparse autoencoder is adept in handling tasks, which need to analyze complex and high-dimensional input data, e.g., videos, images, and motion sensor data. Using the sparsity term, the representation of general features can be learned. In addition, the trained model is linearly separable, robust, and invariant to displacements, distortion, changes, and learning applications [232]. Thus, the sparse autoencoder model is very effective in acquiring low-dimensional features from high-dimensional input data and performing compact interpretation of complicated input data by supervised learning method.

A study proposed a contractive autoencoder [162], which can effectively represent features by introducing a penalty term of partial derivative. For the size of the input data, the square sum of all the partial derivatives is used for the eigenvectors, so that the feature is located in the neighborhood of the input data. Besides, the penalty term cuts down the feature space of dimension by training the data to make the change and distortion of model invariants. Compared with the denoising autoencoder, contractive autoencoder applies penalty terms to small damaged data sample. While it is different from denoising autoencoders, the contractive autoencoder penalizes aggregate data rather than encoded input samples.

4.3 Sparse Coding

Sparse coding is an ML technique first proposed by Olshausen and Field [144], applied for overcomplete learning and producing efficient characterization of data. Sparse coding decreases the data dimension effectively and describes the data dynamically as the linear combination of base vectors, which makes it possible for the model of sparse coding to acquire the data structure and to ascertain the relationship between different input vectors [109]. In recent years, many studies have put forward sparse coding methods for learning data characterization, particularly for the recognition of human activity, such as sparse fusion and shift-invariant method [50]. These algorithms provide the reduction strategies of feature dimensions for reducing the complexities in WHM computation.

4.4 CNNs

Convolution was first proposed for the first time to detect image modes layer-by-layer from the simple features to complex features [95]. The basic visual features with low level, such as edge and corners, can be detected by the deep layers, and the higher-level features can be detected by subsequent layers observed, which consists of simple features with low level. CNN [120] is a deep NN with the structures that are interconnected and the convolution operation heuristics (Fig. 15).

CNN convolution of original data (such as sensor values) is one of the most studied mature DL techniques. CNNs have a wide range of applications in ad speech recognition, sentence modelling, and image classification and have been widely used recently in the recognition of human activity based on wearable and mobile sensors [73, 120, 167]. The CNN model generally comprises a pooling layer, convolutional layer, together with fully connected layer (Fig. 16). It is stacked of these layers to develop a deep structure for automatic feature acquisition from the original sensor data [146]. The convolutional layer acquires feature maps with various step sizes and kernel sizes and then cuts down the connection number between the pooling and convolutional layers by concentrating together the features maps. The pooling layer

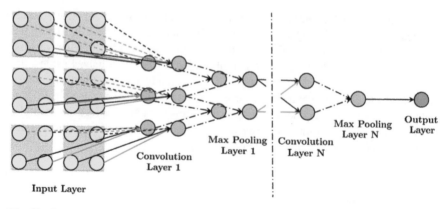

Fig. 15 CNN architecture

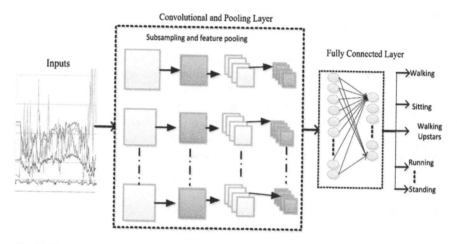

Fig. 16 Deep convolutional neural network for WHM [120]

reduces the number of parameters and feature maps and enables the network to keep constant transnationally to distortion and changes. Researchers have proposed various pooling strategies on multiple applications of CNN implementations, which include spatial, stochastic, average, and max pooling units [73]. Recently, performance estimation and theory analysis of the pooling strategies have instructed that the max-pooling strategies exhibit superior performance than all other strategies. Thus, the maximum pool strategy has been widely used in DL training.

What's more, the recent WHM studies related to the recognition of human activity have applied maximum pool strategies because of the robustness in detecting minor changes [100]. Nevertheless, the investigations including time series analysis and DL showed that the discriminative ability of maximum pool strategy decreases [100]. Thus, experimental evaluation and analysis are further needed on pooling strategies in recognition of human activities and applications in time series to confirm the effectiveness. An inference engine, e.g., a HMM, a SVM, or SoftMax, is integrated in the fully connected layer, that uses eigenvectors of sensor data to identify activities [33, 53, 166]. In CNN, the activation unit values of each area of the network are calculated for learning the patterns in the input data [146]. The output of the convolutional operation is computed as $C_i^{l,j} = \alpha\left(b_j^l + \sum \omega_m^{l,j} x_{i+m-1}^{l-1,j}\right)$, where l is the layer index, α is the activation function, b is the offset term of the feature mapping, W is the feature map weight, and M is the size of kernel/filter. Weights can be shared in order to make complexity reduction and make it easy to train the network. The concept of CNN was obtained from a study by Hubel et al. [88]. They analyzed the structure of the human visual cortex and found that the cortex comprised of map of local receptive field whose granularity values decrease as the cortex moves along receptive fields. Since then, several other CNN patterns have been proposed, such as GoogLeNet [94], VGG [105], and AlexNet [88].

Recently, the CNN architectures which unite DL techniques of various CNN patterns were also proposed [94, 146]. For instance, DeepConvLSTM was developed to replace the CNN pooling layer which has the long short-term memory (LSTM) of a recursive NN (RNN) [94]. Moreover, convolutional DBNs (CDBNs) were developed to use the capabilities of discriminative CNNs and pretraining technique of DBN [110]. Furthermore, Masci et al. (2011) combine convolutional NN with online stochastic gradient descent optimization training of autoencoder and propose a deep convolution autoencoder for feature learning [132]. The deep CNN framework for WHM is displayed in Fig. 16.

4.5   RNN

RNNs were proposed for modelling series data, such as original sensor data or as time series. The architecture of an ANN is illustrated in Fig. 17. RNN combines a time layer for acquiring sequence information, and then it learns complicated changes by hidden units of recursive units. Hidden units can be changed according to the available information on the network, and the information is constantly updated for reflecting the present network state. RNN calculates the present hidden state through evaluating the next hidden state as the activation function of the previous hidden state. However, this model is challenged in training and including exploding or vanishing gradients, which limits the application in the modelling of long-term activity sequence and time correlation in the sensor data [143]. RNN variation, such as gated recursive unit (GRU) and LSTM, integrate a large number of memory cells and gates to acquire the time activity sequence [71]. LSTM [83] merges memory storage units to reserve contextual information; thus, it can control the flow of information into the network. Because it contains memory cell with learnable weights, such as input gate, output gate, and function gate, LSTM can model temporal correlation in time series data and fully capture global features to improve the recognition accuracy.

Although LSTM has many advantages, Cho et al. (2014) pointed out that several parameters are needed to be updated during training, which increases the LSTM computational complexity [39]. In order to reduce the complexity due to the requirement of updating parameters, Cho et al. introduced GRUs with fewer parameters

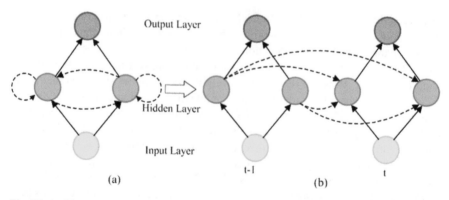

Fig. 17 Architectures of (**a**) of RNN and (**b**) RNN across a time step [230]

that made the implementation faster and simpler. GRU and LSTM are different in the method of updating the hidden state of next one and the exposure mechanism content [200]. The LSTM updates the next hidden state through a summation operation, and the GRU updates the state through confirming the correlation on basis of the time that makes to keep the information in memory. In addition, a recent contrastive analysis of the performance of GRU and LSTM shows that GRU is slightly better than LSTM in most applications of ML [41]. This paper attempts to improve GRU by cutting down the gate number in the network and introducing only multiplication gates for controlling the flow of information [66]. Through comparing with GRU and LSTM, this algorithm is superior to other algorithms in memory requirement together with computing time. In recent, Chung et al. [40] proposed a gating feedback RNN (GF-RNN) for solving the learning problem in multiplicative scale. The learning process is very challenging in the application fields of the language modeling and the sequence evaluation of programming language. Specifically, GF-ANN was proposed by superimposing multiple recursive layers and allowing the signal control of the flow, which is from the upper layer to lower one. The process is based on the previous hidden state to control information flow adaptively and assign different layers in various time scales. Nevertheless, the GF-RNN has not been applied in the recognition of human activity of WHM. Among all the reviewed investigations, the specific study, which applies GF-RNN for WHM, has not been found.

4.6 Generative Adversary Network

Goodfellow et al. [89] proposed the generative adversary network (GAN) in 2014. The network became one of the most encouraging breakthroughs quickly in ML field. GAN consists of two portions—a function discriminator (FD) and a function generator (FG)—as described in Fig. 18. In a GAN, the FG and FD compete with each other. That is, the FG tries to confuse the FD, and the FD tries to differ between

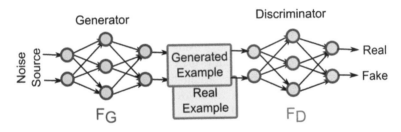

Fig. 18 The architecture of GAN [89]

the samples that are generated by the FG and those samples that are obtained from the raw data. GANs have a pattern of zero-sum game, in which both FD and FG complete to obtain a better capacity of imitating the raw data and distinguishing iteratively between the samples, respectively.

Categorical adversarial autoencoder (CatAAE) [75], a new GAN framework, was proposed. In this framework, an autoencoder is automatically trained by a training process with antagonism; meanwhile, the prior distribution is applied on the potential coding domain. Next, the classifier clusters the input sample units through balancing the reciprocal information between the sample units and their class distribution that is predicted. The potential training process and coding space were utilized to study the model advantages. Experiments under various ratios of signal-to-noise and motor loads fluctuations show that the proposed CatAAE framework has advantages in terms of useful characteristics.

GANs have been extensively applied in the fault diagnosis of machines in real-world applications. Because the operation conditions vary, the general assumption that the test set and training set are distributed in the same form is usually invalid. Some advanced GANs were developed [75] and inspired by GAN. These GANs included adversarial adaptive one-dimensional CNN model (A2CNN) and deep convolution GAN (DCGAN) [16], which exhibited better performance in terms of the training and testing accuracies. However, GANs have not been used for healthcare monitoring and illness diagnosis. Among all the studies reviewed, no study applied a GAN for WHM.

5 Algorithms, Application, and Frameworks of Different ML Methods for WHM

5.1 Comparison of Different DL Algorithms for WHM

In this part, the methods mentioned above are compared in terms of the advantages and disadvantages in WHM. Different DL methods mentioned in the paper bring the latest performances of WHM in human activity and diseases. The main DL advantage is that it can automatically study capacity from original sensor data that is unlabeled. Nevertheless, different capabilities are provided by these methods for the sensor stream processing. For example, RBM algorithms can efficiently transform the sensor data into eigenvectors through using unlabeled data for a layer-by-layer training. Moreover, the algorithms allow the extraction of robust feature vectors. However, RBMs exhibit high parameter initialization, which is a major drawback and makes training computationally expensive. Supporting real-time and onboard activity recognition is challenging due to the computing power of wearable sensor and mobile devices [216].

Auto depth encoder is an effective method, which can automatically convert unsupervised features into lower eigenvectors from original sensor data. A greedy layer-by-layer learning method is adopted by deep autoencoder methods to learn unsupervised features by continuous sensor streams. Auto depth encoder algorithm is robust to noise sensor data, and it can learn complex and hierarchical features from the sensor data. However, the main weaknesses of deep automatic encoders are that it is impossible to find the optimal solution and the calculation time is long owing to the high requirements of parameter setting. The sparse coding method can efficiently simplify the sensor data in high dimension into feature vectors with linear combination and ensure the simplicity of feature representation.

In addition, sparse coding is invariant to sensor localization and transformation, and it can effectively simulate the changes in the active process [229]. Changes in the sensor orientation pose significant challenges in the WHM system, especially for smartphone accelerometers [90]. In this case, the accelerometer signals produced by smartphones and wearable sensor devices will change with the direction and location of the accelerometer.

However, the use of sparse coding for effectively performing unsupervised feature learning is still challenging. CNNs are able to learn eigenvectors from the data of sensor for the high dimension and complex sensor data modeling. The major advantage of CNNs is that it can use the pool layer for reducing the training data dimensions and making the data translation invariant to the distortions and changes [167]. The algorithms can learn repetitive and remote activities by the multi-channel method [231]. CNN is mainly used to process images; so, sensor data is converted into image description for supporting extraction of distinguishing features [176]. CNN can solve the problem of uncertainty of sensor measurement and inconsistency of high-dimensional sensor data correlation. However, in order to obtain optimal features, multiple hyperparameters must be adjusted in CNN.

Besides, supporting the identification of complex activity details on board is a challenge. Finally, RNNs can be applied to time dynamics modeling in sensor data, so that complex activity details can be modeled. RNNs, such as LSTM, are effective for creating global time correlation in sensor data. The primary problem of RNNs, especially LSTM, is the high computation time required because many parameters are required to be updated. The techniques such as high throughput parameter update method can help to decrease computation time. Table 4 summarizes the latest applications of WHM and the advantages and disadvantages of each DL methods, focusing on the processing of sensor data.

Table 4 A summary of various DL architectures

Architecture	Description	Characteristics
	CNN Well-suited for 2D data, i.e., images Inspired by the neural-biological model of the visual cortex [88]. Every hidden convolutional filter transforms its input to a 3D output volume of neuron activation	*Pros:* Few neuron connections required for a typical ANN Many variants have been proposed: AlexNet [105], Clarifai [225], and GoogLeNet [80] *Cons:* May require many layers to find an entire hierarchy of visual features May require a large dataset of labeled data
	Deep autoencoder Mainly designed for feature extraction or dimension reduction Has the same number of input and output nodes Unsupervised learning method aiming to recreate the input vector	*Pros:* Does not require labeled data Many variations have been proposed to make the representation more noise-resilient and robust: Sparse AutEnc [154], Denoising AutEnc [201], Contractive AutEnc [162], Convolutional AutEnc [132] *Cons:* Requires a pretraining stage Training may suffer from the vanishing of errors
	DBN Composed of RBMs where each subnetwork's hidden layer serves as the visible layer for the next Has undirected connections just at the top two layers Allows unsupervised and supervised training of the network	*Pros:* Proposes a layer-by-layer greedy learning strategy to initialize the network Tractable inferences minimize the likelihood directly *Cons:* Training may be computationally expensive due to the initialization process and sampling

Table 4 (continued)

Architecture	Description	Characteristics
	RNN An ANN capable of analyzing data streams LSTM revibrated the application of RNNs Suitable for applications where the output depends on the previous computations Share the same weights across all steps	*Pros:* Memorizes sequential events Models time dependencies Has shown great success in many applications: speech recognition, natural language processing, video analysis *Cons:* Learning issues are frequent due to gradient vanishing/exploding
	GAN Mainly designed to generate photographs that look superficially authentic to human observers. Implemented by a system of generative and discriminative networks. Semi-supervised learning method aiming to recreate the input vector.	*Pros:* Requires almost no modifications transferring to new applications Requires no Monte Carlo approximations to train Does not introduce deterministic bias *Cons:* GAN training is unstable as it requires finding a Nash equilibrium of a game Hard to learn to generate discrete data, like text
	DNN The general deep framework usually used for classification or regression Made of many hidden layers (more than two) Allows complex (nonlinear) hypotheses to be expressed	*Pros:* Widely used with successes in many areas *Cons:* Training is not trivial because once the errors are backpropagated to the first few layers, they become minuscule The learning process can be prolonged

Architecture	Description	Characteristics
Visible Layer Hidden Layer 1 Hidden Layer N-1 Hidden Layer N	*DBM* Proposed in [174] is another approach based on the Boltzmann family Possesses undirected connections (conditionally independent) between all layers of the network Uses a stochastic maximum likelihood [224] algorithm to maximize the lower bound of the likelihood	*Pros:* Incorporates top-down feedback for a more robust inferences with ambiguous inputs *Cons:* The time complexity for the inference is higher than DBN Optimization of the parameters is not practical for large datasets

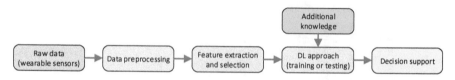

Fig. 19 Integration of wearable sensor data in DL method

Table 5 Overview of different DL methods of wearable medicine. Acc, accuracy; BA, Bland-Altman slope (systematic error); P, precision

Data	Application	Network type	Ref. no	Results
EEG	Recognition of cognitive activities	DBN CNN	207	Acc: 91.15% Acc: 91.63%
	Sleep stage scoring	DBN	208 209	Acc: 91.33% Acc: 91.31%
		LSTM	210	Acc: 85.92%
	Anomaly detection	DBN	211	P: 0.1920 High performance
	Classification of motor imagery	CNN Autoencoder	212	Acc: 77.6%
		Frequency DBN	213	Acc: 84%
	Feature extraction of motor-onset visual evoked potential	CNN	214	Acc: 87.5%
EMG	Hand movement classification	DBN	215	Acc: 66.59% (healthy) 38.09% (amputees)
ECG	Arrhythmia classification	DBN	216	Acc: 98.83%
	Abnormal ECG recognition	DNN	217	Acc: 85.52%
	Biometric user identification	CNN-LSTM	218	Acc: 99.54%
	Diabetes detection	CNN	219	Acc: 95.1%
PPG	Monitoring and detecting of atrial fibrillation	DBN	220	Acc: 91.8%
	Biometric user identification	DBN	221	Acc: 96.t1%
	Blood pressure monitoring	CNN, LSTM- RNN	222	BA: 0.47 (systolic) 0.16 (diastolic)
Motion	Human activity recognition	CNN, LSTM	178	Acc: 95.8%
	Closed loop for human activity recognition	DBN	223	Acc: 90%
	Mobile applications on activity recognition	DBN CNN	224 28 225	Acc: 73–94% Acc: 95.75% Acc: 91.5–98.2%
	Movement disorder	CNN	226	Acc:90.9%

5.2 Different DL Applications in WHM Systems

Some comprehensive comments on the increase of wearable sensors and the importance of utilizing data science methods to improve WHM systems have been found
in the documents [7, 183]. These reviews highlight the growing trend of continuous
multimodal sensing in the early diagnosis of diseases, rapid response to emergencies, prevention of chronic disease, and monitoring of physical activity. Gravina
et al. [72] delivered a global overview of multisensor information fusion in the
network of body sensors. Banaee et al. [19] reviewed a data mining of healthcare
and wearable sensors under life signals: blood pressure, heart rate, electrocardiogram, respiratory rate, blood glucose, photoplethysmography, and oxygen saturation. In this part, we will concentrate on the DL methods used in WHM for the
recognition of physiological activities or human motion analysis. The general concept of DL method for wearable sensor data is shown in Fig. 19. The first step of DL
method is to acquire original data from various wearable sensors. The next is data
preprocessing (such as normalization, filtering, all data synchronization, denoising),
then feature acquisition (with nonlinear features, or in time or frequency domain),
and the selection of most useful features to train or test the DL model. The result of
feature acquisition and selection as well as additional knowledge, e.g., study metadata, patient metadata, and expert opinion, are inputs that are used to train or test the
algorithm of DL. The algorithm ultimately determines the interested medical phenomenon (prediction, detection, etc.).

A summary of the possible application of DL algorithms in WHM is presented
in Table 5 with a comparison of the accuracies of the algorithms.

Sarkar et al. [175] proposed a pattern using DL algorithms, which combines
multiplicate EEG sensors in an unconstrained environment for recognizing human
cognitive activities in the real time, and picked a smaller sensor suite that is suitable
for wearable sensor systems. DBN and CNN were used to classify the two important activities—"watching" and "listening" (91.63% and 91.15%, respectively). A
two layer of DBN was tested by Langkvist et al. [108], and each layer has 200 hidden units. They pointed out that in contrast to other manual approaches, the DBN
improves sleep score accuracy (91.33%) by about 3%. It is concluded by the authors
that the separated DBNs should be applied for each signals of multimodal data.
Besides, their outputs should be combined using a secondary DBN. Zhang et al.
[228] used the sparse version DBN (SDBN) in the classification of sleep stage. A
voting principle was also used on basis of classification entropy utilizing SDBN and
a classifiers combination, such as HMM, k-NN, and SVM, and it attained 91.31%
accuracy. Dong et al. [51] applied LST network to learn sequence data and optimized classification performance with the single channel EEG. Single channel EEG
(Fp2-EOG left and F4-EOG left) of the forehead were measured. According to
494 hours of sleep, 62 people were evaluated. Compared with the existing vertex or
pillow electrode placements methods, this method has a higher algorithm performance. Classification accuracy of the LST network was 85.92%. The value was
relatively higher than that of the MLP (81.43%), random forest (RF, 81.67%), and

SVM (79.7%) methods. Wulsin et al. [213] used DBN in the semi-supervised paradigm to simulate EEG waveform for anomaly detection and classification. An anomaly is a small isolated set of waveform patterns, e.g., eye blinks, seizures, spikes, and other noise or artifacts. The results show that the performance of DBN is equivalent to that of standard classifiers (k-NN, SVM, and decision trees); meanwhile, the classification time is faster than other high-performing classifiers with 1.7 to 103.7 times. Compared with other common techniques, DBNs with original data inputs can be more efficient in automatically identifying anomalies online. Tabar et al. [194] improved the classification of EEG motion images using DL method for BCI. They used CNN and an automatic encoder network for classifying moving images from EEG. A new deep network was proposed to classify the features extracted by CNN by the autoencoder network. Besides, the average error of classification was 77.6%. They improved by 9% over the winner of the fourth BCI competition (Berlin, 2008). Lu et al. [122] evaluated the frequency-domain characterization of motor imaginary EEG signals obtained by wavelet package decomposition and fast Fourier transform and trained three RBMs. These RBMs were superimposed with additional output layer to develop a four layer NN called frequential DBN (FDBN). The output layer is classified by SoftMax regression, and the FDBN is fine adjusted by backpropagation method and conjugate gradient method. When FDBN was used, the results of benchmark data showed statistically a remarkable improvement in classification (84% vs. 73–80%) compared with the most advanced methods selected. Ma et al. [126] combined DBN and compressed sensing to extract the multimodal features generated by the sensing method, which improved the BCI accuracy by about 3.5%. Compared with the traditional mVEP features, the proposed method achieves higher classification accuracy (87.5% vs. 84%). The result was applicable to subjects, which have the relatively poor performance.

A CNN is applied by Atzori et al. [14] to categorize 50 hand movements with surface EMG signals. They used the NinaPro open database, which included data from 78 subjects—67 healthy subjects and 11 transradial amputees. The average classification accuracies obtained utilizing a simple CNN and various classical classification methods (such as the random forest, k-NN, SVM, and linear discriminant analysis methods) were comparable (66.59% vs. 62.06% for dataset 1 comprising data of healthy participants, 60.27% vs. 60.28% for dataset 2 comprising data of healthy participants, and 38.09% vs. 38.82% for the dataset comprising the data of participants who underwent amputation).

Yan et al. [217] used the MIT-BIH standard ECG signal database to train the RBM. Among it, half of the data was utilized for RBMs training, 30% for DBN fine-tuning, and the remaining 20% for testing. The results showed that the specificity, sensitivity, and accuracy of two kinds of ECG were 96.05%, 99.83%, and 98.83%, respectively. Ripol et al. [163] compared the effectiveness of DBN in identifying abnormal 12 lead ECG data from a large group of patients (1390 patients from Clinic of Barcelona Hospital) and compared with the professional algorithm of extreme learning machines, k-NN, SVM, and dedicated heart disease system. Both DBN (specificity 78.27% and accuracy 85.52%) and SVM (specificity 73.46%

and accuracy 84.76%) were better than other methods with the higher specificity and accuracy. Page et al. [149] utilized a deep NN network to the QRS segments of 90 resting participants for identifying their biometrics. Optimal accuracy, sensitivity, and specificity of the applied NN were 99.54%, 99.49%, and 99.55%, respectively. Ashiquzzaman et al. [12] utilized a CNN-LSTM to detect diabetes by heart rates that were obtained from ECG signals. The method exhibited an accuracy of 95.1%. Thus, this method is promising for noninvasive diabetes detection.

Shashikumar et al. [181] conducted atrial fibrillation detection on patients in real time. The continuous wavelet transform of PPG signal, which is recorded by the Simband smartwatch, is applied to obtain features used in training CNN. The accuracy of the method was 91.8%, and it was equivalent to that based on ECG. Jindal et al. [93] compared the DBN performance with classic fuzzy and k-NN classifiers in biometric user recognition. The DBN method consists of clustering step, forming subgroups before data preprocessing through DBN and RBM fine-tuning. The accuracy rate of the combination of clustering and DL is 96.1%, which was more than 10% higher than the classical method. Ruiz et al. [169] recorded both noninvasive (through light plethysmograph) and invasive blood pressure (through the radial artery catheter) simultaneously. RBM training was carried out in 572 patients with stable blood pressure, which was measured by the PPG signal. Systematic errors (Bland-Altman slope) of the diastolic and systolic arterial pressure were 0.16 and 0.47, respectively.

The DL-based WHM systems has been used by different authors to identify human physical activity. In this systems, the input signals applied for DL training come from motion sensors (such as gyroscopes and accelerometers). Ordóñez et al. [146] reported that the combination of CNN and RNN can effectively identify human activities for18 gesture tasks, and the accuracy of this method is 95.8%. Using the concept of closed loop proposed by Saeedi et al. [171], the robustness of activity identification can be improved. In this case, the accuracy of activity recognition could reach 90%. Some authors have proposed a framework for activity identification using the mobile devices, thus demonstrating the possibility of commercial applications [167]. Bhattacharya et al. [27] proposed a simple RBM solution for smartwatch processor (Qualcomm Snapdragon 400). The prototype of smartwatch includes the following sensors: gyroscope, accelerometer, magnetometer, barometer, and temperature and light sensors. Three different RBM patterns were tested for supporting three daily scenarios, physical activities, transportation, and gestures, and the transition between outdoor and indoor environments. The results of classification that were obtained by RBM have higher accuracy than that obtained by traditional methods (decision trees, RF, and SVC). On basis of the RBM model, test results showed that the life of battery was between 6 and 52 hours. Ronao et al. [167] reported the results of an investigation of 30 volunteers who executed different physical activities, e.g., standing, lying walking, and sitting with the smartphone in pockets to collect gyroscope and accelerometer data. They reported that the classification accuracy of CNN for human activity identification was 95.75%. In addition, Ravi et al. [159] also introduced another solution to effectively implement CNN for the recognition of human activities (such as cycling, jogging, and walking) with a low power device. Eskofier et al. [54] explicated the superiority and clinical application of deep CNN in the diagnosis of motor retardation in patients with Parkinson's disease (on basis of the data of accelerometers located in the forearm), and it is contrasted with the classical methods (such as PART, k-NN, SVM, and Ada Boost M1; 90.9% vs. 81.7%, 67.1%, 85.6%, and 86.3%, respectively).

5.3 Hardware and Software Frameworks for DL Implementation

Table 6 provides a list of the most fashionable packages that allow custom DL method on basis of the method described in this article. All the software that are listed in the Table 6 can use CUDA (NVIDIA) for improving performance by GPU acceleration. Because of the increasing trend to transform proprietary DL patterns into the open-source projects, the companies like Nervana Systems [133] and Wolfram Mathematica [34] have made a decision to provide cloud-based services to help researchers expedite training process. The new acceleration hardware of GPU includes microprocessors that are built specifically for DL, like NVIDIA DGX-1 [184]. Other feasible solutions are neural morphological electronic systems, which are commonly used in the simulations of computational neuroscience. These hardware patterns are intended to execute artificial synapses and neurons in the chip. Some of the popular hardware components include Spinnaker [212], IBM TrueNorth, Intel Curie, and NuPIC.

Other patterns to simplify DL implementation across heterogeneous devices and platforms are still under development. For example, Convent, DIGIT, and the MATLAB-based CNN toolbox are being developed for feature acquisition. Besides, CNN's implementation of CUDA, Cudanet, and C++ is being fine-tuned for achieving the DL development. Recently, some estimations of the frameworks have been reported [100, 120] using parameters such as documentation, language support, extension speed, development environment, GPU support, training speed, model library, and maturity level. In these frameworks, TensorFlow has the highest interest and contribution to GitHub, surpassing Caffe and CNTK. Besides, some patterns support GPU or have limited support for GPU, and GPU must reside on the workstation (such as MXNet).

Owing to the development of DL-based recognition of human activities, these patterns have become the main choices for researcher and developers based on mobile and wearable sensor applications. Because of various implementation frameworks and different programming support, the framework choice relies on the user's technical and programming ability. Recent software frameworks for mobile-based human activity recognition include Theano, TensorFlow, Lasagne, Keras, and Caffe [54, 100, 146, 167, 221]. Other researches use MATLAB [27, 53] and other programming platforms such as C++ [50] to develop algorithms.

Table 6 Popular software packages of DL implementation

Name	Creator	License	Platform	Interface	OpenMP support	Supported techniques RNN	CNN	DBN	Cloud computing
Caffe [70]	Berkeley Center	FreeBSD	Linux, Win, OSX, Andr.	C++, Python, MATLAB	X	✓	✓	X	X
CNTK [199]	Microsoft	MIT	Linux, Win	Command-line	✓	✓	✓	X	X
Deeplearning4jK [155]	Skymind	Apache 2.0	Linux, Win, OSX, Andr.	Java, Scala, Clojure	✓	✓	✓	✓	X
Wolfram Math. [34]	Wolfram Research	Proprietary	Linux, Win, OSX, Cloud	Java, C++	X	X	✓	✓	✓
TensorFlow [62]	Google	Apache 2.0	Linux, OSX	Python	X	✓	✓	✓	X
Theano [140]	Universite´ de Montre´al	BSD	Cross-platform	Python	✓	✓	✓	✓	X
Torch [142]	Ronan Collobert et al.	BSD	Linux, Win, OSX, Andr., iOS	Lua, LuaJIT, C	✓	✓	✓	✓	X
Keras [106]	Franois Chollet	MIT license	Linux, Win, OSX	Python	X	✓	✓	✓	X
Neon [133]	Nervana Systems	Apache 2.0	OSX, Linux	Python	✓	✓	✓	✓	✓

6 Challenges and Open Directions in WHM Based on ML or DL Methods

6.1 Challenges of ML- or DL-Based WHM

In this part, some research challenges which need to be further discussed are listed. Some of the areas that require further study are as follows: collection of a large dataset, real-time and onboard implementation on WHM devices, class imbalance problems, data preprocessing and evaluation, and the many research issues in the field of sensor fusion. Here, related research directions are discussed on basis of seven important themes:

- *Implementation of DL algorithm in real time and onboard for WHM:* The onboard implementation of DL algorithms in mobile and wearable devices will help in reducing the computation complexity on data storage and transfer. However, this technique is restricted by data acquisition and memory constraints in the current mobile and wearable sensor devices.
- Moreover, *the tuning and initialization of many parameters* in DL increases the computational time and is not suitable for low-energy mobile devices. Therefore, methods such as optimal compression and mobile-phone-enabled GPU should be utilized to minimize the computation time and resource consumptions. Other methods for real-time implementation include mobile cloud computing platforms for training to reduce the training time and memory usage. By using this type of implementation, the system can become self-adaptive and can require minimal user inputs for a new information source.
- *A comprehensive evaluation of preprocessing and hyperparameter settings on learning algorithms:* Preprocessing and dimensionality reduction are essential aspects of the human activity recognition process. Dimensionality reduction provides a mechanism to minimize the computational complexity, especially for mobile and wearable sensor devices with limited computation ability and memory, by projecting high- dimensional sensor data into lower-dimensional vectors. However, the method and extent of preprocessing for the performance of DL is an open research topic. Many preprocessing techniques such as normalization, standardization, and different dimensionality reduction methods should be investigated to know their effects on the performances, computational time, and accuracy of DL methods. Aspects such as learning rate optimization to accelerate computation and reduce model and data size, kernel reuse, filter size, computation time, memory analysis, and learning process still require further research because current studies depend on heuristics methods to apply these hyperparameters. Moreover, the use of grid search and evolutionary optimization methods for mobile-based DL methods that support lower-energy consumption, dynamic and adaptive applications, and new techniques that enable mobile GPUs to reduce the computational time are very significant research directions [146].

- *Large-sensor dataset collection for evaluation of DL methods:* The training and evaluation of DL techniques require large datasets obtained from different sensor-based Internet of things (IoT) devices and technologies. The current review indicates that most studies on DL implementation for mobile and wearable sensor-based health monitoring depend on benchmark dataset from conventional ML algorithms, such as OPPORTUNITY, Skoda, and WSDM, for evaluation. Data collection methods use cyber-physical systems and mobile crowdsourcing to leverage data pertaining to smart homes, mobile location (for determining the transportation mode), smart home environment (for elderly care and monitoring), and GPS (for conducting context-aware location recognition and other essential applications). Therefore, the collection of large datasets through the synergy of these technologies are crucial for performance improvement.
- *Transfer learning for using DL algorithms for realizing mobile and wearable sensor devices:* Transfer-learning-based activity recognition is a challenging task. Transfer learning leverages the experience acquired from different domains to improve the performance of new areas that is yet to be experienced by the system. Transfer learning is mainly used to reduce training time, provide robust and versatile activity details, and reuse existing knowledge for new domains (a critical issue in activity recognition). Further research in the areas related to kernels, convolutional layers, interlocation transferability, and intermodality transferability would improve implementation of DL-based WHM [146]. In addition, the transfer learning in the recognition of human activities on basis of the mobile wearable sensor can minimize environment, target, and source-specific application implementation that haven't received due attention.
- *Implementing decision fusion of WHM based on DL:* Decision fusion is an important step to further improve the diversity and performance of recognition systems of human activities and is key step to combine multiple classifiers, sensors, and architectures into one decision. Moreover, heterogeneous sensor fusion requires further study as the typical area, and it combines expert knowledge with the DL algorithms as well as various unsupervised feature-learning methods for improving the activity recognition system's performance.
- *Solving the class imbalance problem of DL in WHM:* During the abnormal activity of WHM, the class imbalance problems can be discovered in the dataset. It is very important to solve the problem of class imbalance in medical monitoring, especially when the real fall is very steep. In human activity recognition based on mobile and wearable sensors, due to the distortion of dataset and the calibration of sensor data, performance generalization will be reduced, resulting in class imbalance. Previous studies have developed a series of solutions, such as the cost-sensitive learning strategy and weighted extremum based on hybrid kernel. However, there is no study to find out the impact of class imbalance on DL implementation, especially for the mobile wearable sensors. Thus, strategies of reducing class imbalance using DL methods can improve WHM significantly.
- *Enhancing WHM to improve DL performance:* Another aspect to be studied is to utilize data enhance technology to improve the DL performance for motion sen-

sors (gyroscopes, accelerometer, etc.) of WHM with CNN. The data expansion methods use limited wearable and mobile sensor data to generate new data by converting existing data of training sensors. The processes are important owing to that they help to generate enough training data for avoiding overfitting and improving translation invariance in sensor variation, distortion, and orientation, especially in CNN models. Data enhancement is the joint training strategy in the image categorization [73]. In WHM based on wearable and mobile sensors, the performance and impact of data expansion need to be evaluated for generating more training instances and prevent overfitting caused by small datasets. Different data expansion methods, such as arbitrary rotations, sensor position change, position arrangement with sensor events, scaling, and time warping, provide effective method to improve the WHM performance based on DL [229].

6.2   Open Research Directions of ML-/DL-Based WHM

To monitor human activities and health conveniently and smartly, high-performance and high-reliability WHM devices based on ML or DL approaches should be developed urgently. Four research directions should be considered in future studies.

- The exploration of a novel data acquisition system based on DL algorithm is one primary direction that should be considered to ensure rapid and real-time data collection of all signals with less signal loss. In particular, the development of a wireless data acquisition system by adopting wireless transmission technology is crucial for collecting remote signal data from human bodies more conveniently and rapidly.
- The transfer system of signals should be investigated by using DL algorithms for developing an intelligent transfer model for accurately and rapidly transmitting signals from the transmission terminal to the receiving terminal wirelessly.
- The method of adopting the DL approach to process the signal data should be urgently investigated. When signals are used, the feature extraction of these signals is a crucial research direction. The feature extraction techniques have to be developed in ML- or DL-based WHM devices for the precise identification of different classes of signals that are obtained for different health and illnesses conditions. How to acquire enough data to cater for the use of DL approach is very important to structure database. Use of DL in WHM needs large-scale data to training DL model. Therefore, the collections and buildup of the database of the human-body-related bio-characteristics is highly needed for the application of the ML-/DL-based WHM device. In this case, it is necessary to develop more efficient methods to replenish the insufficient database and to build big database. For example, collaboration with related hospitals, healthcare centers, clinics, or interdisciplinary research teams would be possible approaches.
- The interoperability of WHM system is a challenge in information exchange among different populations and subsystems in WHM system (or device). The

development of the fifth-generation wireless network technology (5G) makes connecting more devices in hospital into the network on the spot and obtaining remote access at home possible. Thus, how to adopt 5G technology to transmit important activity and signals information to the home computer and how to send data to appropriate medical professionals by telephone line and the internet with a miniature, wearable, and low-power radio are the key technologies of the interoperability of WHM system. Besides, the use of 5G technology is also promising to advance the new devices of the WHM system.

7 Conclusions

Automatic feature learning in WHM has been developed rapidly in terms of feature extraction and processing of the data or signals pertaining to the activities of individuals who are monitored. The development has benefited from the steady development of computing infrastructure capabilities and access to large datasets by wearable and mobile sensing technologies, crowd sourcing, and IoT. In the research, we reviewed multiple ML methods, including manual feature acquisition from data signals. To conduct automatic feature extraction in WHM, DL methods, such as RBMs, autoencoders, CNNs, and RNNs, were presented. What's more, their advantages, characteristics, and disadvantages were introduced in detail. The DL method can be divided into discriminative, generative, and mixed methods. We used these categories for reviewing and summarizing DL implementation of WHM. The generative DL methods include RBMs, autoencoders, sparse coding, and deep mixture models. In addition, the discrimination methods include RNNs, CNNs, hydrocarbons, and deep neural model. It is similar that the hybrid method combines discriminant and generative model for enhancing feature learning. Currently, such combinations are mainly used in the studies pertaining to DL for WHM. The hybrid method combines different generation models (such as RBM and autoencoder) with a CNN or combines the discriminative model (such as LSTM and CNN). These methods are the key steps to realize automatic feature learning and improve performance generalization across activities and datasets.

The DL implementation is supported by the software framework and high-performance computing GPU. As open-sources project, a number of these software frameworks have been released to research communities recently. These software frameworks were discussed by considering the cognizance of their characteristics and the information provided by developers'selection of particular frameworks. Besides, the evaluation, classification, and training of DL algorithms for WHM are not trivial all the time. In order to provide the best categorizations and comparisons of recent events in research communities, we reviewed the optimization and training strategies used by different recently proposed studies of human activities recognition that are based on wearable and mobile sensors.

Performance and classification metrics obtained by various validation techniques are critical for ensuring generalization across the datasets. The methods can avoid the overfitting on training sets. It provided an open dataset for identifying and modelling human activities. Some of the extensively applied datasets are PAMAP2, Skoda, and OPPORTUNITY. Besides, the datasets are popular in classic ML algorithms as well.

To further understand the direction of research progress, we put forward the relevant challenges to be overcome and need researchers' attention. For example, the decision fusion based on DL, the implementation of DL mobile devices, class imbalance, and transfer learning make the WHM implementation achieve higher performance accuracy. With the further development of wearable computing technology and wearable devices, people are looking forward to the further development of digital learning technology. In addition, many meaningful research directions are proposed to guide future research.

Acknowledgments This work was supported in part by the Innovation and Technology Fund of the Hong Kong SAR government (Grant no. ITP/097/18TP), University Grants Committee of the Hong Kong SAR government (Grant no. UGC-UAHB), the National Natural Science Foundation of China (Grant no. 51975127), Shanghai International Cooperation Project of One Belt and One Road of China (Grant No. 20110741700), Aerospace Science and Technology Fund of China (Grant no. AERO201937), and Fudan Research Start-up Fund (Grant no. FDU38341). The authors would like to thank them.

Conflicts of Interest The authors declare that there is no conflict of interests regarding the publication of this article.

References

1. © Polar Electro 2016. H7 Heart Rate Sensor. Available online: www.polar.com.
2. Ahmad, N.F., Hoang, D.B., Phung, M.H. (2009) Robust Preprocessing for Health Care Monitoring Framework. In: the 11th International Conference on E-Health Networking, Applications and Services, Sydney, Australia, pp. 169–174.
3. Ahrens, T. (2008) The most important vital signs are not being measured. Aust. Crit Care 21:3–5.
4. Alaiad, A., Zhou, L. (2014) The determinants of home healthcare robots adoption: an empirical investigation. Int. J. Med. Inf. 8(3):825–840.
5. Al-Hajji, A.A. (2012) Rule-Based Expert System for Diagnosis and Symptom of Neurological Disorders "Neurologist Expert System (NES)". In: the 1st Taibah University International Conference on Computing and Information Technology, Al-Madinah Al-Munawwarah, Saudi Arabia, pp. 67–72.
6. Andreoni, G., Standoli, C.E., Perego, P. (2016) Defining requirements and related methods for designing sensorized garments. Sensors 16:769.
7. Andreu-Perez J, Leff DR, Ip HM, Yang GZ. (2015) From wearable sensors to smart implants—toward pervasive and personalized healthcare. IEEE Trans. on Biomed. Eng. 62(12):2750-2762.
8. Anguita, D., Ghio, A., Oneto, L., Parra, X., & Reyes-Ortiz, J. L. (2012) Human activity recognition on smartphones using a multiclass hardware-friendly support vector machine. In Int. Workshop on Ambient Assisted Living 216-223.
9. Apiletti, D., Baralis, E., Bruno, G., Cerquitelli, T. (2009) Real-time analysis of physiological data to support medical applications. Trans. Info. Tech. Biomed. 13:313–321.

10. Appelboom, G., Camacho, E., Abraham, M.E., Bruce, S.S., Dumont, E.L., Zacharia, B.E., D'Amico, R., Slomian, J., Reginster, J.Y., Bruyere, O., et al. (2014) Smart wearable body sensors for patient self-assessment and monitoring. Arch. Public Health 72:28.
11. Asensio, A., Marco, A., Blasco, R., Casas, R. (2014) Protocol and architecture to bring things into internet of things. Int. J. Distrib. Sens. Netw.
12. Ashiquzzaman A, Tushar AK, Islam MR, Shon D, Im K, Park JH et al. (2018) Reduction of Overfitting in Diabetes Prediction Using Deep Learning Neural Network. In: IT Convergence and Security 2017. Singapore: Sringer, pp. 35–43.
13. Atallah, L., Lo, B., Yang, G.Z. (2012) Can pervasive sensing address current challenges in global healthcare? J. Epidemiol. Glob. Health 2:1–13.
14. Atzori M, Cognolato M, Müller H. (2016) Deep learning with convolutional neural networks applied to electromyography data: a resource for the classification of movements for prosthetic hands. Frontiers in Neurorobotics. 10(9): 1–8.
15. Avci, A., Bosch, S., Marin-Perianu, M., Marin-Perianu, R., Havinga, P. (2010) Activity Recognition Using Inertial Sensing for Healthcare, Wellbeing and Sports Applications: A Survey. In: the 23th International Conference on Architecture of Computing Systems, Hannover, Germany, pp. 167–176.
16. B. Zhang, W. Li, J. Hao, X.-L. Li, and M. Zhang. (2018) Adversarial adaptive 1-D convolutional neural networks for bearing fault diagnosis under varying working condition eprint arXiv:1805.00778.
17. Bae, J., Tomizuka, M. (2011) Gait phase analysis based on a Hidden Markov Model. Mechatronics 21:961–970.
18. Baig, M., Gholamhosseini, H. (2013) Smart health monitoring systems: An overview of design and modeling. J. Med. Syst. 37:1–14.
19. Banaee, H., Ahmed, M.U., Loutfi, A. (2013) Data mining for wearable sensors in health monitoring systems: A review of recent trends and challenges. Sensors 13:17472–17500.
20. BASIS. PEAK—The Ultimate Fitness and Sleep Tracker. Available online: https://www.mybasis.com/.
21. Bellazzi, R., Zupan, B. (2008) Predictive data mining in clinical medicine: Current issues and guidelines. Int. J. Med. Inform. 77:81–97.
22. Bellazzi, R., Ferrazzi, F., Sacchi, L. (2011) Predictive data mining in clinical medicine: A focus on selected methods and applications. Wiley. Interdiscip. Rev.: Data. Min. Knowl. Discov. 1:416–430.
23. Belle, A., Thiagarajan, R., Soroushmehr, S., Navidi, F., Beard, D.A., Najarian, K. (2015) Big data analytics in healthcare. BioMed Res. Int. 2015 370194.
24. Bellos, C.C., Papadopoulos, A., Rosso, R., Fotiadis, D.I. (2010) Extraction and Analysis of Features Acquired by Wearable Sensors Network. In: the 10th IEEE International Conference on Information Technology and Applications in Biomedicine, Corfu, Greece, pp. 1–4.
25. Bellos, C., Papadopoulos, A., Rosso, R., Fotiadis, D.I. (2012) A Support Vector Machine Approach for Categorization of Patients Suffering from Chronic Diseases. In Wireless Mobile Communication and Healthcare, Nikita, K.S., Lin, J.C., Fotiadis, D.I., Arredondo Waldmeyer, M.T., Eds., Springer: Berlin, Germany, Volume 83, pp. 264–267.
26. Bengio, Y. (2009) Learning deep architectures for AI. Foundations and trends® in Machine Learning, 2:1-127.
27. Bhattacharya S, Lane ND. From smart to deep: Robust activity recognition on smartwatches using deep learning. In: IEEE International Conference on Pervasive Computing and Communication Workshops (PerCom Workshops), Sydney, Australia, pp. 1–6. (2016)
28. Bieber, G., Haescher, M., Vahl, M. (2013) Sensor requirements for activity recognition on smart watches. the 6th Int Conf. on PErvasive Technol. Relat. to Assist. Environ. 29–31.
29. Biodevices, S.A. VitalJacket®. Available online: http://www.vitaljacket.com/.
30. Blonde, L., Karter, A.J. (2005) Current evidence regarding the value of self-monitored blood glucose testing. Am. J. Med. 118:20–26.
31. Bluetooth SIG, "Health Device Profile Specification Vol. 1.0," http://www.bluetooth.org/.

32. Bsoul, M., Minn, H., Tamil, L. (2011) Apnea medassist: Real-time sleep apnea monitor using single-lead ECG. IEEE Trans. Inf. Technol. Biomed. 15:416–427.
33. Bulling, A., Blanke, U., & Schiele, B. (2014) A tutorial on human activity recognition using body-worn inertial sensors. Acm Comput. Surv. 46:1-33.
34. Center Berkeley, Caffe, 2016. [Online]. Available: http://caffe.berkeley vision.org/
35. Chan, M., Esteve, D., Fourniols, J.Y., Escriba, C., Campo, E. (2012) Smart wearable systems: Current status and future challenges. Artif. Intell. Med. 56:137–156.
36. Chaovalit, P., Gangopadhyay, A., Karabatis, G., Chen, Z. (2011) Discrete Wavelet transform-based time series analysis and mining. ACM Comput. Surv. 43:6:1–6:37.
37. Chatterjee, S., Dutta, K., Xie, H.Q., Byun, J., Pottathil, A., Moore, M. (2013) Persuasive and Pervasive Sensing: A New Frontier to Monitor, Track and Assist Older Adults Suffering from Type-2 Diabetes. In: the 46th Hawaii International Conference on System Sciences, Grand Wailea, Maui, HI, USA, pp. 2636–2645.
38. Cho, K., Raiko, T., & Ihler, A. T. (2011) Enhanced gradient and adaptive learning rate for training restricted Boltzmann machines. In: the 28th International Conference on Machine Learning (ICML-11) pp. 105–112.
39. Cho, K., Van Merriënboer, B., Gulcehre, C., Bahdanau, D., Bougares, F., Schwenk, H., & Bengio, Y. (2014) Learning phrase representations using RNN encoder-decoder for statistical machine translation. arXiv preprint arXiv:1406.1078.
40. Choi, J., Ahmed, B., Gutierrez-Osuna, R. (2012) Development and evaluation of an ambulatory stress monitor based on wearable sensors. IEEE Trans. Inf. Technol. Biomed. 16:279–286.
41. Chung, J., Gulcehre, C., Cho, K., & Bengio, Y. (2014) Empirical evaluation of gated recurrent neural networks on sequence modeling. arXiv preprint arXiv:1412.3555.
42. Chung, J., Gülçehre, C., Cho, K., & Bengio, Y. (2015) Gated Feedback Recurrent Neural Networks. In ICML. pp. 2067–2075.
43. Clifton, L., Clifton, D.A., Pimentel, M.A.F., Watkinson, P.J., Tarassenko, L. (2013) Gaussian processes for personalized e-health monitoring with wearable sensors. IEEE Trans. Biomed. Eng. 60:193–197.
44. Continua Health Alliance, "Version2010 Design Guidelines," http://www.continuaalliance. org/products/design-guidelines.html.
45. Cortes, C., Vapnik, V. (1995) Support-vector networks. Mach. Learn. 20:273–297.
46. Cunha, J.P.S., Cunha, B., Pereira, A.S., Xavier, W., Ferreira, N., Meireles, L. (2010) Vital-Jacket®: A wearable wireless vital signs monitor for patients' mobility in cardiology and sports. 4th Int. Conf. on Pervasive Comput. Technol. for Healthc. 1–2.
47. Custodio, V., Herrera, F.J., Lopez, G., Moreno, J.I. (2012) A review on architectures and communications technologies for wearable health-monitoring systems. Sensors 12:13907–13946.
48. Danie G. Krige (1951) A statistical approach to some basic mine valuation problems on the Witwatersrand, J. Chem. Metall. Min. Soc. S. Afr. 52:119–139.
49. Ding, H., Sun, H., mean Hou, K. (2011) Abnormal ECG Signal Detection Based on Compressed Sampling in Wearable ECG Sensor. In: the International Conference on Wireless Communications and Signal Processing, Nanjing, China, pp. 1–5.
50. Ding, X., Lei, H., & Rao, Y. (2016) Sparse codes fusion for context enhancement of night video surveillance. Multimed. Tools and Appli., 75:11221–11239.
51. Dong H, Supratak A, Pan W, Wu C, Matthews PM, Guo Y. (2018) Mixed neural network approach for temporal sleep stage classification. IEEE Trans. on Neural Syst. and Rehabil. Eng. 26:324–333.
52. Elliott, M.C.A. (2012) Critical care: The eight vital signs of patient monitoring. Br. J. Nurs. 21: 621–625.
53. Erfani, S. M., Rajasegarar, S., Karunasekera, S., & Leckie, C. (2016) High-dimensional and large-scale anomaly detection using a linear one-class SVM with deep learning. Pattern Recognit. 58:121–134.
54. Eskofier BM, Lee SI, Daneault JF, Golabchi FN, Ferreira-Carvalho G, Vergara-Diaz G. et al. Recent machine learning advancements in sensor-based mobility analysis: deep learning

for Parkinson's disease assessment. In: IEEE 38th Annual International Conference of the Engineering in Medicine and Biology Society (EMBC), Lake Buena Vista, Orlando, USA, pp. 655–658. (2016)

55. Fei, C.W., Bai, G.C. (2013) Wavelet correlation feature scale entropy and fuzzy support vector machine approach for aeroengine whole-body vibration fault diagnosis. Shock and Vib. 20(2):341–349.

56. Fei, C.W., Bai, G.C., Tang, W.Z., Ma, S. (2014) Quantitative diagnosis of rotor vibration fault using process power spectrum entropy and support vector machine method. Shock and Vib. 2014:957531.

57. Fei CW, Lu C, Liem R.P. (2019) Decomposed-coordinated surrogate modelling strategy for compound function approximation and a turbine blisk reliability evaluation. Aerosp. Sci. Technol. 95: UNSP105466.

58. Figo, D., Diniz, P. C., Ferreira, D. R., & Cardoso, J. M. (2010) Preprocessing techniques for context recognition from accelerometer data. Personal and Ubiquitous Computing. 14:645–662.

59. Fischer, A., & Igel, C. (2014) Training restricted Boltzmann machines: An introduction. Pattern Recognition. 47:25–39.

60. Fraile, A.J., Javier, B., Corchado, J.M., Abraham, A. (2010) Applying wearable solutions in dependent environments. IEEE Trans. Inf. Technol. Biomed. 14(6):1459–1467.

61. Frank, M. (2015) Your Head Is Better for Sensors than Your Wrist, Outside-Live Bravely: Santa Fe, NM, USA.

62. Franois Chollet, Keras, 2016. [Online]. Available: https://keras.io/.

63. Frantzidis, C.A., Bratsas, C., Klados, M.A., Konstantinidis, E., Lithari, C.D., Vivas, A.B., Papadelis, C.L., Kaldoudi, E., Pappas, C., Bamidis, P.D. (2010) On the classification of emotional biosignals evoked while viewing affective pictures: An integrated data-mining-based approach for healthcare applications. Trans. Inf. Tech. Biomed. 14:309–318.

64. G. Matheron (1963) Principles of geostatistics, Econ. Geol. 58:1246–1266.

65. G. Matheron (1973) The intrinsic random functions and their applications, Adv. Appl. Probab. 5(3):439–468.

66. Gao, Y., & Glowacka, D. (2016) Deep Gate Recurrent Neural Network. arXiv preprint arXiv:1604.02910.

67. Garmin Ltd. HRM-Tri™. Available online: https://buy.garmin.com.

68. Gialelis, J., Chondros, P., Karadimas, D., Dima, S., Serpanos, D. (2012) Identifying Chronic Disease Complications Utilizing State of the Art Data Fusion Methodologies and Signal Processing Algorithms. In Wireless Mobile Communication and Healthcare, Nikita, K.S., Lin, J.C., Fotiadis, D.I., Arredondo Waldmeyer, M.T., Eds., Springer: Berlin, Germany, Volume 83, pp. 256–263.

69. Giri, D., Rajendra Acharya, U., Martis, R.J., Vinitha Sree, S., Lim, T.C., Ahamed VI, T., Suri, J.S. (2013) Automated diagnosis of Coronary Artery Disease affected patients using LDA, PCA, ICA and Discrete Wavelet Transform. Know. Based Syst. 37:274–282.

70. Google, Tensorflow, 2016. [Online]. Available: https://www.tensorflow.org/.

71. Graves, A. (2013) Generating sequences with recurrent neural networks. arXiv preprint arXiv:1308.0850.

72. Gravina R, Alinia P, Ghasemzadeh H, Fortino G. (2017) Multi-sensor fusion in body sensor networks: State- of-the-art and research challenges. Inf. Fusion. 35:68–80.

73. Guo, Y., Liu, Y., Oerlemans, A., Lao, S., Wu, S., & Lew, M. S. (2016) Deep learning for visual understanding: A review. Neurocomputing 187:27–48.

74. Guyon, I., Gunn, S., Nikravesh, M., Zadeh, L.A. (2006) Feature Extraction: Foundations and Applications (Studies in Fuzziness and Soft Computing), Springer: Secaucus, NJ, USA.

75. H. Liu, J. Zhou, Y, Xu, Y, Zheng, X. Peng, and W. Jiang (2018) Unsupervised fault diagnosis of rolling bearings using a deep neural network based on generative adversarial networks, Neuro comput. 315:412–424.

76. Hakonen, M., Piitulainen, H., Visala, A. (2015) Current state of digital signal processing in myoelectric interfaces and related applications. Biomed. Signal Process. Control 18:334–359.

77. HealthWatch Technologies Ltd. Available online: http://www.personal-healthwatch.com/.

78. Hexoskin. Available online: http://www.hexoskin.com/.

79. Hinton, G. E., & Salakhutdinov, R. R. (2006) Reducing the dimensionality of data with neural networks. Science. 313:504-507.

80. Hinton, G. E., Osindero, S., & Teh, Y.-W. (2006) A fast learning algorithm for deep belief nets. Neural comput. 18:1527–1554.

81. Hinton, G. E., Srivastava, N., Krizhevsky, A., Sutskever, I., & Salakhutdinov, R. R. (2012) Improving neural networks by preventing co-adaptation of feature detectors. arXiv preprint arXiv:1207.0580.

82. Hjalmarson, A. (2007) Heart rate: An independent risk factor in cardiovascular disease. Eur. Heart J. Suppl. 9:F3–F7.

83. Hochreiter, S., & Schmidhuber, J. (1997) Long short-term memory. Neural Comput. 9:1735–1780.

84. Hongxia Li, Tao Liu, Minjie Wang, Danyang Zhao, Aike Qiao, Xue Wang, Junfeng Gu, Zheng Li, Bao Zhu (2017) Design optimization of stent and its dilatation balloon using kriging surrogate model, Biomed. Eng. Online 16(13):1–17.

85. http://www8.cao.go.jp/kourei/whitepaper/index-w.html

86. Hu, F., Jiang, M., Celentano, L., Xiao, Y. (2008) Robust medical ad hoc sensor networks (MASN) with wavelet-based ECG data mining. Ad Hoc Netw. 6:986–1012.

87. Huang, G., Zhang, Y., Cao, J., Steyn, M., Taraporewalla, K. (2013) Online mining abnormal period patterns from multiple medical sensor data streams. World Wide Web 2013, doi:https://doi.org/10.1007/s11280-013-0203-y.

88. Hubel, D. H., & Wiesel, T. N. (1962) Receptive fields, binocular interaction and functional architecture in the cat's visual cortex. The J. of physiol. 160:106–154.

89. I. J. Goodfellow, J. Pouget-Abadie, M. Mirza, B. Xu, D. Warde-Farley, S. Ozair, A. C. Courville, Y. Bengio, Generative adversarial nets, in Advances in Neural Information Processing Systems 27: Annual Conference on Neural Information Processing Systems 2014, December 8-13 2014, Montreal, Quebec, Canada, pp. 2672–2680.

90. Incel, O. (2015) Analysis of Movement, Orientation and Rotation-Based Sensing for Phone Placement Recognition. Sensors, 15:25474.

91. J. Sacks, W.J. Welch, T.J. Mitchell, H.P. Wynn (1989) Design and analysis of computer experiments, Stat. Sci. 4:409–423.

92. J. Tian, C. Morillo, M. H. Azarian and M. Pecht (2016) Motor bearing fault detection using spectral Kurtosis-based feature extraction coupled with K-nearest neighbor distance analysis. IEEE Trans. Ind. Electron. 63(3):1793–1803.

93. Jindal V, Birjandtalab J, Pouyan MB, Nourani M, An adaptive deep learning approach for PPG-based identification. In: 38th Annual International Conference of the Engineering in Medicine and Biology Society (EMBC), Lake Buena Vista, Orlando, USA, pp. 6401–6404. (2016)

94. Jing, L., Wang, T., Zhao, M., & Wang, P. (2017) An Adaptive Multi-Sensor Data Fusion Method Based on Deep Convolutional Neural Networks for Fault Diagnosis of Planetary Gearbox. Sensors. 17:414.

95. K. Fukushima. (1980) Neocognitron: A self-organizing neural network model for a mechanism of pattern recognition unaffected by shift in position. Biolog. Cybernetics. 36:193–202.

96. Kaewwichian, P., Tanwanichkul, L., Pitaksringkarn, J. (2019) Car ownership demand modeling using machine learning: decision trees and neural networks. Int. J. of Geomate. 17(62):219–230.

97. Kalagnanam, J., Henrion, M. (2013) A comparison of decision analysis and expert rules for sequential diagnosis. arXiv:1304.2362.

98. Karabadji, N.E., Khelf, I., Seridi, H., Aridhi, S., Remond, D., Dhifli, W. (2019) A data sampling and attribute selection strategy for improving decision tree construction. Expert Syst. with Appli. 129:84–96

99. Karlen, W., Mattiussi, C., Floreano, D. (2009) Sleep and wake classification with ECG and respiratory effort signals. IEEE Trans. Biomed. Circuits Syst. 3:71–78.

100. Kautz, T., Groh, B. H., Hannink, J., Jensen, U., Strubberg, H., & Eskofier, B. M. (2017) Activity recognition in beach volleyball using a Deep Convolutional Neural Network. Data Min. and Knowl. Discov. 1–28.
101. Khan, Z.A., Sivakumar, S., Phillips, W., Robertson, B. (2014) ZEQoS: A New Energy and QoS-Aware Routing Protocol for Communication of Sensor Devices in Healthcare System. Int. J. Distrib. Sens. Netw. 1–18.
102. Khan, S., Yairi, T. (2018) A review on the application of deep learning in system health management, Mech. Syst. and Signal Process. 107:241–265.
103. Kharel, J., Reda, H.T., Shin, S.Y. (2018) Fog Computing-Based Smart Health Monitoring System Deploying LoRa Wireless Communication. IETE Tech. Rev. 1–14.
104. Kim, Y., & Ling, H. (2009) Human activity classification based on micro-Doppler signatures using a support vector machine. IEEE Trans. on Geosci. and Remote Sens. 47:1328–1337.
105. Krizhevsky, A., Sutskever, I., & Hinton, G. E. (2012) Imagenet classification with deep convolutional neural networks. In Adv. in Neural Inf. Process. Syst. pp. 1097–1105.
106. L. A. Pastur-Romay, F. Cedrón, A. Pazos, and A. B. Porto-Pazos. (2016) Deep artificial neural networks and neuromorphic chips for big data analysis: Pharmaceutical and bioinformatics applications, Int. J. Molecular Sci., vol. 17, no. 8, Art. no. 1313.
107. L. Zhao, K.K. Choi, I. Lee (2011) Metamodeling method using dynamic Kriging for design optimization, AIAA J. 49(9):2034–2046.
108. Längkvist M, Karlsson L, Loutfi A. (2012) Sleep stage classification using unsupervised feature learning. Adv. in Artif. Neural Syst. 2012:1-9.
109. LeCun, Y., Bengio, Y., & Hinton, G. (2015) Deep learning. Nature. 521:436–444.
110. Lee, H., Grosse, R., Ranganath, R., & Ng, A. Y. (2009) Convolutional deep belief networks for scalable unsupervised learning of hierarchical representations. In: the 26th annual international conference on machine learning, pp. 609-616. ACM.
111. Lee, K.H., Kung, S.Y., Verma, N. (2012) Low-energy formulations of support vector machine kernel functions for biomedical sensor applications. J. Signal Process. Syst. 69:339–349.
112. Lee, Y.D., Chung, W.Y. (2009) Wireless sensor network based wearable smart shirt for ubiquitous health and activity monitoring. Sensor. Actuator. B 140:390–395
113. Li, G., Deng, L., Xu, Y., Wen, C., Wang, W., Pei, J., & Shi, L. (2016) Temperature based Restricted Boltzmann Machines. Sci. Rep. 6.
114. Li, H., Wu, J., Gao, Y.W., Shi, Y. (2016) Examining individuals' adoption of healthcare wearable devices: an empirical study from privacy calculus perspective. Int. J. Med. Inf. 88:8–17.
115. Li, Q., Clifford, G.D. (2012) Dynamic time warping and machine learning for signal quality assessment of pulsatile signals. Physiol. Meas. 33:1491–1501.
116. Li, X., Porikli, F. (2010) Human State Classification and Predication for Critical Care Monitoring by Real-Time Bio-signal Analysis. In: the 20th International Conference on Pattern Recognition, Istanbul, Turkey, pp. 2460–2463.
117. Liddy, C., Dusseault, J.J., Dahrouge, S., et al. (2008) Telehomecare for patients with multiple chronic illnesses: pilot study. Can. Fam. Physician 54:58–65.
118. Lin, L., Wang, K. Z., Zuo, W. M., Wang, M., Luo, J. B., & Zhang, L. (2016) A Deep Structured Model with Radius-Margin Bound for 3D Human Activity Recognition. Int. J. of Comput. Vis. 118:256–273.
119. Liou, C.-Y., Cheng, W.-C., Liou, J.-W., & Liou, D.-R. (2014) Autoencoder for words. Neurocomputing. 139:84–96.
120. Liu, G., Liang, J., Lan, G., Hao, Q., & Chen, M. (2016) Convolution neutral network enhanced binary sensor network for human activity recognition. In SENSORS, 2016 IEEE (pp. 1–3): IEEE.
121. López-Vallverdú, J.A., Riaño, D., Bohada, J.A. (2012) Improving medical decision trees by combining relevant health-care criteria. Expert Syst. Appl. 39:11782–11791.
122. Lu N, Li T, Ren X, Miao H. (2017) A deep learning scheme for motor imagery classification based on restricted boltzmann machines. IEEE Trans. on Neural Syst. and Rehabil. Eng. 25: 566–576.

123. Lukowicz, P., Anliker, U., Ward, J., Troster, G., Hirt, E., Neufelt, C. (2002) AMON: A wearable medical computer for high risk patients. The 6th Int. Symp. on Wearable Comput. 133–134.
124. Lymberis, A.G.L. (2006) Wearable health systems: From smart technologies to real applications. In: the Annual International Conference of the IEEE Engineering in Medicine and Biology Society, New York, NY, USA, pp. 6789–6792.
125. M. Li, G. Li, S. Azarm (2008) A Kriging metamodel assisted multi-objective genetic algorithm for design optimization, J. Mech. Des. 130(3):031401.
126. Ma T, Li H, Yang H, Lv X, Li P, Liu T, et al. (2017) The extraction of motion-onset VEP BCI features based on deep learning and compressed sensing. J. of Neurosci. Methods. 275: 80–92.
127. Ma, J., Sheridan, R. P., Liaw, A., Dahl, G. E., & Svetnik, V. (2015) Deep neural nets as a method for quantitative structure–activity relationships. Journal of Chemical Information and Modeling, 55:263–274.
128. Majumder, S., Mondal, T., Deen, M.J. (2017) Wearable sensors for remote health monitoring. Sensors 17:130.
129. Mao, Y., Chen, W., Chen, Y., Lu, C., Kollef, M., Bailey, T. (2012) An Integrated Data Mining Approach to Real-Time Clinical Monitoring and Deterioration Warning. In: the 18th ACM SIGKDD International Conference on Knowledge Discovery and Data Mining, Beijing, China, pp. 1140–1148.
130. Marc'Aurelio Ranzato, C. P., Chopra, S., & LeCun, Y. (2007) Efficient learning of sparse representations with an energy-based model. In: NIPS.
131. Marco Di Rienzo, G.P., Brambilla, G., Ferratini, M., Castiglioni, P. (2005) MagIC System: A New Textile-Based Wearable Device for Biological Signal Monitoring. Applicability in Daily Life and Clinical Setting. In: the 2005 IEEE, Engineering in Medicine and Biology 27th Annual Conference 2005, Shangai, China, pp. 7167–7169.
132. Masci, J., Meier, U., Cire

an, D., & Schmidhuber, J. (2011) Stacked convolutional auto-encoders for hierarchical feature extraction. In: International Conference on Artificial Neural Networks, pp. 52–59. Springer.
133. Microsoft, Cntk, 2016. [Online]. Available: https://github.com/Microsoft/CNTK.
134. Montavon, G., & Müller, K.-R. (2012) Deep Boltzmann machines and the centering trick. In Neural Networks: Tricks of the Trade pp. 621–637: Springer.
135. Mukherjee, A., Pal, A., Misra, P. (2012) Data Analytics in Ubiquitous Sensor-Based Health Information Systems. In: the 2012 6th International Conference on Next Generation Mobile Applications, Services and Technologies, Paris, France, pp. 193–198.
136. Murnane, E.L., Cosley, D., Chang, P., Guha, S., Frank, E., Gay, G., Matthews, M. (2016) Self-monitoring practices, attitudes, and needs of individuals with bipolar disorder: implications for the design of technologies to manage mental health. J. Am. Med. Inf. Assoc. 23(3):477–484.
137. Nair, V., & Hinton, G. E. (2010) Rectified linear units improve restricted boltzmann machines. In: the 27th international conference on machine learning (ICML-10) pp. 807–814.
138. Nangalia, V., Prytherch, D., Smith, G. (2010) Health technology assessment review: Remote monitoring of vital signs—current status and future challenges. Crit. Care 14:1–8.
139. Naraharisetti, K.V.P., Bawa, M, Tahernezhadi, M. (2011) Comparison of Different Signal Processing Methods for Reducing Artifacts from Photoplethysmograph Signal. In: the IEEE International Conference on Electro/Information Technology, Mankato, MN, USA, pp. 1–8.
140. Nervana Systems, Neon, 2016. [Online]. Available: https://github.com/NervanaSystems/neon.
141. Niemela, M., Fuentetaja, R.G., Kaasinen, E., Gallardo, J.L. (2007) Supporting independent living of the elderly with mobile-centric ambient intelligence: user evaluation of three scenarios. Lect. Notes Comput. Sci. 4794:91–107.
142. NVIDIA Corp., Nvidia dgx-1, 2016. [Online]. Available: http://www.nvidia.com/object/deep-learning-system.html.

143. Nweke, H.F., Teh, Y.W., Ai-garadi, M.A., & Aio, U.R. (2018) Deep learning algorithms for human activity recognition using mobile and wearable sensor networks: State of the art and research challenges. Expert Syst. with Appli. 105:233–261.
144. Olshausen, B. A., & Field, D. J. (1997) Sparse coding with an overcomplete basis set: A strategy employed by V1? Vis. Res. 37:3311–3325.
145. OM Signal Inc. OM Smart Shirt. Available online: http://omsignal.com.
146. Ordóñez, F. J., & Roggen, D. (2016) Deep Convolutional and LSTM Recurrent Neural Networks for Multimodal Wearable Activity Recognition. Sensors. 16:115.
147. Ordonez, P., Armstrong, T., Oates, T., Fackler, J. (2011) Classification of Patients Using Novel Multivariate Time Series Representations of Physiological Data. In: the 10th International Conference on Machine Learning and Applications, Honolulu, HI, USA, pp. 172–179.
148. Oyedotun, O. K., & Khashman, A. (2016) Deep learning in vision-based static hand gesture recognition. Neural Comput. and Appli. 1–11.
149. Page A, Kulkarni, A, Mohsenin T. (2015) Utilizing deep neural nets for an embedded ECG-based biometric authentication system. In: Biomedical Circuits and Systems Conference (BioCAS), Atlanta, GA, USA, pp. 1–4.
150. Paliwal, M., Kumar, U.A. (2009) Neural networks and statistical techniques: A review of applications. Expert. Syst. Appl. 36:2–17.
151. Pantelopoulos, A., Bourbakis, N.G. (2010) A Survey on Wearable Sensor-Based Systems for Health Monitoring and Prognosis. IEEE Trans. Syst. Man Cybern. Part C Appl. Rev. 40:1–12.
152. Podgorelec, V., Kokol, P., Stiglic, B., Rozman, I. (2002) Decision trees: An overview and their use in medicine. J. Med. Syst. 26:445–463.
153. Postema, T., Peeters, J.M., Friele, R.D. (2012) Key factors influencing the implementation success of a home telecare application. Int. J. Med. Inf. 8(5):415–423.
154. Poultney, C., et al., (2006) Efficient learning of sparse representations with an energy-based model, in Proc. Adv. Neural Inf. Process. Syst., pp. 1137–1144.
155. R. Collobert, K. Kavukcuoglu, and C. Farabet, Torch, 2016. [Online]. Available: http://torch.ch/.
156. Rabiner, L., Juang, B.H. (1986) An introduction to hidden Markov models. IEEE ASSP Mag. 3:4–16.
157. Rahhal, M. M. A., Bazi, Y., AlHichri, H., Alajlan, N., Melgani, F., & Yager, R. R. (2016) Deep learning approach for active classification of electrocardiogram signals. Inf. Sci. 345:340–354.
158. Rault, T., Bouabdallah, A., Challal, Y., Marin, F. (2017) A survey of energy-efficient context recognition systems using wearable sensors for healthcare applications. Pervasive Mob. Comput. 37:23–44.
159. Ravi D, Wong C, Lo B, Yang GZ. cs. In: 13th International Conference on Wearable and Implantable Body Sensor Networks (BSN), San Francisco, CA, USA, pp. 71–76. (2016)
160. Ravì, D., Wong, C., Deligianni, F., Berthelot, M., Andreu-Perez, J., Lo, B., & Yang, G. Z. (2017) Deep Learning for Health Informatics. IEEE J. of Biomed. and Health Inf. 21:4–21.
161. Rhea P. Liem, Charles A. Mader, Joaquim R.R.A. Martins (2015) Surrogate models and mixtures of experts in aerodynamic performance prediction for mission analysis, Aerosp. Sci. Technol. 43:126–151.
162. Rifai, S., Vincent, P., Muller, X., Glorot, X., & Bengio, Y. (2011) Contractive auto-encoders: Explicit invariance during feature extraction. In: the 28th international conference on machine learning (ICML-11), pp. 833–840.
163. Ripoll VJR, Wojdel A, Romero E, Ramos P, Brugada J. (2016) ECG assessment based on neural networks with pretraining. Appli. Soft Comput. 49: 399–406.
164. Rita Paradiso, G.L., Taccini, N. (2005) A Wearable Health Care System Based on Knitted Integrated Sensors. IEEE Trans. Inf. Technol. Biomed. 337–344.
165. Rodriguez, M., Orrite, C., Medrano, C., & Makris, D. (2016) One-Shot Learning of Human Activity With an MAP Adapted GMM and Simplex-HMM. IEEE Trans. Cybern. 1–12.

166. Ronao, C. A., & Cho, S.-B. (2015) Evaluation of deep convolutional neural network architectures for human activity recognition with smartphone sensors. In Proc. of the KIISE Korea Computer Congress 858–860.
167. Ronao, C. A., & Cho, S.-B. (2016) Human activity recognition with smartphone sensors using deep learning neural networks. Expert Syst. with Appli. 59:235–244.
168. Rosenbloom, S.T. (2016) Person-generated health and wellness data for health care. J. Am. Med. Inf. Assoc. 23(3):438–439.
169. Ruiz-Rodríguez JC, Ruiz-Sanmartín A, Ribas V, Caballero J, García-Roche A, Riera J et al. (2013) Innovative continuous non-invasive cuffless blood pressure monitoring based on photoplethysmography technology. Intensive Care Med. 39(9): 1618–1625.
170. S. Lu and X. Wang (2004) PCA-based feature selection scheme for machine defect classification. IEEE Trans. Instrum. Mea., 53(6):1517–1525.
171. Saeedi R, Norgaard S, Gebremedhin AH. A closed-loop deep learning architecture for robust activity recognition using wearable sensors. In: IEEE International Conference on Big Data. Boston, MA, USA, pp. 473–479. (2017)
172. Safi, K., Mohammed, S., Attal, F., Khalil, M., & Amirat, Y. (2016) Recognition of different daily living activities using hidden Markov model regression. In Biomedical Engineering (MECBME) 16–19.
173. Salakhutdinov, R., & Larochelle, H. (2010) Efficient Learning of Deep Boltzmann Machines. In AISTATs 693–700.
174. Salakhutdinov, R., & Hinton, G. (2012) An efficient learning procedure for deep Boltzmann machines. Neural comput. 24:1967–2006.
175. Sarkar S, Reddy K, Dorgan A, Fidopiastis C, Giering M. (2016) Wearable EEG-based activity recognition in PHM-related service environment via deep learning. Int. J. Progn. Health Manag. 7:1–10.
176. Sathyanarayana, A., Joty, S., Fernandez-Luque, L., Ofli, F., Srivastava, J., Elmagarmid, A., Taheri, S., & Arora, T. (2016) Impact of Physical Activity on Sleep: A Deep Learning Based Exploration. arXiv preprint arXiv:1607.07034.
177. Schmidhuber, J. (2015) Deep learning in neural networks: An overview. Neural Netw. 61:85–117.
178. Scully, C., Lee, J., Meyer, J., Gorbach, A.M., Granquist-Fraser, D., Mendelson, Y., Chon, K.H. (2012) Physiological parameter monitoring from optical recordings with a mobile phone. IEEE Trans. Biomed. Eng. 59:303–306.
179. Seoane, F., Mohino-Herranz, I., Ferreira, J., Alvarez, L., Buendia, R., Ayllon, D., Llerena, C., Gil-Pita, R. (2014) Wearable biomedical measurement systems for assessment of mental stress of combatants in real time. Sensors. 14:7120–7141.
180. Shao, H., Jiang, H., Zhao, H. and Wang, F. (2017) A novel deep autoencoder feature learning method for rotating machinery fault diagnosis, Mech. Syst. Signal Process. 95:187–204.
181. Shashikumar SP, Shah AJ, Li Q, Clifford GD, Nemati S, A deep learning approach to monitoring and detecting atrial fibrillation using wearable technology. In: IEEE EMBS International Conference of Biomedical & Health Informatics (BHI), 4–7 March, Las Vegas, Nevada, USA, pp. 141–144.
182. Shoaib, M., Bosch, S., Incel, O. D., Scholten, H., & Havinga, P. J. (2016) Complex human activity recognition using smartphone and wrist-worn motion sensors. Sensors 16:426.
183. Simpao AF, Ahumada LM, Gálvez JA, Rehman MA. (2014) A review of analytics and clinical informatics in healthcare. J. Med. Syst. 38(4):1–7.
184. Skymind, Deeplearning4j, 2016. [Online]. Available: http://deeplearning4j.org/.
185. Solmitech. Pacth-type SHC-U7. Available online: http://www.solmitech.com/.
186. Song, Q., Zheng, Y. J., Xue, Y., Sheng, W. G., & Zhao, M. R. (2017) An evolutionary deep neural network for predicting morbidity of gastrointestinal infections by food contamination. Neurocomputing 226:16–22.
187. Sow, D., Turaga, D., Schmidt, M. (2013) Mining of Sensor Data in Healthcare: A Survey. In Managing and Mining Sensor Data, Aggarwal, C.C., Ed., Springer: Berlin, Germany, 459–504.

188. Stacey, M., McGregor, C. (2007) Temporal abstraction in intelligent clinical data analysis: A survey. Artif. Intell. Med. 39:1–24.
189. Stowe, S., Harding, S. (2010) Telecare, telehealth and telemedicine. Eur. Geriatr. Med. 1:193–197.
190. Sun, F.T., Kuo, C., Cheng, H.T., Buthpitiya, S., Collins, P., Griss, M. (2012) Activity-Aware Mental Stress Detection Using Physiological Sensors. In Mobile Computing, Applications, and Services, Gris, M., Yang, G., Eds., Springer: Berlin, Germany, Volume 76, pp. 211–230.
191. Sutskever, I., Vinyals, O., & Le, Q. V. (2014) Sequence to sequence learning with neural networks. In Adv. Neural Inf. Process. Syst. pp. 3104–3112
192. Szegedy, C., Liu, W., Jia, Y., Sermanet, P., Reed, S., Anguelov, D., Erhan, D., Vanhoucke, V., & Rabinovich, A. (2015) Going deeper with convolutions. In: the IEEE Conference on Computer Vision and Pattern Recognition, pp. 1–9
193. T.W. Simpson, T.M. Mauery, J.J. Korte, F. Mistree (2001) Kriging metamodels for global approximation in simulation-based multidisciplinary design optimization, AIAA J. 39(12):2233–2241.
194. Tabar YR, Halici U. (2016) A novel deep learning approach for classification of EEG motor imagery signals. J. Neural Eng. 14:016003.
195. Taylor, G. W., Hinton, G. E., & Roweis, S. T. (2007) Modeling human motion using binary latent variables. Adv. Neural Inf. Process. Syst. 19:1345.
196. Tennina, S., Di Renzo, M., Kartsakli, E., Graziosi, F., Lalos, A.S., Antonopoulos, A., Mekikis, P.V., Alonso, L. (2014) WSN4QoL: A WSN-Oriented Healthcare System Architecture. Int. J. Distrib. Sens. Netw. 503417.
197. Thakker, B., Vyas, A.L. (2011) Support vector machine for abnormal pulse classification. Int. J. Comput. Appl. 22:13–19.
198. Thomas, O., Sunehag, P., Dror, G., Yun, S., Kim, S., Robards, M., Smola, A., Green, D., Saunders, P. (2010) Wearable sensor activity analysis using semi-Markov models with a grammar. Pervasive Mob. Comput. 6:342–350.
199. Universite de Montreal, Theano, 2016. [Online]. Available: http://deeplearning.net/software/theano/.
200. Valipour, S., Siam, M., Jagersand, M., & Ray, N. (2016) Recurrent Fully Convolutional Networks for Video Segmentation. arXiv preprint arXiv:1606.00487.
201. Vincent, P., Larochelle, H., Bengio, Y., & Manzagol, P.-A. (2008) Extracting and composing robust features with denoising autoencoders. In: the 25th international conference on Machine learning, pp. 1096–1103.
202. Vincent, P., Larochelle, H., Lajoie, I., Bengio, Y., & Manzagol, P.-A. (2010) Stacked denoising autoencoders: Learning useful representations in a deep network with a local denoising criterion. J. of Mach. Learn. Res. 11:3371–3408.
203. Vital Connect. HealthPatch® MD. Available online: http://www.vitalconnect.com/.
204. Vivonoetics. ActiWave Cardio. Available online: http://vivonoetics.com/.
205. Vivonoetics. Smartex WWS. Available online: http://vivonoetics.com/.
206. VPMS Asia Pacific. V-Patch. Available online: http://www.vpatchmedical.com/.
207. Vu, T.H.N., Park, N., Lee, Y.K., Lee, Y., Lee, J.Y., Ryu, K.H. (2010) Online discovery of Heart Rate Variability patterns in mobile healthcare services. J. Syst. Softw. 83:1930–1940.
208. Wang, L. (2016) Recognition of human activities using continuous autoencoders with wearable sensors. Sensors. 16:189.
209. Wang, W., Wang, H., Hempel, M., Peng, D., Sharif, H., Chen, H.H. (2011) Secure stochastic ECG signals based on gaussian mixture model for e-healthcare systems. IEEE Syst. J. 5:564–573.
210. Widodo, A., Yang, B.S. (2007) Application of nonlinear feature extraction and support vector machines for fault diagnosis of induction motors. Expert Syst. Appl. 33:241–250.
211. Withings—Inspire Health. Pulse Ox—Track. Improve. Available online: http://www.withings.com/eu/withings-pulse.html.

212. Wolfram Research, Wolfram math, 2016. [Online]. Available: https://www.wolfram.com/mathematica/.
213. Wulsin D, Gupta J, Mani R, Blanco J, Litt B. (2011) Modeling electroencephalography waveforms with semi-super- vised deep belief nets: fast classification and anomaly measurement. J. Neural Eng. 8(3):1–28.
214. X. Xue and J. Zhou (2017) A hybrid fault diagnosis approach based on mixed-domain state features for rotating machinery. ISA Trans. 66:284–295.
215. Xu, P.J., Zhang, H., Tao, X.M. (2008) Textile-structured electrodes for electrocardiogram. Text. Prog. 40:183–213.
216. Yalçın, H. (2016) Human activity recognition using deep belief networks. In 2016 24th Signal Processing and Communication Application Conference (SIU) pp. 1649–1652.
217. Yan Y, Qin X, Wu Y, Zhang N, Fan J, Wang L. (2015) A restricted Boltzmann machine based two-lead electrocardiography classification. In: 12th International Conference on Wearable and Implantable Body Sensor Networks (BSN), Cambridge, Massachusetts, pp. 1–9.
218. Yang, J. B., Nguyen, M. N., San, P. P., Li, X. L., & Krishnaswamy, S. (2015) Deep convolutional neural networks on multichannel time series for human activity recognition. In: the 24th International Joint Conference on Artificial Intelligence (IJCAI), Buenos Aires, Argentina, pp. 25–31.
219. Yeh, J.Y., Wu, T.H., Tsao, C.W. (2011) Using data mining techniques to predict hospitalization of hemodialysis patients. Decis. Support Syst. 50:439–448.
220. Yilmaz, T., Foster, R., Hao, Y. (2010) Detecting vital signs with wearable wireless sensors. Sensors 10837–10862.
221. Yin, W., Yang, X., Zhang, L., & Oki, E. (2016) ECG Monitoring System Integrated With IR-UWB Radar Based on CNN. IEEE Access, 4:6344–6351.
222. Yoo, I., Alafaireet, P., Marinov, M., Pena-Hernandez, K., Gopidi, R., Chang, J.F., Hua, L. (2012) Data mining in healthcare and biomedicine: A survey of the literature. J. Med. Syst. 36:2431–2448.
223. Yoon, J. (2013) Three-Tiered Data Mining for Big Data Patterns of Wireless Sensor Networks in Medical and Healthcare Domains. In: the 8th International Conference on Internet and Web Applications and Services, Rome, Italy, pp. 18–24.
224. Younes, L. (1999) On the convergence of Markovian stochastic algorithms with rapidly decreasing ergodicity rates. Stochastics: An Int. J. Probab. Stoch. Process. 65:177–228.
225. Zeiler, M. D., and Fergus, R. (2014) Visualizing and understanding convolutional networks, in Proc. Eur. Conf. Comput. Vision, pp. 818–833.
226. Zephyr Performance Systems. BioHarness™ 3. Available online: http://www.zephyranywhere.com/products/bioharness-3.
227. Zephyr Technology Corp. Available online: http://zephyranywhere.com/.
228. Zhang J, Wu Y, Bai J, Chen F. (2016) Automatic sleep stage classification based on sparse deep belief net and combination of multiple classifiers. Trans. of the Institute of Meas. and Control. 38: 435–451.
229. Zhang, M., & Sawchuk, A. A. (2013) Human daily activity recognition with sparse representation using wearable sensors. IEEE J. Biomed. Health Inf. 17: 553-560.
230. Zhang, S., Zhang, S., Wang, B., Habetler, T.C., Machine Learning and Deep Learning Algorithms for Bearing Fault Diagnostics – A Comprehensive Review, https://arxiv.org/pdf/1901.08247.pdf.
231. Zheng, Y.-J., Ling, H.-F., & Xue, J.-Y. (2014) Ecogeography-based optimization: enhancing biogeography-based optimization with ecogeographic barriers and differentiations. Comput. & Oper. Res. 50:115-127.
232. Zhou, X., Guo, J., & Wang, S. (2015) Motion recognition by using a stacked autoencoder-based deep learning algorithm with smart phones. In Int. Conf. on Wirel. Algorithm., Syst., and Appli., pp. 778–787: Springer.
233. Zhu, Y. (2011) Automatic detection of anomalies in blood glucose using a machine learning approach. J. Commun. Netw. 13:125–131.

Characterization of Signals of Noncontact Respiration Sensor for Emotion Detection Using Intelligent Techniques

P. Grace Kanmani Prince, R. Rajkumar Immanuel, B. Revathy, B. Jeyanthi, J. Premalatha, and A. Sivasangari

Abstract Emotion detection has been carried out through various techniques such as EEG, image and video recording of facial expressions, body gestures, text-based emotion identification, and so on. In this work, a noncontact temperature sensor is used to detect the pattern of breathing for various emotions. The emotions that are considered for this work are happy, surprise, sad, and angry. The wavelet transform of the signal has been acquired, and the wavelet features are taken for classification. Twelve features are taken from the wavelet transformed signal. Feature reduction is done using principal component analysis. Four principal component analysis features are obtained. These PCA features are given to the classifiers which uses intelligent techniques. Both supervised and unsupervised learning methods have been employed to characterize the signals. KNN classifier has given the maximum accuracy of 91% for approximation and ensemble learning 91% for features from detail.

Keywords Respiration · Emotion detection · Noncontact respiration detector · Wavelet transform · Classifiers

1 Introduction

The emotion sensors are used for various purposes and have found a variety of applications such as detection of emotions in coma patients, behavioral studies, etc. It has found its application to develop humanoid robot which can depict the emotions of human being. Emotions are studied for the purpose of producing successful advertisements. It is also used in the field of education to assess the processing of learning and to find how efficiently the knowledge has been transferred. Emotions

P. G. K. Prince (✉) · R. R. Immanuel · B. Revathy · B. Jeyanthi
J. Premalatha · A. Sivasangari
Sathyabama Institute of Science and Technology, Chennai, India

© The Author(s), under exclusive license to Springer
Nature Switzerland AG 2021
A. K. Manocha et al. (eds.), *Computational Intelligence in Healthcare*, Health
Information Science, https://doi.org/10.1007/978-3-030-68723-6_7

161

are studied using various means such as electroencephalogram (EEG), electrocardiogram (ECG), Galvanic skin resistance (GSR), photoplethysmography (PPG), respiration rate analysis (RR), skin temperature measurement (STM), electrooculogram (EOG), etc. [1]. Numerous methods are used for detection of emotions. The emotion sensor is either contact type which is not comfortable to the person wearing it or it is quite costly. But the technique used for emotion detection in this work is done by using a simple noncontact temperature sensor. The sensor is placed near the nostrils to sense the pattern of breathing. It is hoped to be an inexpensive but an effective tool for determining the emotions of persons who are not able to express themselves. For example, a coma patient or a critically ill patient may not be able to outwardly express pain or anguish. In such a case, based on the breathing patterns the emotions can be predicted to certain extent. It can be noted that during strong emotions like anger and excitement, the respiration rate is much higher. Its signal slope is higher. Whereas for emotions like sadness and calmness, the signal varies slowly with lesser slope and hence lesser respiration rate. This same setup can also be effectively used for detection of various respiratory abnormalities like asthma, bronchitis pneumonia, or any other breathing problems.

2 Physiological Aspects of Emotion and Respiration

The brain is responsible for emotion and also plays a vital role in respiration. In this section, a run-through of how respiration and emotion are related with each other is presented. Also how the brain is responsible in connecting these two parameters is discussed below.

2.1 Brain and Emotion

Of all the four lobes of the brain, temporal lobe is more related to the development of emotions. Patterns of behavior, memory, smell, and motivation are generated in this region of the brain. Another important structure in the anatomy of the brain which consists of the end of the frontal lobe and the temporal lobe is the limbic system. It is termed as the emotional nervous system. It takes care of patterns of behavior, long-term memory, sense of smell, etc. Limbic system has a part called as amygdala which initiates changes in the body parameters when it comes across various types of emotions [2]. It is joined with the autonomous nervous system [3]. Hence respiration rate is one of the parameters which gets altered during different emotions.

2.2 Brain and Respiration

The brain centers responsible for vital body parameters such as heart rate, respiration rate, etc. are medulla oblongata and pons. These regions act as a bridge between the brain and the spinal cord. The medulla oblongata has two respiratory groups called dorsal respiratory group and ventral respiratory group, and pons has one respiratory group called as the pontine respiratory group. This dorsal respiratory group is responsible for the rhythmicity of respiration, and the pontine respiratory group is responsible for altering the respiration with respect to the stimulus that is received from the external environment and voluntary alteration in the inhalation and exhalation of air [4, 5].

2.3 Relation Between Respiration and Emotion

The pontine region of the brain changes the respiration rate depending on the stimulus that has been got from the external environment. For example, if a person hears a loud sound and is shocked by hearing such a sound which was unexpected will definitely experience a change in the respiration rate since gasping would be present. The person would be taking short breaths in a faster rate and would be perturbed. But if the person is relaxed, then the breathing will be slower and rhythmic. Hence respiration can be used as one of the important markers for determining and analyzing emotions.

3 Noncontact Respiration Rate Detector and Data Acquisition

A number of methods are used for detection of respiration. Resistance temperature detector, Thermistor [6], microphone to detect the sound produced by inhalation and exhalation [7], airflow-measuring sensor [8], pressure sensor, video camera [9], ECG electrodes, and many other types are used for measuring the respiration rate.

In this work infrared sensor is used to measure the temperature of the air that comes out of the nostrils. The air that is coming from within the body has temperature higher than the ambient temperature. Hence as the exhalation starts, the temperature around the nostrils gets increased gradually, and while inhaling the temperature decreases gradually. Hence the rate of variation of temperature per minute is calculated, which gives the breath rate. The breathing pattern also can be vividly seen from the output of the sensor. The sensor that is used is **MLX90614 DAA** which is a medical-grade sensor. Figure 1 shows the simple setup required of

Fig. 1 MLX90614 DAA
with data
acquisition system

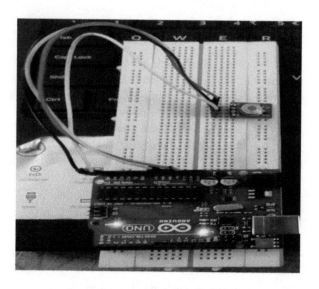

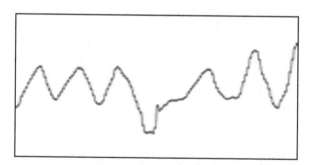

Fig. 2 Signal acquired from MLX90614 DAA from an angry person

the noncontact infrared temperature sensor with data acquisition system. This sensor is kept near the nostrils, or it can be fitted as in an oxygen face mask. The data is acquired through ATMega328P. Figure 2 shows the signal acquired from a subject who simulated the feeling of anger. Figure 3 shows the signal acquired from the sensor when the subject simulates a feeling of happiness. Samples for study were taken from 50 subjects who were asked to simulate four emotions: anger, surprise, happy, and sad. The data was used for further analysis through wavelet transform. From the data that is collected, it is observed that the signals follow different patterns for different emotions. For example, for a person who simulated anger, the waveform obtained had higher frequency and amplitude. If the person is happy, the waveform that is obtained is slowly varying. Hence the signal has lower frequency.

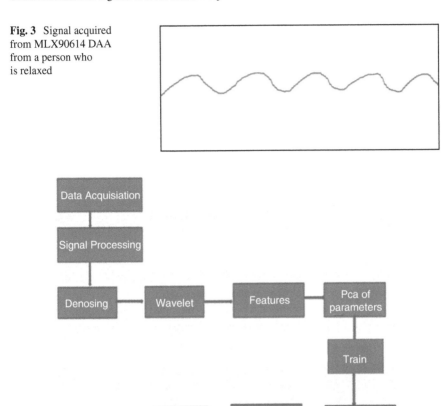

Fig. 3 Signal acquired from MLX90614 DAA from a person who is relaxed

Fig. 4 Block diagram of classification of respiration measurement for detection of emotion

4   Methodology

The time frequency analysis is done using wavelet transform. Daubechies wavelet is used in this work. İt is used for noise removal [10] and splitting the input signals into approximations and details [11]. From the approximation and details of wavelet, the features are extracted. Twelve features are extracted from approximation and details. The features that are obtained from the wavelet transform are mean, median, maximum, minimum, range, standard deviation, median absolute deviation, mean absolute deviation, L1 normal, L2 normal, and maximum normal. These 12 features are then reduced through principal component analysis (PCA). Not all the obtained features are useful for classification. When applying the given features to principal component analysis, the features are reduced to four. The PCA features are normalized and hence would prove advantageous for classification. Figure 4 shows the flowchart of the overall process that is being carried out in this study.

5   Results and Discussion

In this section, the results obtained from wavelet denoising, wavelet decomposition, feature extraction from the approximation, and detail wavelets are presented. Feature reduction using principal component analysis is done. These PCA features are given to classifiers or classification and prediction.

5.1   Wavelet Transform

Daubechies wavelet is used as the mother wavelet. The noise present in the signal is rectified using wavelet denoising. Figure 5 shows the denoising of the signal through wavelet. Then the signals are decomposed into approximation and two details. The statistical parameters that are mentioned above are taken from the approximation and the details of the wavelet-decomposed signal. Figure 6 shows the decomposition of the signal into approximation and details.

The wavelet decomposition used a high-pass filter and low-pass filter. The output of the low-pass filter is approximation, and the output of high-pass filter is further

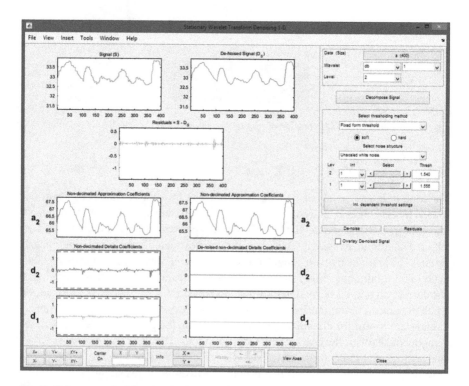

Fig. 5 Noise removal of the signal using wavelet transform

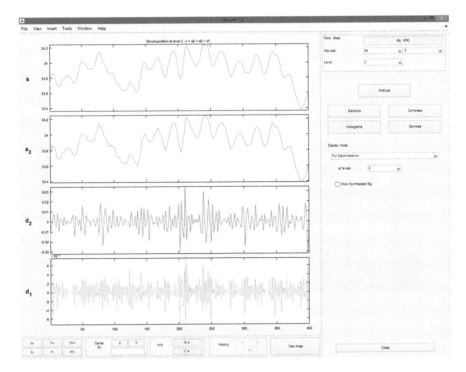

Fig. 6 Decomposing the signal into approximation and decimations

given to a high-pass and a low-pass filter which gives the detailed information of the signal. The 12 parameters are retrieved from the approximations and details as shown in Fig. 7 which shows the histogram of the approximation and all the statistical parameters for approximation for one subject.

Table 1 displays the statistical parameters of a subject from whom signals for all four emotions such as happy, sad, and angry are retrieved. The parameters got from the approximation of a subject are given in Table 1.

5.2 Principal Component Analysis

The number of features taken up for training and prediction is large, and the time taken to train with many number of features is also large. Principal component analysis is used for reducing the number of features and it considers taking the features that contribute to successful classification and the selected features are normalized. Hence when principal component analysis is done for the 12 features, it was reduced to 4 principal component parameters. Hence these are taken as features for prediction and classification (Table 2).

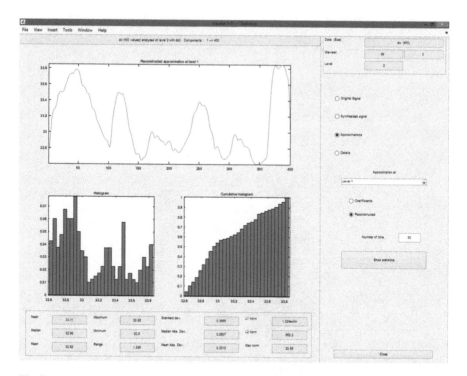

Fig. 7 Approximation and its histogram

Table 1 A sample of the features obtained from the approximation of a signal

Parameters	Happy	Surprise	Sad	Angry
Mean	35.3	35.03	31.75	34.3
Median	35.25	34.97	31.89	34.3
Maximum	37.41	35.71	32.51	34.62
Minimum	33.32	34.57	30.21	34.04
Range	4.09	1.141	2.298	0.5807
Standard deviation	1.044	0.231	0.6006	0.1188
Median absolute deviation	0.8591	0.141	0.2392	0.6177
Mean absolute deviation	0.8947	0.1856	0.4253	0.08927
L1 normal	7060	7006	6351	6860
L2 normal	499.4	495.4	449.1	485.1
Maximum normal	37.41	35.71	32.51	34.62

5.3 Classification of Signals Based on the Signals

The PCA features are fed into classifiers such as tree method, linear discriminant, quadratic discriminant, SVM, KNN, and ensemble learning in MATLAB application for classifier. The samples from 50 subjects with 4 PCA features were used for

Table 2 A sample of the features obtained from principal component analysis

Features	Happy	Surprise	Sad	Angry
PCA 1	0.9872	−0.1594	−0.0105	−0.0005
PCA 2	0.0087	−0.0027	0.8856	−0.4644
PCA 3	0.1594	0.9872	0.0021	0.0011
PCA 4	0.0050	−0.0027	0.4644	0.8856

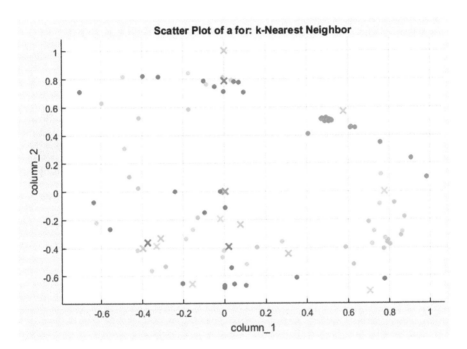

Fig. 8 Accuracy for approximation samples using KNN

classification. The approximation and detail for all the 50 samples were considered to find whether approximation or detail gives better result and to conclude which classifier algorithm would suit the best for emotion detection using noncontact respiration sensor. When approximation is considered, tree method gave an accuracy of 78%. Linear discriminant produced an accuracy of 57%. Quadratic discriminant has an accuracy of 65%. The performance of SVM is better and gave an accuracy of 84%. The highest accuracy is produced by KNN method which is 91% accurate, and ensemble learning produced an accuracy of 89.0%. The accuracy for KNN is the highest, and it is best suited for emotion detection when approximation is considered. Figure 8 shows the scatterplot and their classification for approximation for all four emotions.

The confusion matrix for KNN classifier is given in Fig. 9. The ROC curve is given in Fig. 10.

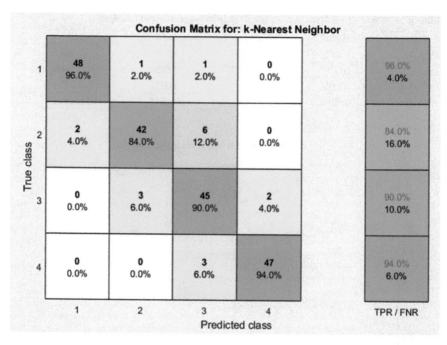

Fig. 9 Confusion matrix for KNN classifier

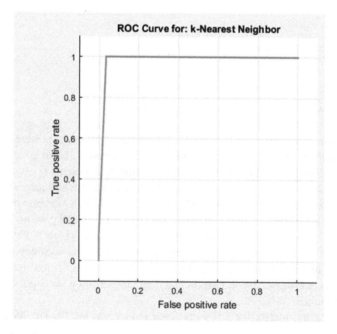

Fig. 10 Region of convergence curve for KNN

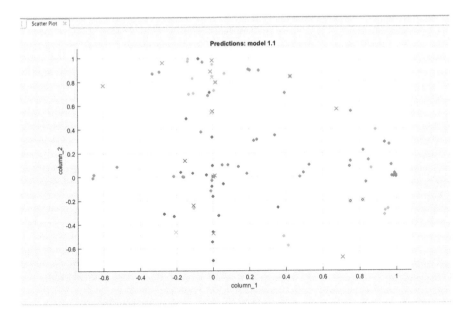

Fig. 11 Accuracy for approximation samples using KNN

When detail is considered, tree method gave an accuracy of 85.9%. Linear discriminant produced an accuracy of 61.8%. Quadratic discriminant has an accuracy of 79.9%. The performance of SVM is better and gave an accuracy of 88.4%. The accuracy is produced by KNN method which is 89.9% accurate, and ensemble learning with subspace KNN produced the highest accuracy of 91.0%. The accuracy for ensemble learning is the highest, and it is best suited for emotion detection when detail is considered. Figure 11 shows the scatterplot and their classification for approximation for all four emotions. The blue denotes happy, red denotes values for surprise, orange represents sad, and purple denotes sadness (Figs. 12 and 13).

Hence it is seen that an accuracy of 91% is got for approximation features using K-nearest neighbor and 91% of accuracy for ensemble learning when applying the details.

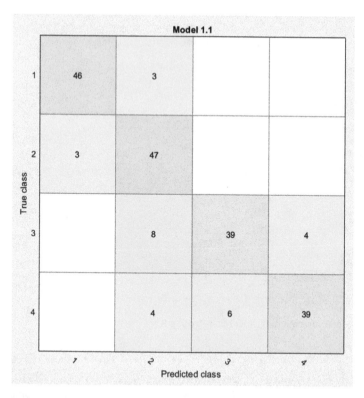

Fig. 12 Confusion matrix for ensemble classifier

6 Conclusion

Thus a real-time system for detecting emotion by observing the patterns of respiration has been developed. Physiological sensors have found to be the best approach to recognize emotional changes, as they provided information about changes that take place physiologically and are out of a person's control. The noncontact temperature sensor used in this project has the capability of monitoring real-time breath rate and obtaining reliable data output. Preprocessing is used to reduce the noise in the input of the sample reading by adding statistics coefficient parameters. The filtered data has been sent to machine leaning. The KNN network algorithm used in this work for data clustering has shown a result of 91% for approximation, and ensemble learning also produces an accuracy of 91% for detail. This same setup can be used for diagnosis of respiration system diseases based on data provided by

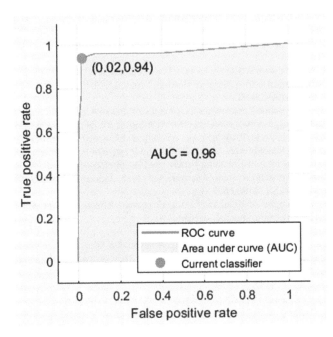

Fig. 13 Region of convergence curve for ensemble learning classifier

physiological sensor. It can also be used for COVID-19 patients to continuously monitor their breathing pattern.

References

1. Karinna Vazqueza, Jonathan Sandlera, Alejandro Interianb, Jonathan M. Feldman,: Emotionally triggered asthma and its relationship to panic disorder, ataques de nervios, and asthma-related death of a loved one in Latino adults. Journal of Psychosomatic Research. Volume 93, February (2017), Pages 76–82
2. Anna Llorca, Elisabeth Malonda and Paula Samper.: The role of emotions in depression and aggression. Med Oral Patol Oral Cir Bucal. (2016) Sep; 21(5): e559–e564.
3. Bahremand M, Alikhani M, Zakiei A, Janjani P, Aghei A. Emotion Risk-Factor in Patients with Cardiac Diseases: The Role of Cognitive Emotion Regulation Strategies, Positive Affect and Negative Affect (A Case-Control Study). Glob J Health Sci. 2015;8(1):173–179. Published (2015) May 15. doi:https://doi.org/10.5539/gjhs.v8n1p173
4. University of Illinois at Urbana-Champaign. (2014, June 25). People with tinnitus process emotions differently from their peers, researchers report. ScienceDaily. Retrieved July 1, (2019) from www.sciencedaily.com/releases/2014/06/140625184901.htm
5. K.C Horner.: The emotional ear in stress. Neuroscience & Biobehavioral Reviews, Volume 27, Issue 5, August 2003, Pages 437–446.

6. Arti Sawant et al: Respiratory Monitor with Corrective Measure System Using Thermistor, At Mega 328 and GSM. International Journal of Innovative Research in Computer and Communication Engineering (An ISO 3297: 2007 Certified Organization) Vol. 4, Issue 3, March (2016).

7. Yunyoung Nam, Bersain A Reyes, Ki H. Chon: Estimation of Respiratory Rates Using the Built-in Microphone of a Smartphone or Headset. September 2015 IEEE Journal of Biomedical and Health Informatics 20(99)

8. Tiina M Seppanen, Janne Kananen, Kai Noponen, Olli-Pekka Alho, Tapio Seppanen: Accurate measurement of respiratory airflow waveforms using depth data, Annu Int Conf IEEE Eng Med Biol Soc. (2015) Aug;2015:7857–60. doi: https://doi.org/10.1109/EMBC.2015.7320213

9. Carlo Massaroni, Daniel Simões Lopes, Daniela Lo Presti, Emiliano Schena, Sergio Silvestri, "Contactless Monitoring of Breathing Patterns and Respiratory Rate at the Pit of the Neck: A Single Camera Approach", Journal of Sensors, vol. 2018, Article ID 4567213, 13 pages, 2018. https://doi.org/10.1155/2018/4567213

10. Md. Mamun, Mahmoud Al-Kadi, Mohd. Marufuzzaman: Effectiveness of Wavelet Denoising on Electroencephalogram Signals. Journal of Applied Research and Technology, Volume 11, Issue 1, February (2013), Pages 156-160

11. Xinyang Yu, Pharino Chum, Kwee-Bo Sim: Analysis the effect of PCA for feature reduction in non-stationary EEG based motor imagery of BCI system. Optik journal, 125 (2014) 1498–1502.

Benefits of E-Health Systems During COVID-19 Pandemic

Amandeep Kaur, Anuj Kumar Gupta, and Harpreet Kaur

Abstract E-health means the availability of various health facilities electronically without going anywhere. In rural areas there is a great demand of implementing such techniques because this is a time of the spreading COVID-19 pandemic. Patients and disabled people from villages are facing many difficulties due to the closure of transportation facilities during this lockdown period. For this there is a major requirement to develop the—connected—network that consists of various medical devices, Such type of E-health systems will fulfill the needs of the people who live in rural areas. In this research work, a multilayer- and multiprotocol-based E-health system is proposed. This is done on the basis of review and feedback from the health industry facing new challenges such as COVID-19 pandemic. This model attempts to overcome the challenges faced by COVID-19 patients and health workers. The proposed system helps to further propagate DIY revolution happening all over the world, but here the focus is doing DIY with the help of medical instrumentation. The proposed system will help communities at large to monitor their health status and at the same time maintain social distancing.

Keywords E-health framework · DIY instruments · Connected

1 Introduction

At present the whole world is under the threat of COVID-19. It originated in consequence of the intense respiratory syndrome coronavirus 2 (SARS-CoV-2) [9]. Firstly it was identified in December 2019 in Wuhan, China, and has spread all over the whole world [1, 2]. More than 4.02 million cases have been reported across 187 countries from 10 May 2020. As a result of which more than 279,000 people have

A. Kaur
IKGPTU, Kapurthala, India

A. K. Gupta (✉)
Department of CSE, Chandigarh Group of Colleges, Mohali, India

H. Kaur
Department of Applied Science, SBBS University, Jalandhar, India

© The Author(s), under exclusive license to Springer
Nature Switzerland AG 2021
A. K. Manocha et al. (eds.), *Computational Intelligence in Healthcare*, Health
Information Science, https://doi.org/10.1007/978-3-030-68723-6_8

175

died, and more than 1.37 million people have recovered. The common symptoms for COVID-19 are cough, fever, shortness of breath, fatigue, and loss of taste and smell [3, 4]. The exposure time to onset of symptoms is normally 5 days, but it may also range from 2 to 14 days [5, 6].

As declared by the World Health Organization (WHO), its expanse is so large that is has been declared as a global pandemic. Due to this, medical facilities all over the world are in great stress and demand. The reason is no vaccine or proper treatment is available till now. And new infected persons are increasing day by day. Under these circumstances it becomes very difficult for hospitals to handle these patients. Implementation and explanation of E-health monitoring framework is the solution to handle this pandemic. By using these types of online systems, doctors, nurses, and health workers can monitor more number of patients without the fear of infection that is created by the gathering of huge number of patients in the hospital. The advantage of this E-health framework is it maintains social distancing; avoids touching; provides health security for nurses, doctors, and health workers; and solves the problem of overcrowding in health centers.

2   Literature Survey

This paper aims to analyze the various health monitoring techniques, which are introduced in the recent years for building reliable and flexible E-healthcare monitoring framework. Different types of designs have been used in the implementation of healthcare framework to meet the demands of patients. Table 1 describes the summary of techniques, designs, and models used for healthcare framework.

It can be observed that most frequently used methods in E-health systems are using machine learning algorithms such as SVM and ANN and some are using statistical methods such as regression analysis.

3   E-Health Methods and System Study

This paper comprises of various types of designs and techniques that can be used for the E-health monitoring framework, which will be very helpful for the diagnosis of COVID-19 patients during this pandemic period. The methodology used for this paper is based on the combination of various E-health designs—connected network—which uses different E-health monitoring techniques.

Table 1 Summary of the literature survey

Reference paper type		Objective	Method used	Key findings
[7]	Machine learning	Hybrid machine Learning algorithm	ACO, DT, SVM, KNN	ACO and SVM has a accuracy of 62.58
[8]	Statistics	A comprehensive guide for E-health	Systematic study E-health industry	Gives lessons on hypothesis testing, reegression models, etc.
[9]	Review paper design of E-health	A systematic review of mobile and GIS-based technologies	Draws statistics-based influences and conclusions	Integration of GIS technologies
[10]	Design of E-health system (book)	Describe the architectural models that characterize HCIS, HIS, HCO	Case studies in the context of the design of HCIS, HIS, HCO	Improve capacities of HCIS
[11], [12]	Design of E-health systems	Develop use cases for building shared data models in E-healthcare	DICOM, HL7, FHIR	Medical standards need to be adopted
[13]	Design of E-health systems	Propose a comprehensive design of systems	A systematic study of industrial 4.0 systems	The highly responsive and reactive E-healthcare
[14]	Design of E-health systems	Use of blockchain technology in healthcare	A systematic study on emerging opportunities in health-care	Adopt blockchain technology for better traceability
[15]	Machine learning-based	Study of machine learning healthcare models	A systematic study of AI, machine learning projects	Machine learning modeling is a need of the hour
[16]	Design of E-healthcare	Evaluate technologies related to mobile apps	A study of mobile apps, social media that can form the E-healthcare	Healthy behavior re-enforcement can be done with E-health platform integration
[17]	Integration of E-health technologies	Integrate Big Data, wearable devices and mobile technologies	Big Data is created with the help of wearable and mobile technology	Of Big data, IOT, mobile technologies, etc.
[18]	Review paper	Survey the ROC analysis	A study of classification, ROC	ROC and AUC metrics must be used for the optimization of classifier

3.1 Techniques that Are Used to Build E-Health Framework

3.1.1 Health Monitoring and Detection Using Statistics

From multiple books and journals, it can be observed that in many health-related computations such as epidemic spread, finding a degree of association between the variables and for predicting the growth pattern of a particular outbreak, counting

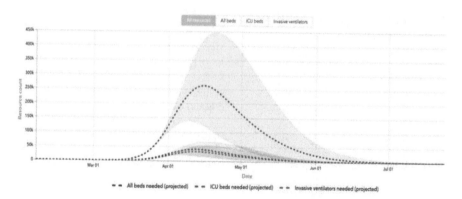

Fig. 1 Frequency Count Graph of the Resources required during Corona pandemic

how many resources are required for handling epidemics and pandemics (Fig. 1), etc., statistical methods play a major role. It can be observed in the present context of the coronavirus spread that many mathematicians and researchers working in this field are making frequency tables and histograms and many of them are trying to find a pool of variables that are acting together when the coronavirus is spreading. For this, they are using well-established methods such as Pearson correlation to identify. Researchers are using multiple visualization methods to show interesting statistics about a particular phenomenon. In Fig. 2, a geographic graph is been visualized to show the spread of coronavirus.

This graph has been developed using cumulative frequency statistics of corona cases.

3.1.2 Health Detection Using Machine Learning

In the current context of the problems faced by the health industry, many researchers are using machine learning models. Using data from the publicly available X-ray data of coronavirus diseases, many researchers have developed systems of detection by using machine learning algorithms. Similarly to other diseases such as heart, liver, kidney, and eye and many kinds of ailments, researchers are employing machine learning algorithms. Taking a clue from the current world health crisis, it can be observed that researchers are using machine learning in the following four areas to build E-health monitoring and detecting system that tracks issues such as corona:

1. Predict the structure of proteins and their interactions for building drugs. This is done with the help of protein sequencing and clustering algorithms such as ANN and K-means.
2. Deep learning-based drug screening. Many researchers are applying deep learning methods shown in Fig. 3 for ruling out potential drugs for building a robust

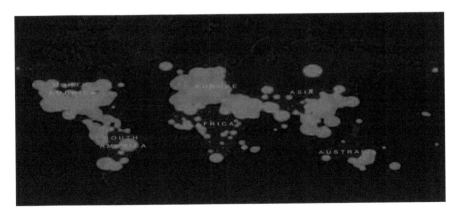

Fig. 2 Visualization of cumulative frequency tables (coronavirus spread)

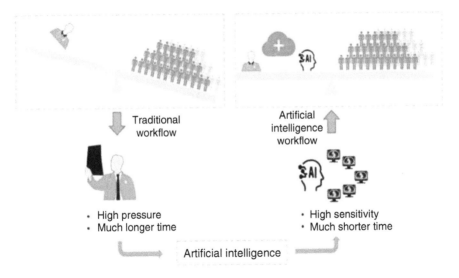

Fig. 3 Workflow using ANN for detecting diseases as compared to traditional workflow

medicine system for many types of ailments such Ebola, corona, and even for other diseases such as heart attack.

3. Predicting existing drug efficacy for the treatment of novel coronavirus: building a vaccination process takes a long time. Many researchers are using deep learning CNN algorithms to find how existing drugs or a combination of drugs can help to solve the problem of coronavirus.

4. DeepMind: Using libraries and API of DeepMind algorithms, many research organizations have predicted the protein structure of the coronavirus.

5. The forecasting infection rate has been done using machine learning algorithms as well as using statistical methods.

3.1.3 Health Monitoring Using Deep Learning

From Fig. 4, one can observe the full process of how coronavirus, in fact in other diseases such as flu, pneumonia, etc., a similar process is followed when deep learning is used for building E-health systems. It can be seen that the first step is to preprocess the corona patient X-rays so that they become suitable for running in supervised learning machine learning algorithms. The region of interest or the region that gives maximum hints on the presence and absence of respiratory stress (which means there is pneumonia or coronavirus) is segmented. Then, this image matrix is subjected to the CNN model, and after multiple evaluations, a CNN model is finalized for detection of the coronavirus.

3.2 Techniques Used for Online Monitoring

The motivation for the adoption of a new type of health monitoring systems and algorithms can be visualized from the facts, hereunder.

3.2.1 Continuous Patient Monitoring (CPM)

With time, new vectors of diseases are coming in to play. The pharmacological treatments are becoming complex and long duration day by day. For this reason, the patients and doctors need to work together, in the long run, to avoid readmission to the hospital. Developments in cloud and IoT technologies can help solve the

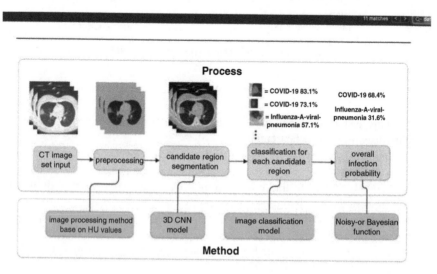

Fig. 4 Full process of Health Monitoring Using Deep learning

problem of tracking medical protocol adherence for both patients and doctors that took continuously 24 hours a day. Medical history records can be maintained forever and can be made available for exchange with the help of standards such as HL7, FHIR, etc.

3.2.2 Remote Patient Monitoring (RPM)

The outbreak of pandemic such as COVID-19 warrants for unprecedented measures for the healthcare industry. This pandemic has made the whole world how vulnerable aged people are. Hence, there is an urgent need to develop a mechanism that can support remote healthcare systems. The healthcare system now needs to keep pre- and post-monitoring and detection of the health issues a priority.

3.2.3 Early Detection of Onset of Health Issues

Early detection refers to the mechanism by which the identification of the diseases is done in the phase when the treatment of the health issue is easy. Remote medical sensors and instruments along with shared data models, data mining, and machine learning can help in this process. The need is to integrate a stack of technologies that support early detection. Early detection is also related to the sensitivity and accuracy of the algorithms for identifying small changes from which early signs of the health problem can be detected.

3.2.4 Shared Data Models

It can be observed from the ongoing COVID-19 crisis that multiple clinical research initiatives have been taken by countries to find a solution to contain the COVID-19 virus. Sharing of medically accurate data must reach the medical specialist and to the providers of healthcare; only then solutions to the healthcare problems can be found. Hence, there is an urgent need to take such initiatives.

3.2.5 DIY Medical Instrumentation

The current market trends show that people now prefer to buy portable medical and fitness devices rather than go to a hospital or clinic for getting periodic checkups. Blood pressure, glucose, oxygen, and many medical DIY kits are available for home use. People at large are now storing their health and medical data with cloud-based healthcare services. There is an urgent need to build extensions and novel solutions so that people may not only analyze the data but store as well.

3.2.6 Machine Learning Modeling

Recent developments in machine learning show that multiple machine learning models can be leveraged for building the onset of health issue applications. Now, libraries such as tens flow. It can deliver all kinds of results and outcomes from machine learning models to mobile apps.

For this research work, it is assumed that all technology stacks are working together for providing better health management. The next section focuses on giving information on the use of algorithms to improve the effectiveness of such systems in real-time conditions.

4 E-Health Framework Designs and Architectures

In this section, we discuss the various possible design options that are already in use in the medical industry. It presents information on the progression of the E-health systems until now. And the last section discusses an aggregated E-health system that can be assumed for building an algorithmic centric E-health system.

4.1 E-Health System Design I

Figure 5 shows a basic design, with which an E-health system may be designed. It can be seen from Fig. 5 that it is primarily client-server architecture. This arrangement consists of big fat servers and client machines. The client machines are connected with some medical devices such as glucometer. This may require serial to Ethernet connectors as shown in Fig. 6. It can be observed from Fig. 6 [https://www.edn.com/getting-medical-devices-onto-the-lan/] and Fig. 7 the installation of the device that can be done close to the patient's bed, and this arrangement can do the

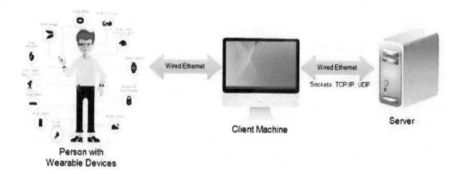

Fig. 5 E-health system design I

Fig. 6 Anesthesia care unit

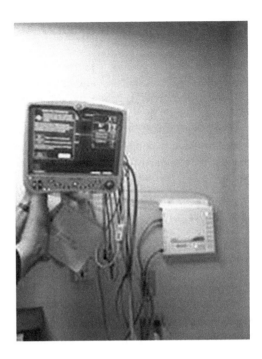

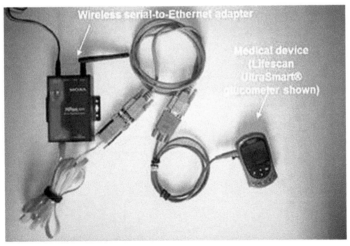

Fig. 7 Installation of the device

raw data transmission and translation. Figure 6 shows the use of the anesthesia care unit. Figure 7 gives images of the cables and adaptors that require making such arrangements.

4.2 E-Health System Design II

In case the medical facility is in a remote area, the same E-health network needs to be extended with the help of radio links as shown in Fig. 8. The antenna is the physical link to the network connectivity for almost all kinds of medical instruments. Instruments such as the insulin pump and a defibrillator can be connected using specially built antenna that can get connected to large-size radio links. For an automated decision-making, the clients and server machine must carry soft components that use regression and machine learning algorithms (Fig. 9).

4.3 E-Health System Design III

The architecture shown in Fig. 8 gives information on Wi-Fi-enabled healthcare system that can be constructed. This arrangement supports the medical telemetry with the help and use of Internet service providers (ISP).

The Wi-Fi-enabled health management systems are more widely supported by the technical and medical communities simply because the penetration of the Wi-Fi technologies is increasing day by day. This arrangement required the use of a router and switches that are multiprotocol enabled.

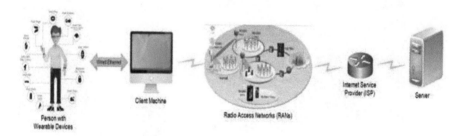

Fig. 8 E-health system design II

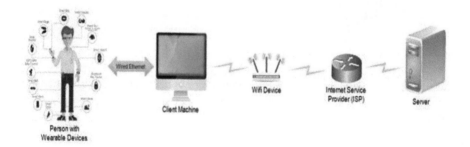

Fig. 9 E-health system design III

4.4 E-Health System Design IV

The design and architecture of the group of remotely administrated devices are different from the in-house hospital use. It is even different from the common IoT devices. The E-health systems are put in place to support mission-critical actions that correlate with the life and death of the patients.

Hence, in extraordinary conditions, satellite communication may be helpful, especially in cases like the coronavirus worldwide epidemic.

4.5 E-Health System Design V

The design of the remotely controlled devices based facilities different from the telematics or systems of security. Some of the medical devices contain high-powered electronics that may even interfere with the radio's device performance.

Hence, the electronic hardware of the medical and communication devices needs special technical approach. Moreover, with the increase in several hospitalization cases, the existing health systems are already under stress. There is an urgent need for argumentation of the health systems. The existing systems must leverage all kinds of protocols and the latest in algorithms for building a reliable healthcare system. Figure 10 shows the use of blue tooth, Wi-Fi, satellite, and RFID technologies working together seamlessly.

5 Proposed Architecture

It is assumed the health monitoring system consists of multiple technological stacks that are working together for the exchange of data with the health monitoring system. The system will not only have medical sensors connected with radio links but

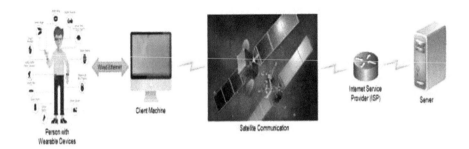

Fig. 10 E-health system design IV

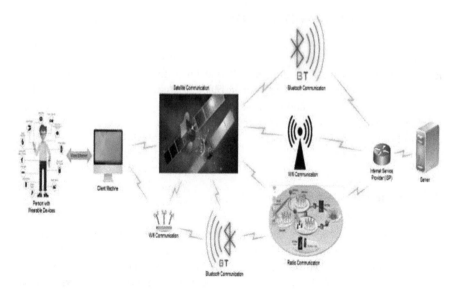

Fig. 11 E-health system design V

also with other communication methods such as Bluetooth, Wi-Fi, etc. All the components of the system will be connected with the health cloud and even with other industries such as fitness, insurance, etc.

Figure 11 shows the model that integrates modern generation of health sensors and biomedical instruments. Another thing that it takes into consideration is the use of knowledge discovery and data mining as the main components of electronics health monitoring system. The main advantage of this healthcare system will be to provide extended service to the E-health system. By using this platform, insurance industry will be able to customize their policies, and the healthcare management unit will become more accurate. The following are the components and layers of healthcare management system (Fig. 12).

5.1 E-Healthcare Service Interface

All the health sensor devices in this module are configured to a common platform to provide the facility of interoperability. The data that is obtained during this process will be stored in the database server that contains unprocessed data collected from different geo-locations of health sensor devices. The large part of this module consists of interfaces for the system administrators, insurance persons, and a person under observation for configuring the time schedule, sensors, and fine-tuning parameters.

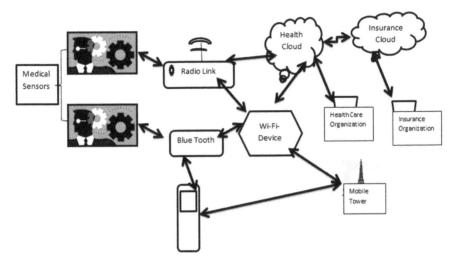

Fig. 12 Our proposed E-health system

5.2 E-Healthcare Data Processing

This module consists of health data, e.g., body temperature, blood pressure patterns, heart monitoring, physical and mental state, falls, etc., that will be processed for monitoring and analyzing for health as well as to build models of insurance premiums for insurance industry. Format of fields may be used for BLE profile standards. All types of data will be collected for real-time processing as mentioned in Table 1 in chapter "Realization of Carry-Free Adder Circuit Using FPGA". These real-time fitness data, which are subjected under continuous health monitoring, will be stored in the database for further analysis using fog computing.

5.3 E-Healthcare Business Logic and Rules

In this phase, E-health business policies and logic are being constructed for sending the alert messages to the patients based on the data collected from the various health sensors. These alert messages can also be exchanged with sports clubs, fitness centers, and medical support centers. The data is stored temporarily on local machines, and some processing may be done before sending to the server. The alert in medical field must be able to support common alerting protocol (CAP) and HL7 message format for exchanging the medical reports. The exchange of messages will be based on well-defined rules and policies based on events such as pain. This would help in obtaining health status information to performing a specific action like alerting a patient's relative and the hospital for some medical emergency.

5.4   E-Healthcare Data Analytics Monitoring

This module will analyze the health data to be sent to the extended E-healthcare services based on the business policies. An interface for analyzing and monitoring the statistical data of a person will be provided to the healthcare facilities. In this module, various algorithms for computing the estimation of health status will be executed. Further, the module will also consist of different types of machine learning algorithms that will be applied to the different types of health problems and issues that are to be solved using the health sensor data that is being collected in real time.

5.5   Extended E-Health Services Platform

This module relates to the open marketing services, which may be in the form of apps, API, etc., and patients can use these apps as well as insurance companies, hospitals, different health organizations, and doctors for making better decisions in medical fields. The proposed model is based on coherent technologies such as XML/JSON and is simple and scalable to implement.

6   Comparative Study

In this section, we compare the outcome of the study carried out for familiarizing the functioning of the various E-healthcare systems in terms of technology stacks and its impact on the healthcare systems. Table 2 describes various parameters that give comparative view of various designs.

7   Conclusion

This paper proposed a design for E-health monitoring framework that can be adopted during COVID-19 pandemic where doctors, nurses, and health workers can remotely monitor the patients. Additionally, the new model integrates various types of health sensors that allow the uploading of patient's vitals over the system. At last doctors will be able to monitor the health status of patients online and can remotely diagnose the disease. Another advantage of this E-health system is that it will provide extended service. By using this extended service, the insurance industry will be able to personalize their policies, and the healthcare management will become more targeted and accurate. It should support multiple technological stacks (legacy as well as current systems). The E-health framework follows dominant standards such as HIIPA, HL7, and FHIR.

Table 2 E-health design comparison

Parameters	Design I	Design II	Design III	Design IV	Proposed V
Ease of implementation	Easy	Easy	Complex	Complex	Complex
Mobility [19]	No	Limited	Medium	Highest	Yes
Portability [20]	No	Limited	Yes	Yes	Yes
In-hospitable	Yes	Yes	Yes	Yes	Yes
At home	No	Yes	Yes	Very low	Yes
Adoption rate	Low	Low	Medium	Very low	Low
Internet ready	Low	Medium	Medium	High	High
Interoperability	No	Fair	Good	Good	Excellent
Availability	Low	Fair	Good	Low	Excellent
Scalability [21]	Not much	Fair	Medium	High	High
Remote facilitation factor	No	Fair	Medium	High	High
Connected CT scanners	Not possible	Limited	Limited	Limited	High
Connected MRI	Not possible	Limited	Limited	Limited	High
Connected hospital beds	Not possible	Limited	Limited	Limited	High
Connected nurse	Not possible	Limited	Limited	Limited	High
Connected physicians	Not possible	Limited	Limited	Limited	High
Health access	Limited	Limited	Limited	Limited	High

The system should have the capacity to incorporate machine learning modeling for a better degree of automation and statistical modeling for building long-term health issue detection models. The systems must incorporate elements of remote patient management and supervision through algorithms, especially in situations such as COVID-19 pandemic.

References

1. B. M. C. Staff, Knuth: coronavirus disease 2019-symptoms and causes. URL https://www.mayoclinic.org/diseases-conditions/coronavirus/symptoms-causes/syc-20479963
2. D. S. Hui, E. I. Azhar, T. A. Madani, F. Ntoumi, R. Kock, O. Dar, G. Ippolito, T. D. Mchugh, Z. A. Memish, C. Drosten, et al., The continuing 2019-ncov epidemic threat of novel coronaviruses to global health—the latest 2019 novel coronavirus outbreak in wuhan, china, International Journal of Infectious Diseases 91 (2020) 264–266.
3. S. Murthy, C. D. Gomersall, R. A. Fowler, Care for critically ill patients with covid-19, Jama 323 (15) (2020) 1499–1500.
4. M. Cascella, M. Rajnik, A. Cuomo, S. C. Dulebohn, R. Di Napoli, Features, evaluation and treatment coronavirus (covid- 19), in: Statpearls [internet], StatPearls Publishing, 2020.
5. B. Bikdeli, M. V. Madhavan, D. Jimenez, T. Chuich, I. Dreyfus, E. Driggin, C. Der Nigoghossian, W. Ageno, M. Madjid, Y. Guo, et al., Covid-19 and thrombotic or thromboembolic disease: Implications for prevention, antithrombotic therapy, and follow-up: Jacc state-of-the-art review, Journal of the American College of Cardiology 75 (23) (2020) 2950–2973.
6. T. Velavan, C. Meyer, La epidemia de covid-19, Trop Med Int Health (2020).
7. S. S. Shrivastava, V. Choubey, A. Sant, Classification based pattern analysis on the medical data in health care environment, International Journal of Scientific Research in Science, Engineering and Technology 2 (1) (2016).

8. T. E. Melander, Statistics from scratch: An introduction for health care professionals, Journal of Quality Technology 29 (4) (1997) 491.
9. J. A. Nhavoto, Å. Grönlund, Mobile technologies and geographic information systems to improve health care systems: a literature review, JMIR mHealth and uHealth 2 (2) (2014) e21.
10. S. U. Amin, M. S. Hossain, G. Muhammad, M. Alhussein, M. A. Rahman, Cognitive smart healthcare for pathology detection and monitoring, IEEE Access 7 (2019) 10745–10753.
11. M. S. Islam, M. M. Hasan, X. Wang, H. D. Germack, et al., A systematic review on health-care analytics: application and theoretical perspective of data mining, in: Healthcare, Vol. 6, Multidisciplinary Digital Publishing Institute, 2018, p. 54.
12. P. D. Kaur, I. Chana, Cloud based intelligent system for delivering health care as a service, Computer methods and programs in biomedicine 113 (1) (2014) 346–359.
13. V. M. Tovarnitchi, Designing distributed, scalable and extensible system using reactive architectures, in: 2019 22nd International Conference on Control Systems and Computer Science (CSCS), IEEE, 2019, pp. 484–488.
14. R. Krawiec, D. Housman, M. White, M. Filipova, F. Quarre, D. Barr, A. Nesbitt, K. Fedosova, J. Killmeyer, A. Israel, et al., Blockchain: Opportunities for health care, in: Proc. NIST Workshop Blockchain Healthcare, 2016, pp. 1–16.
15. M. A. Sarwar, N. Kamal, W. Hamid, M. A. Shah, Prediction of diabetes using machine learning algorithms in healthcare, in: 2018 24th International Conference on Automation and Computing (ICAC), IEEE, 2018, pp. 1–6.
16. D. Arigo, D. E. Jake-Schoffman, K. Wolin, E. Beckjord, E. B. Hekler, S. L. Pagoto, The history and future of digital health in the field of behavioral medicine, Journal of behavioral medicine 42 (1) (2019) 67–83.
17. S. Chakraborty, V. Bhatt, T. Chakravorty, Big-data, iot wearable and mhealth cloud platform integration triads-a logical way to patient-health monitoring, International Journal of Engineering and Advanced Technology 9 (3) (2020) 388–394.
18. M. Pooja, D. Das, Comparative analysis of iot based healthcare architectures, International Journal of Computer Applications 975 (2017) 8887.
19. S. González-Valenzuela, M. Chen, V. C. Leung, Mobility support for health monitoring at home using wearable sensors, IEEE Transactions on Information Technology in Biomedicine 15 (4) (2011) 539–549.
20. K. Mahato, A. Srivastava, P. Chandra, Paper based diagnostics for personalized health care: Emerging technologies and commercial aspects, Biosensors and Bioelectronics 96 (2017) 246–259.
21. A. Lounis, A. Hadjidj, A. Bouabdallah, Y. Challal, Healing on the cloud: Secure cloud architecture for medical wireless sensor networks, Future Generation Computer Systems 55 (2016) 266–277.

Low-Cost Bone Mineral Densitometer

Riddhi Vinchhi, Neha Zimare, Shivangi Agarwal, and Bharti Joshi

Abstract Osteoporosis is a common disease prevalent mostly among the elderly individuals. The characteristics of osteoporosis include increased fragility which is caused due to the reduction of the bone's absorption capability. This leads to increase in the porosity and reduction in the elastic stiffness of the bone and causes thinning of the cortical wall. Osteoporosis increases the risk of fractures and hence can cause suffering and also leads to the economic loss. The current existing standard method of detecting osteoporosis is dual energy X-ray absorptiometry (DXA) which cannot reliably predict whether a person is suffering from porous bones. Also, the devices which use DXA are expensive. Hence there is a call for alternative techniques for measuring the bone mineral density. Quantitative ultrasound (QUS) methods have shown a rapid and promising development of new alternative methods for reliable and inexpensive diagnosing of osteoporosis. Hence as a part of this progress, this work focuses on the development of a new machine which is low-cost and uses ultrasonic transducers for generating ultrasonic waves instead of using X rays. In this paper, a low-cost bone mineral density machine has been designed.

Keywords Bone mineral density · Osteoporosis · Pulser-receiver · Piezoelectric ultrasonic transducer · Velocity and attenuation

R. Vinchhi · N. Zimare
Ramrao Adik Institute of Technology, Nerul, Navi Mumbai, India

S. Agarwal (✉)
Department of Electronics Engineering, Ramrao Adik Institute of Technology,
Nerul, Navi Mumbai, India

B. Joshi
Department of Computer Engineering, Ramrao Adik Institute of Technology,
Nerul, Navi Mumbai, India

© The Author(s), under exclusive license to Springer
Nature Switzerland AG 2021
A. K. Manocha et al. (eds.), *Computational Intelligence in Healthcare*, Health
Information Science, https://doi.org/10.1007/978-3-030-68723-6_9

1 Introduction

Bone density, or bone mineral density which is abbreviated as BMD, is defined as the amount of bone mineral present in bone tissue. It refers to the concept of mass of the mineral per volume of bone. Incorrect bone mineral density can create osteoporosis, i.e. it leads to porous bones. Under a microscope, a healthy bone looks like a honeycomb. While in case when the person has osteoporosis, it is observed that the holes and spaces of the honeycomb like image are much bigger. This indicates a reduced bone mineral density. Bones are broken easily if they are less dense. The reports till now indicate that osteoporosis has caused 3–4 million fractures each year due to fragility. Hence, osteoporosis has become a significant health problem. Therefore, there is a great need to take measures for detecting osteoporosis at an early stage and also for the prevention and treatment of it. The imbalance between generation of new bone and the capability of the bone to produce new bone causes osteoporosis. Phosphate and calcium are the two main minerals for normal bone generation. If the calcium intake is insufficient or if the body does not absorb enough calcium from the diet, then the bone tissue or bone generation will suffer. Due to this the bones may become weaker which further results in fragile and brittle bones, and these bones tend to break easily. Present existing system for bone density scanning uses X-rays which is expensive. Also such systems are bulkier. Person's body may have some side effects in using X-rays. So, a novel idea of using ultrasound to measure the bone density is used. Bone density can be evaluated using the difference between sound intensity at two different locations and then finding Net Time Delay (NTD) using linear regression. This system can be made portable. Also, X-ray-based systems are more complex compared to this setup.

2 Literature Survey

In applied acoustics field, a lot of recognition is being amassed by the Ultrasonic technique. A study done by Joanne Homik and David Hailey shows that quantitative calcaneal ultrasound appears to be promising diagnostic technology [1]. Also, the development and installation of the details of various modules of a C-scan ultrasonic facility ULTIMA 200M2 is done at the Indira Gandhi Centre for Atomic Research, Kalpakkam [2]. Day by day, the applications of ultrasound have increased in the field of medicine and military [3]. As the quantitative ultrasound technique is emerging at a fast pace, design and development of low-cost pulser-receivers are gaining importance. Hence, the work done shows the design of Low Cost Broadband Ultrasonic Pulser-Receiver [4]. Also, a new technology for ultrasonic phase velocity evaluation in liquids [5], attenuation [6] and power measurement in pulse-echo setup has been designed [7]. The transducer is excited, ultrasonic waves are transmitted in the bone, the reflected waves are received to produce echoes and then these ultrasonic echoes are further analysed in the method of ultrasonic testing which is reported in the international standard ASTM, E 494 [8]. Single transducer systems have been also asserted by this standard, which is more suitable for measurements of the velocity [9]. In order to develop a multimode quantitative ultrasound (QUS) assessment which is employing both photo-acoustic skeletal (FAS) as well as fundamental flexural-guided wave (FFGW), measurements of ultrasound in bone were performed by using an Array Transducer [10].

3   Methodology

3.1   Quantitative Ultrasound (QUS) and Its Basic Physics

Ultrasound is referred as the mechanical vibration which has a frequency which cannot be detected by human ears as this frequency is too high, i.e. the frequencies greater than 20 kHz are ultrasonic frequencies. Similar to the other sound vibrations, ultrasound propagates in an innate isotropic medium. When a particle in a medium is disturbed, this force propagates to the neighbouring particles through the connections. This propagation carries the information available in the ultrasonic wave across the bone tissues. In this system, one of the method of quantitative ultrasound called as pulse-echo method [11] is used. It uses the same operating principle as used in sonar for locating an obstacle in the path. In this method, a pulser-receiver transmits a pulse. Then the ultrasound wave passes through tissues and is scattered from cancellous bone, and then the reflected ultrasound wave called as echo is read shortly. Considering the properties and working of the ultrasound, the device tracks the attenuation and time of flight of the pulse to obtain information about the structure being investigated.

3.2   System Description

It is a device to measure the bone density in order to monitor the calcium content in the bone which is being tested (Fig. 1). Pair of ultrasonic transducers of 1 MHz which are spaced oppositely are placed in a clamping apparatus which is closely attached to the bone which is under examination. These ultrasonic transducers contain piezoelectric crystal which is used to pass signals through the bone which is circumscribed in the finger and heel of the subject which is being tested. A pulser-receiver is coupled to one of the transducers, and then it produces an electric pulse allowing the transducers to produce an ultrasonic sound wave which is directed through the bone structure to the other transducer. The signals are coupled by an electric circuit along with an amplifier and a band pass filter from the receiver transducer back to the pulse generator for retriggering the pulse generator at a frequency which is proportional to the duration taken by the ultrasonic wave to travel through

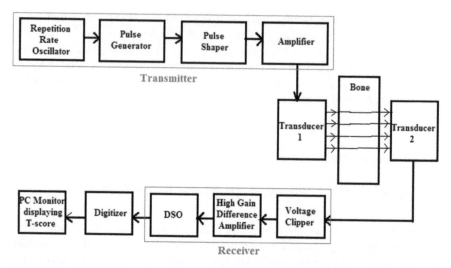

Fig. 1 System block diagram

the bone structure being examined. The received data is collected via a digitizer using PyUsb and is then connected to computer for computing the Net Time Delay (NTD) and for calculating the bone density to find the T-score.

3.3 Pulse Generator

The transmitter is the first part to be designed to generate the driver frequency. A square signal of 5 MHz frequency is constantly provided by the LM555 timer. This signal is then applied to the monostable multivibrator 74121 which generates a pulse width of 3 μs. 500 Hz is the sample rate of the output signal generated by the monostable multivibrator which is then fed to IRF530 Power MOSFET for amplification of the signal. 15–20 V peak-to-peak amplitude of the output pulse is used, which is sent to sender transducer (Tx). The pulse generator circuit is shown in the Fig. 2.

3.4 Receiver

In practice, the signal intensity of the received echo can be less than 1% of that of the signal which is sent out from the transducer. In order to strengthen the echo signal, a high-gain amplifier is required. Receiver circuit diagram is shown in the Fig. 3, in which a single-stage amplifier is assembled with the dual-precision AD822. Maximum output dynamic range is provided by output voltage swing when it ranges to within 10 mV of each rail. The maximum offset voltage is 800 μV, drift

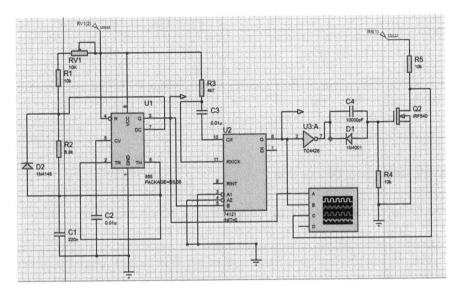

Fig. 2 Transmitter circuit

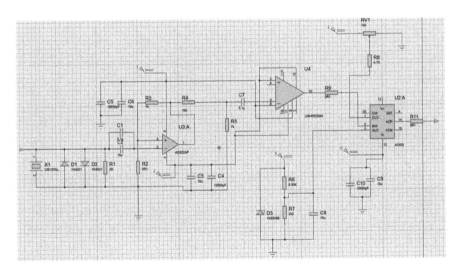

Fig. 3 Receiver circuit

of offset voltage is 2 V/C, input bias current is below 25 pA and noise of input voltage is low which gives dc precision along with the source impedance up to giga-ohm. The unity-gain bandwidth is 1.8 MHz, slew rate is 3 V/s and total harmonic distortion (THD) is 93 dB at 10 kHz which are given per amplifier with a low supply current of 800 μA. The output from AD822 is then fed to LH0002 which is a general purpose buffer. Low output impedance is provided for both the positive as well as negative slopes of output pulses by the symmetrical output portion of the circuit. At the output, the signal to noise ratio (SNR) is improved because of lower gain of the AD602. However, 1.4 nV/Hz is the input noise spectral density for both products.

A linear regression model is used for calculating the value of bone density (BD) when the Net Time Delay (NTD) is known. Further, T-score is calculated based on the obtained value of bone density from the regression model. For this, any operating system with Python support can be used. Linear regression (LR) model can be implemented in Python 3.5 or above versions.

4   Results and Discussion

The following Table 1 shows the calculated bone density depending on the Net Time Delay obtained from the difference between the transmitted and received ultrasonic waves using linear regression model.

The graph of obtained bone density against Net Time Delay is plotted as shown in the Fig. 4.

Thus the prediction about bone density for given NTD can be obtained. T-score is calculated using the following formula:

$$T\text{-score} = \frac{\bar{x}\mu_0}{s\sqrt{n}}$$

where

$\bar{x}$ = sample mean
μ_0 = population mean
s = sample standard deviation
n = sample size

T-score of a healthy 30-year-old adult as per World Health Organization (WHO) is shown in Table 2.

A low T-score indicates a lower bone density. Hence, based on the calculated T-score, detection of the level of bone density can be done for the given bone sample; hence chance of Osteoporosis can be predicted.

Table 1 Comparison of the predicted and calculated bone density when the Net Time Delay (NTD) is known

NTD	Predicted bone density	Actual bone density
1.10110	0.571144214843	0.61111
1.51211	0.779640913428	0.79211
1.90232	0.986363580424	0.99213
2.10000	1.08892875335	1.09000
2.70000	1.40023542957	1.40000

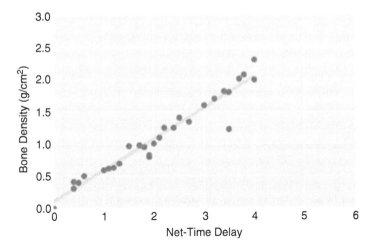

Fig. 4 Linear regression plot

Table 2 Bone density level indicator (*T*-score)

Bone density level	*T*-scores	Examples
Normal	−1 or above	0.9, 0 and −0.9
Low or osteopenia	−1 and −2.5	−1.1, −1.6 and −2.4
Osteoporosis	−2.5 or below	−2.6, −3.3 and −3.9

5 Conclusion

The objective of the proposed low-cost setup can be accomplished using the above low-cost hardware circuit. Also, osteoporosis can now be predicted by a low-cost well-trained system. Linear regression algorithm used for prediction of *T*-score facilitates the ease of calculation. Hence, to assist and improvise doctor's diagnostics, early diagnosis of osteoporosis can be performed easily.

References

1. Homik Joanne and Hailey David: Quantitative ultrasound for bone density measurement, Alberta Heritage Foundation for Medical Research (1998)
2. Kumar, A., Patankar, V., Joshi, V., Lande, B.: Development and application of C-scan ultrasonic facility, BARC News 285 (2006) 49–57
3. Lewis Jr, K.G., Olbricht W.L.: Development of a portable therapeutic high intensity ultrasound system for military medical and research use, Rev. Sci. Instrum 2008 Nov;79(11):114302. doi: https://doi.org/10.1063/1.3020704
4. Sharma, K., Singh, S., Dubey, P.K.: Design of Low Cost Broadband Ultrasonic Pulser–Receiver, MAPAN-Journal of Metrology Society of India, (June 2017) 32(2):95–100

5. Joshi, D., Bhatnagar, D., Kumar, A., Gupta, R.: Direct measurement of acoustic impedance in liquids by a new pulse echo technique, MAPAN-J. Metrol. Soc. India 24 (2010) 215–224
6. Dubey, P.K., et al: High resolution ultrasonic attenuation measurement in pulse-echo setup, MAPAN-J. Metrol. Soc. India, 23(4) (2008) 245–252
7. Dubey, P.K., Jain, A., Singh, S.: Improved and automated primary ultrasonic power measurement setup, CSIR-NPL, India, MAPAN-J. Metrol. Soc. India,30(4) (2015) 231–237
8. ASTM, E 494, Standard practice for measuring ultrasonic velocity in materials (1995)
9. Joshi, D., Gupta, R., Kumar, A., Kumar, Y., Yadav, S.: A precision ultrasonic phase velocity measurement technique for liquids, MAPAN-Journal of Metrology Society of India, 29 (2014) 09–17
10. Kilappa Vantte: Ultrasound Measurements in Bone Using an Array Transducer, University of JYVÄSKYLÄ,(June 2017) 32(2):95–100
11. Abarkane Chihab, Galé-Lamuela David, Benavent-Climent Amadeo, Suárez Elisabet, Gallego Antolino: Ultrasonic Pulse-Echo Signal Analysis for Damage Evaluation of Metallic Slit-Plate Hysteretic Dampers Metals-Open Access Metallurgy Journal 7(12):526-November 2017

Smart Infusion Pump Control:
The Control System Perspective

J. V. Alamelu and A. Mythili

Abstract Smart infusion pump utilization is grown significantly in hospitals. An infusion is a mechanism by which an infusion system is used to administer fluids or medications via the intravenous, subcutaneous, epidural, or enteral path to the patient in solution. For the healthcare drug delivery devices, exact dosing is crucial. The use of smart pumps may avoid errors resulting from an incorrect dose, dose rate, or solution concentration resulting from the ordering provider, as well as errors resulting from human failures in the programming of pumps. Even though programming is performed with smart alarms, the accurate flow with motor control has to be focused. In this chapter, a framework on optimal motor control to perform a precise flow of drug to be concentrated to the patient through infusion device is discussed. The framework comprises of the mathematical model of the infusion pump with an electric motor associated with it. The mechanical and electrical parameters of the electric motor is based on the manufacturer specification, further based on these values the control design with Proportional Integral Derivative (PID) controller, PID control with Particle Swarm Optimization (PSO), and Linear Quadratic Gaussian (LQG) are discussed. The comparison of the stability criteria and time response analysis with the help of the mentioned algorithms is contemplated. The motor of the infusion device should have a quick rise time so fast infusion will occur, further reduces the lag time and delay in the infusion of the drug's flow rate.

Keywords Control strategy · Smart infusion pump · Motor actuation · Optimal control

J. V. Alamelu (✉)
SENSE, VIT University Vellore, Vellore, Tamil Nadu, India

Department of Electronics and Instrumentation Engineering, M.S.Ramaiah Institute of Technology, Bangalore, India

A. Mythili (✉)
SENSE, VIT University Vellore, Vellore, Tamil Nadu, India
e-mail: mythili.asaithambi@vit.ac.in

1   Introduction

1.1   *Background and Literature*

Immense technological advances have contributed to advancements in medical device design. Physical devices, such as sensors and actuators, can be connected to the cyber environment, to other devices, and to the entire system connected in a remote location. The application is about healthcare, the system is created as a Medical Cyber Physical System (MCPS) [1]. Almost all medical devices that are standalone are designed to communicate only with physicians, patients, and caregivers. Today's technology has allowed most medical devices to communicate remotely with other devices, medical providers, and caregivers. Communication with medical devices has been improved with operational efficiency. The medical pump, for instance, an infusion pump is considered here for the study.

Medical devices, such as infusion pumps, are standalone devices that interacted with the patient or healthcare personnel. Because of technological advances to enhance patient care, these devices now wirelessly hook up with various systems, networks, and other tools within the Healthcare Delivery Organization (HDO) and ultimately medical aid, eventually contributing to MCPS. MCPS-based devices focus on physical system design, communication with the cyber world, and security systems [2]. Cybersecurity is also an important aspect to consider, as the entire environment is based on cyberspace. The manufacturer is solely responsible for the design and implementation of the device to create an efficient, safe, and compatible environment for the sensors and other components used in MCPS-based infusion pumps.

Accuracy and efficiency are achieved in collaboration with physicians and computers. Nowadays infusion pumps are smart pumps and that they are operated in wireless mode. Data stored within the wireless infusion pump ecosystem face numerous threats, including unauthorized access to Protected Health Information (PHI), changes in prescription drug rates, and pump interference. Except for the safety factor when we consider the MCPS scenario, proper physical design, and implementation of the entire smart infusion pump is imperative. The amount of drug reserve is given based on the available drug cache library [3]. Delivery to the patient is important, and therefore the control and monitoring of the components of the infusion pump must be thoroughly monitored. In this chapter, a detailed overview, classification of an infusion pump, and pumping actuation with control system techniques are discussed.

2 Infusion Pump, Definition, and Classification

Infusion systems are electromechanical systems used to administer anesthetic drugs with moderate accuracy. To ensure reliable delivery of prescribed fluid volumes and assist in effective nursing management, the use of smart infusion pumps over a manual flow control system has been recommended. Nutrients, medications such as insulin, hormones, antibiotics, drugs for chemotherapy, and pain relievers can be delivered. Infusion pumps are commonly used in healthcare settings and home environments [4].

Infusion pumps can be broadly categorized based on function, the volume of the fluid delivered, and mobility. Based on the function, they are piston, peristaltic, gravity feed, and syringe pumps. According to the volume of the fluid and mobility, they are classified as large volume pumps, small, ambulatory, and standalone infusion pumps. The usage, implementation, and advantage vary as per the type of fluid, a drug used to deliver to the patient, and the application of medical devices [5].

2.1 Block Diagram of a Smart Infusion Pump

The generic block diagram of the smart infusion pump is shown below.

The smart infusion pump is shown in Fig. 1 has an infusion set with a smart control unit. The infusion set is connected to the patient, and the control unit has a microprocessor that is interfaced with the infusion pump reservoir, cannula, and to the external world with the inbuilt transceivers. The controller is programmed to handle the optimum flow rate by controlling the motor of the pump by using the smart drug library [6]. The motor control is an important aspect, and hence the control strategies for the actuation of the pump with the motor are discussed in this chapter.

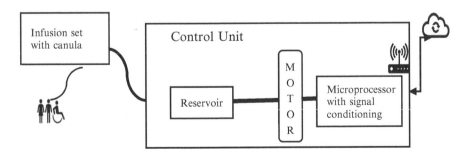

Fig. 1 Block diagram of a smart infusion pump

2.2   Infusion Pump Control Model for Drug Infusion

Drugs are provided by continuous infusion to maintain a constant pharmacody-namic activity. The usage of drug infusions requires information about pharmacoki-netics and pharmacodynamics [7]. Pharmacokinetics is the study of kinetics that deals with drug absorption, distribution, and elimination. Kinetics is the study on analysis of the rate of process and the factors affecting it. The rate of a process is the change in velocity with time [8].

In practice, the pharmacokinetics study includes both practical and computa-tional form. The practical form enables the implementation of biological sampling procedures, systematic strategies for drugs, its metabolism, and methods that assist in data processing; in the computational approach, pharmacokinetic models are designed to facilitate the prediction of drug administration. The process of drug absorption, delivery, and removal is based on the concentration rate which is $\pm \, dC/dt$.

With the formation of the pharmaceutical dosage forms, the drug delivery system is established to guarantee the clinical application in patient care. The investigation of the pharmacokinetics within the body is compartmentalized or non-compartmentalized. The compartmentalized form describes the drug disposition, concentration in plasma, and the elimination process from the central compartment. The non-compartmentalized form is utilized to recognize certain pharmacokinetic parameters without choosing any compartmental model [9].

The modern infusion system is a compartment model that contains a reservoir to store the fluid, tube, catheter, flow control, and pressure control mechanism. The mechanism that drives fluid to the patient is based on gravity, syringe-driven, and mechanical propulsion. In the gravity-based IV setup, the movement of the patient and the variation of the blood pressure affects the constant flow rate even though the clinical settings of the flow rate are done precisely by the nurse. The syringe pumps are widely used for anesthesia drugs, and the mechanical pumps and peristaltic pumps have small mechanical motors and gear arrangement with multiple tubing [10]. These pumps can be used for continuous and intravenous delivery of the fluid also in the multiple infusion scenarios.

The design of medical infusion systems is very important as a medical error should be minimized because it may lead to device failure, and it is fatal [11]. The problems are usually based on the specification of the hardware associated such as the type of sensor, motor, the weight of the device, power supplies, batteries, pump-ing mechanism, program error messages, operator errors, faulty parts, alarms, flow velocity, and drug flow based on the infusion type.

Sophisticated devices are available to meet the criteria for patients who are in the serious disease, need multiple medications to be infused. Providing the right drug with the correct dose at the right time is the crucial factor in infusion pump perfor-mance. Flow rate, start-up delays, dead volume, drug delivery, lag time, valve and in-line filter settings, and drug absorption are the parameters that influence the delivery of the drugs and fluids. Patients treated in clinical and home environs with a continuous infusion system should be provided with a specific medical error-free

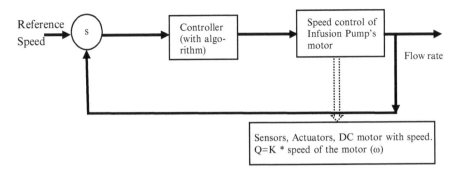

Fig. 2 Block diagram of an infusion pump

device that ensures safety. Therefore, modeling is necessary [12]. The control system block diagram to implement modeling is given in Fig. 2. The set point (s) regarding the flow rate will be considered as the desired input, and control strategy is implemented to perform the complete automated and optimal control system [13].

The block diagram is depicted with the controller and infusion pump's motor. The control of the flow rate is essential for the suitable dosage to be infused to the patient [14]. The reference speed is given to the controller as a set point and further processed. To achieve these different control strategies, they have to be incorporated into the medical grade motor employed to the infusion pump. In this chapter, different control strategies are discussed and compared. These details are discussed in Sects. 3 and 4.

3   Methodology

The control algorithms of the infusion pump are constituted with the speed of the DC motor and flow rate of the infusion pump. The motor considered here for the simulation is the DC motor used widely for the medical applications, and its manufacturer specification for the motor is employed. The classical control algorithms incorporated for the overall pump with the pump actuation unit are:

- Proportional Integral Derivative (PID) controller
- Linear Quadratic Gaussian (LQG)

3.1   PID Controller

The block diagram of the infusion pump with the PID controller is given in Fig. 3.

The transfer function for the operation of the infusion pump is the product of the gain and the speed of the DC motor interfaced. The flow rate Q is identified from u

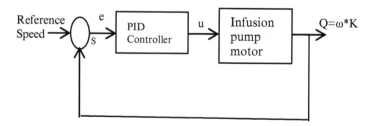

Fig. 3 Control strategy of an infusion pump with a PID controller

and the transfer function of the speed of the motor. Hence the transfer function $Q(s)$ is $Q(s) = k^* \omega(s)$

$$Q(s) = K * \frac{\omega(s)}{e(s)} = K * \frac{K_T}{\left(L_a(s) + R_a\right)\left(Js + B\right) + \left(K_b K_T\right)} \tag{1}$$

In several industrial control applications, to obtain a stable response to the traditional controller, the PID controller is widely implemented. To the infusion pump considered, the process plant is of brushed micro DC motor. Micromotors are prominent in most medical equipment. The transient response of such a motor interfaced with the infusion pump is analyzed [15]. The mathematical representations of the PID controller are given below. Equation 2 shown is used to tune the flow rate $Q(s)$ of the infusion pump:

$$u(t) = K_p e(t) + K_i \int_0^t e(\tau) d(\tau) + K_d \frac{de(t)}{dt} \tag{2}$$

where $u(t)$ is the controller output, $e(t)$ is an error, and K_p, K_i, K_d are the controller gains of the controller and tuned using Z-N method. The time response analysis has been plotted. Time response analyses are important as for the optimal infusion to the patient, the important parameter of the response curve such as rise time and settling time becomes crucial for the optimal infusion. The infusion should be quick infusion; hence the analysis of the quick rise time and optimal settling time is needed for the analysis [16, 17]. The PID controller is suitable for an infusion pump that is not susceptible to disturbances. The response obtained is shown in the results section.

3.1.1 Controller Tuning

In this section, the PID controller tuning is implemented with Particle Swarm Optimization (PSO) algorithm [18]. The PSO algorithm assigns values for K_p, K_i, and K_d and computes the objective function (OF). This process continues until the J exceeds J_{min}. The implementation diagram is shown in Fig. 4.

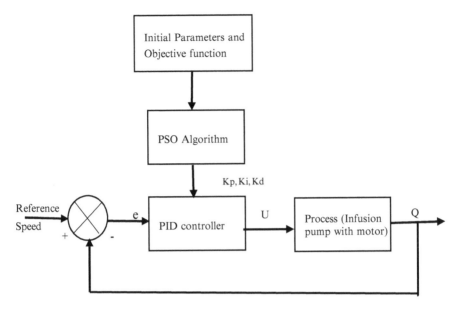

Fig. 4 PID controller with PSO for an infusion pump

PSO

PSO is an optimization algorithm, developed due to the inspiration of social interactions in the behavior of birds and schools of fish. It is widely applied due to its high computational efficiency in several design problems.

Compared to other stochastic optimization approaches, PSO has better search efficiency with faster, stable convergence rates and is considered as an efficient optimal algorithm [19, 20].

The following steps are followed to implement PSO:

1. Initialize swarm: Particles are generated randomly between the minimum and maximum limits of N population size parameter values.
2. Evaluate cost function: Based on the performance criteria, the objective function values are evaluated.
3. Initialize p_{best} and g_{best}: From step 2, initial values of swarm particles are considered as initial p_{best}. The best value among the p_{best} is considered as g_{best}.
4. Evaluate velocity and updating swarm: Computation of new velocity for each particle is carried out. The position of a particle is updated using cost function and on computation; if the new value of p_{best} is better, the new value will be set and g_{best} is updated in correspondence to the p_{best}.
5. Stop conditions: Once the stop conditions are fulfilled, the optimal values are the positions of particles which is p_{best}. The iteration has to be performed until the optimal values are attained.

The performance of PSO algorithm is purely based on the fitness function which controls the optimization. The values are chosen to maximize or minimize the domain and preference constraints. The minimization of J and selection of D in-universe U have to be performed without loss. The fitness function or objective function is set to satisfy the required parameters chosen [21]. In the case of the infusion pump, the parameters concentrated to optimize are rise time t_r and settling time t_s. Further, the optimized values are based on the reduction of t_r; t_s has to obtain as best fit for K_p, K_i, and K_d. The output response obtained is shown in the result section.

3.2   *Linear Quadratic Gaussian*

In practical conditions, the infusion pump is prone to noise. It can be a measurement or process noise. Optimal controllers such as LQG are suitable and efficient where noise and disturbances are always prominent in the system. Linear Quadratic Gaussian (LQG) is an optimal controller that implements Kalman filter to estimate noise [16, 22]. Figure 5 displays the block diagram of the DC motor with LQG. In the block diagram, it is clear that the plant is the electric motor specified for the infusion pump. The manufacturer details of the motor chosen have been considered for the simulation of the required parameters; hence the flow rate Q is achieved. The desired control parameters are verified by monitoring the external noise w and v using LQG optimizer by driving the controller u [23].

Equations involved in LQG are given below.

The cost function for LQG $J(u)$ is written as

$$J(u) = \frac{1}{2}\int_0^\infty \left(x^\mathsf{T} + 2x^\mathsf{T}Nu + u^\mathsf{T}Ru\right)dt \qquad (3)$$

where, N is the value between control effort and the performance of regulation. The state feedback matrix which $u(t)$ is given as $u(t) = -k*x(t)$ is needed to minimize $J(u)$.

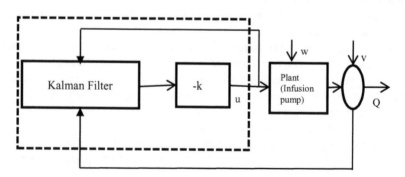

Fig. 5 LQG controller for an infusion pump

Further, k which is the gain matrix should be solved algebraically using Riccati equation. The Riccati equation is given as

$$A^{\mathrm{T}}s + sA - (sB + N)R^{-1}(B^{\mathrm{T}}s + N^{\mathrm{T}}) + Q = 0 \tag{4}$$

where, s is a matrix and k should be obtained from s. The equation is expressed as

$$K = R^{-1}(B^{\mathrm{T}}s + N^{\mathrm{T}}) \tag{5}$$

Further, the Kalman gain has to be determined for the infusion pump. In general, the process noise Q and measurement noise R is obtained as

$$Q = E[ww^{\mathrm{T}}] \quad \text{and} \quad R = E[ww^{\mathrm{T}}]. \tag{6}$$

The next step is to find the Kalman gain for the system model. The predictor, covariance matrix, and the gain value for the Kalman filter will be computed for the infusion pump. The infusion pump model is designed with LQG, and hence the transient response of the plant is plotted. The control parameters such as t_r, t_s have to be analyzed to verify the stability of the infusion pump system. The rise time and settling time are 0.221 s and 0.4 s. The values obtained are better when compared with the traditional PID controller [24, 25].

The following steps are implemented:

- The transfer function for the infusion pump system is designed.
- Linear Quadratic optimal controller implementation in the form of LQG. The cost function J value is minimized based on the Q and R values.
- Identifying P by computing the algebraic Riccati equation.
- Identifying Kalman gain.

4 Results and Discussion

The parameters needed to be analyzed for an infusion pump are optimum flow rate, minimized dead time, and lag time. The dead time and lag time can be identified from the flow rate obtained. If the infusion pump design is based on a regular closed loop control system, the lag time and dead time will be more as the rise time and settling time obtained is more [26]. The comparison of the rise time for different controllers is tabulated, and the plotted graphs are shown in Figs. 6, 7, and 8. Table 1 is provided with the comparison of the control parameters for the infusion pump.

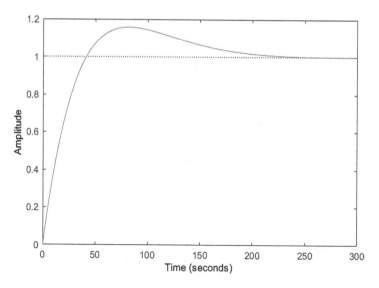

Fig. 6 Time response analysis with PID controller

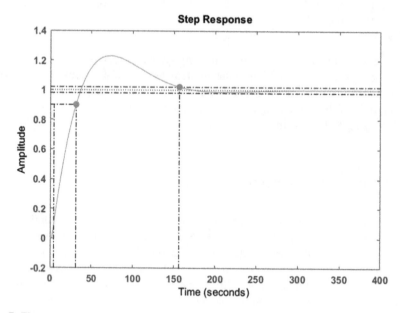

Fig. 7 Time response analysis with PID controller tuned with PSO

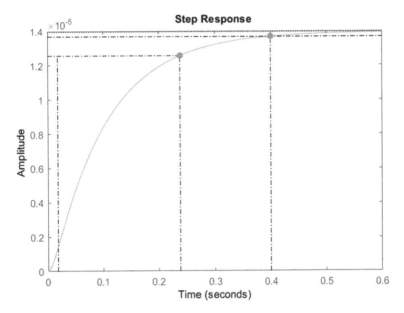

Fig. 8 Time response analysis with LQG

Table 1 Control parameter comparison

Control technique	Rise time t_r (s)	Settling time t_s (s)
PID controller	30.9	194
PID tuned with PSO	26.6	156
LQG	0.221	0.4

5 Conclusion

The performance of an infusion pump is influenced by its optimum flow rate, which depends on the speed of the pump and its motor. Once the optimum speed of the pump based on the flow rate is achieved, other influential parameters such as dead time and lag time are also reduced. The inclusion of a pump with a motor in the pumping system should be controlled with rapid rise time and stability. To achieve these results, a conventional PID controller and PID controller with PSO and LQG an optimum controller are implemented. The results are obtained by the prediction of tuning as required for the system according to the flow rate of the drug to the patient. The time response analysis and stability of the system are verified initially for a closed loop system without any control strategies. The rise time and the settling time with the PID controller are 30.9 and 194s. The PID gain parameters tuned with PSO resulted in 26.6 s and 156 s. For stability attainment, pole replacement has been done and in addition to this, LQG strategy is incorporated and verified that the rise time is 0.221 s and settling time is 0.4 s. Furthermore, the stability is investigated based on the pole-zero plots. Transient response analysis of the LQG based implementation of the infusion pump device infers that the rise time is fast and stable with the optimal flow. The drug is then delivered to the patient more efficiently with minimized dead time and lag time.

References

1. L. Insup and O. Sokolsky, "Medical Cyber Physical Systems," *Control*, no. June, pp. 743–748, 2010, doi: https://doi.org/10.1145/1837274.1837463.
2. T. D. Brown, D. S. Grady, and M. Michael, "Implementation of Smart Pump Technology With Home Infusion Providers," doi: https://doi.org/10.1097/NAN.0000000000000302.
3. I. Lee *et al.*, "Challenges and Research Directions in Medical Cyber-Physical Systems," *Proc. IEEE*, vol. 100, no. 1, pp. 75–90, 2012, doi: https://doi.org/10.1109/JPROC.2011.2165270.
4. B. W. Bequette, "Challenges and progress in the development of a closed-loop artificial pancreas," *Proc. Am. Control Conf.*, vol. 36, no. 2, pp. 4065–4071, 2012, doi: https://doi.org/10.1109/acc.2012.6315593.
5. F. Engbers, "Pump pitfalls and practicalities," *Total Intraven. Anesth. Target Control. Infusions*, pp. 329–340, 2017, doi: https://doi.org/10.1007/978-3-319-47609-4.
6. R. A. Peterfreund and J. H. Philip, "Critical parameters in drug delivery by intravenous infusion," *Expert Opin. Drug Deliv.*, vol. 10, no. 8, pp. 1095–1108, 2013, doi: https://doi.org/10.1517/17425247.2013.785519.
7. M. Baeckert *et al.*, "Performance of modern syringe infusion pump assemblies at low infusion rates in the perioperative setting," *Br. J. Anaesth.*, vol. 124, no. 2, pp. 173–182, 2020, doi: https://doi.org/10.1016/j.bja.2019.10.007.
8. J. Chua and A. Ratnavadivel, "Comparison of flow pressures in different 3-way infusion devices: An in-vitro study," *Patient Saf. Surg.*, vol. 12, no. 1, pp. 1–6, 2018, doi: https://doi.org/10.1186/s13037-018-0165-1.
9. R. Hovorka *et al.*, "Nonlinear model predictive control of glucose concentration in subjects with type 1 diabetes," *Physiol. Meas.*, vol. 25, no. 4, pp. 905–920, 2004, doi: https://doi.org/10.1088/0967-3334/25/4/010.
10. R. A. Snijder, *Physical causes of dosing errors in patients receiving multi-infusion therapy*. 2016.
11. M. A. Lovich, M. E. Kinnealley, N. M. Sims, and R. A. Peterfreund, "The delivery of drugs to patients by continuous intravenous infusion: Modeling predicts potential dose fluctuations depending on flow rates and infusion system dead volume," *Anesth. Analg.*, vol. 102, no. 4, pp. 1147–1153, 2006, doi: https://doi.org/10.1213/01.ane.0000198670.02481.6b.
12. R. Hu and C. Li, "The design of an intelligent insulin pump," *Proc. 2015 4th Int. Conf. Comput. Sci. Netw. Technol. ICCSNT 2015*, no. ICCSNT, pp. 736–739, 2016, doi: https://doi.org/10.1109/ICCSNT.2015.7490848.
13. G. Cocha, J. Rapallini, O. Rodriguez, C. Amorena, H. Mazzeo, and C. E. Drattellis, "Intelligent Insulin Pump Design," *Congr. Argentino Ciencias la Inform. y Desarro. Investig. CACIDI 2018*, pp. 7–10, 2018, doi: https://doi.org/10.1109/CACIDI.2018.8584364.
14. S. Uniyal and A. Sikander, "A Novel Design Technique for Brushless DC Motor in Wireless Medical Applications," *Wirel. Pers. Commun.*, vol. 102, no. 1, pp. 369–381, 2018, doi: https://doi.org/10.1007/s11277-018-5845-8.

15. S. Galijašević, Š. Mašić, S. Smaka, A. Akšamović, and D. Balić, "Parameter identification and digital control of speed of a permanent magnet DC motors," *2011 23rd Int. Symp. Information, Commun. Autom. Technol. ICAT 2011*, no. 1, 2011, doi: https://doi.org/10.1109/ICAT.2011.6102120.

16. M. R. Qader, "Identifying the optimal controller strategy for DC motors," *Arch. Electr. Eng.*, vol. 68, no. 1, pp. 101–114, 2019, doi: https://doi.org/10.24425/aee.2019.125983.

17. T. Kealy and A. O'dwyer, "Analytical ISE calculation and optimum control system design," *Proc. Irish Signals Syst. Conf.*, pp. 418–423, 2003, [Online]. Available: http://arrow.dit.ie/engscheleart.

18. V. Vishal, V. Kumar, K. P. S. Rana, and P. Mishra, "Comparative Study of Some Optimization Techniques Applied to DC Motor Control," *IEEE Int. Adv. Comput. Conf.*, pp. 1342–1347, 2014, doi: https://doi.org/10.1109/IAdCC.2014.6779522.

19. V. Sankardoss and P. Geethanjali, "PMDC Motor Parameter Estimation Using Bio-Inspired Optimization Algorithms," *IEEE Access*, vol. 5, pp. 11244–11254, 2017, doi: https://doi.org/10.1109/ACCESS.2017.2679743.

20. S. Das, S. Das, and K. Maharatna, "Control strategy for anaesthetic drug dosage with interaction among human physiological organs using optimal fractional order PID controller," *Int. Conf. Control. Instrumentation, Energy Commun. CIEC 2014*, pp. 66–70, 2014, doi: https://doi.org/10.1109/CIEC.2014.6959051.

21. A. Madadi and M. M. Motlagh, "Optimal Control of DC motor using Grey Wolf Optimizer Algorithm," *Tech. J. Eng. Appl.*, pp. 373–379, 2014.

22. R. N. Banavar and V. Aggarwal, "A loop transfer recovery approach to the control of an electro-hydraulic actuator," *Control Eng. Pract.*, vol. 6, no. 7, pp. 837–845, 1998, doi: https://doi.org/10.1016/S0967-0661(98)00066-5.

23. M. A. Aravind, N. Saikumar, and N. S. Dinesh, "Optimal position control of a DC motor using LQG with EKF," *2017 Int. Conf. Mech. Syst. Control Eng. ICMSC 2017*, no. 2, pp. 149–154, 2017, doi: https://doi.org/10.1109/ICMSC.2017.7959461.

24. B. A. Angelico, F. Y. Toriumi, F. D. S. Barbosa, and G. P. Das Neves, "On Guaranteeing Convergence of Discrete LQG/LTR When Augmenting It with Forward PI Controllers," *IEEE Access*, vol. 5, pp. 27203–27210, 2017, doi: https://doi.org/10.1109/ACCESS.2017.2768160.

25. J. V. Alamelu and A. Mythili, "Examination of Control Parameters for Medical Grade Insulin Pump," *Int. J. Eng. Adv. Technol.*, vol. 9, no. 1S3, pp. 19–22, 2019, doi: https://doi.org/10.35940/ijeat.a1005.1291s319.

26. J. Brindley, "Undertaking drug calculations for intravenous medicines and infusions," *Nurs. Stand.*, vol. 32, no. 20, pp. 55–63, 2018, doi: https://doi.org/10.7748/ns.2018.e11029.

Automated Detection of Normal and Cardiac Heart Disease Using Chaos Attributes and Online Sequential Extreme Learning Machine

Ram Sewak Singh, Demissie Jobir Gelmecha, Dereje Tekilu Aseffa, Tadesse Hailu Ayane, and Devendra Kumar Sinha

Abstract Cardiovascular diseases (CVDs) are major reason of mortality in the world population, and the numeral of cases is up surging every year. The mortality rate due to coronary artery disease (CAD) and congestive heart failure (CHF) is higher than any other type of CVDs. Therefore, an early detection and diagnosis of CAD and CHF patients are essential. For this, an automated noninvasive approach has been proposed to detect CAD and CHF patients using attributes extracted from heart rate variability (HRV) signal. The automated scheme is based on chaos attributes extracted from heart rate variability signal (HRV), dimension reduction of attributes such as Generalized Discriminant Analysis (GDA) and online sequential extreme learning machine(OSELM). For this study, the HRV database of normal sinus rhythm (NSR), CHF, and CAD subjects have been taken from physionet.org website. The numerical results have shown that GDA with Gaussian kernel function and OSELM with sine activation function achieved accuracy (AC) of 99.34% and sensitivity (SE) of 99.32% for NSR-CAD group, and AC and SE of **100%** were achieved for NSR-CHF group.

Keywords Chaos attributes · Classification performance · Box plot · Activation function

R. S. Singh (✉) · D. J. Gelmecha · D. T. Aseffa · T. H. Ayane
Electronics & Communication Engineering Department, School of Electrical Engineering
& Computing, Adama Science & Technology University, Adama, Ethiopia
e-mail: ram.singh@astu.edu.et

D. K. Sinha
Mechanical Design & Manufacturing Engineering Department, Center of Excellence in
Advanced Manufacturing Engineering, School of Mechanical, Chemical & Material
Engineering, Adama Science & Technology University, Adama, Ethiopia

© The Author(s), under exclusive license to Springer
Nature Switzerland AG 2021
A. K. Manocha et al. (eds.), *Computational Intelligence in Healthcare*, Health
Information Science, https://doi.org/10.1007/978-3-030-68723-6_11

213

1   Introduction

According to reports from World Health Organization (WHO) Fact Sheets [1], cardiac diseases (CDs) are the major cause of death across all regions around the world excluding Africa. An approximate 17.9 million people have died in 2016 from CDs, accounting for 31% of total global deaths, up from 12.3 million in 1990 (25.8%) [2]. The CHF and CAD are two major diseases that constitute 80% of male CD deaths and 75% of female CD deaths [3, 4]. Most of deaths caused by CVDs happen all of a sudden, beginning with a ventricular fibrillation which prompts a heart failure known as sudden cardiac death (SCD) [5]. The WHO has estimated the deaths instigated by CHF to be 180 million in 2009 numbering to 2.39% of total world population of mortality [6]. According to official agencies of Institute of Health Metrics and Evaluation, specifically in India, the years of life lost attributable to CDs increased by 59% from 23.2 million in 1990 to 37 million in 2010 [7]. This figure is predicted to be much greater than the assessments based on statistical data which take into account only death certificate reports and do not consider patients who die from CAD complications [8].

As per the WHO statistical details of heart disease and stroke deaths released in April 2011, it has been able to track the occurrence of CAD worldwide (Table 1). It is noticed that among all other nations in the world, Turkmenistan seemed to have the highest mortality rate (11,665) or 30.86% of deaths worldwide recorded. The death rate is 405, 13 per 100,000 of population; hence Turkmenistan is the world's first rank country in coronary heart disease [9].

Coronary angiography, Computed tomography (CT), electrocardiogram (ECG) stress test, stress echocardiography, and myocardial perfusion imaging are common methods for diagnosis of CADs. Coronary angiography with CT is under heavy development and is expected to play a significant role in CAD diagnosis. Although being invasive, it has a relatively high precision; by analysis it was found that the sensitivity (SE) was 96.12% and the specificity (SP) was 86.98% [10]. The stress test of the ECG is relatively simple assessment for CAD and CHF. It is a simple and inexpensive method, and the results of the test specifically relates to heart functionality. This form, therefore, faced another drawback that it has a low precision as compared to 68% of SE and 77% of SP [11]. The echoes/stress test is an extension of an ECG test phase by evaluating changes in stressed ventricles activity, including exercise [12]. The benefit of this technique is to increase precision rate, but its disadvantages are due to increase in variations in the technicians as well as the system needs highly skilled personnel.

Despite recent medical and treatment advancements, CVDs remains the foremost common risk factor for mortality accounting for nearly one third of deaths worldwide. Robust and efficient diagnosis is essential for improving CVD detection and saving the life from mortality. Signal processing of heart rate variability (HRV) signal (R-R interval consecutive of PQRS morphological of ECG signal) plays a key role in decision making during diagnosis. Present techniques of HRV analysis rely mainly on qualitative visual interpretation of ECG signal and basic quantitative

Table 1 The statistical details of cardiac heart diseases like CAD, CHF, and heart stroke deaths released by WHO in 2011

Country	Deaths	Percentage (%)	Rate	World rank /192
	South America			
Guyana	924	16.41	151.35	50
Venezuela	21,165	17.66	107.26	102
Basil	133,992	13.76	81.18	134
	North America			
Honduras	6168	16.01	152.44	48
Nicaragua	3073	13.93	95.28	119
United states	445,864	21.42	80.48	135
	Australia			
Australia	24,905	21.91	60.34	162
	Africa			
Sudan	39,326	10.67	212	24
Morocco	33,760	24.40	168	36
Nigeria	71,732	4.20	121.6	80
Algeria	14,708	10.63	75.17	145
	Asia			
Turkmenistan	11,665	30.86	405.13	1
Malaysia	22,701	22.18	138.75	57
Korea (North)	27,569	16.35	113.17	91
China	1,040,692	11.71	79.72	137
	Middle East			
Iraq	26,676	14.12	214.13	22
Saudi Arabia	20,877	23.98	180.58	32
Arab Emirates	1161	19.74	94.48	120
	Europe			
Ukraine	338,108	49.36	399.79	2
Romania	56,727	26.16	155.04	45
Poland	79,036	26.93	122.34	78
Switzerland	9804	19.91	52.18	175

measurements of cardiovascular function [13]. To maximize the predictive value of cardiac diseases, more developed HRV signal processing methods are required to allow better quantification of phenotypes in the ECG morphology.

The big data analysis and the availability of high cloud computing in recent years have guided rapid innovation of artificial intelligence (AI) technology in cardiac disease prediction and detection [14]. Machine learning (ML) strategies based on features extracted from HRV, treatment rely on optimization techniques/modeling techniques which learn from the past experiment was conducted to find by recognizing hidden and multiple concerns of HRV signal. Many authors already demonstrated the ECG-based cardiovascular diseases diagnosis like detection and prediction of CAD and CHF with ML. The ML detection and prediction efficiency

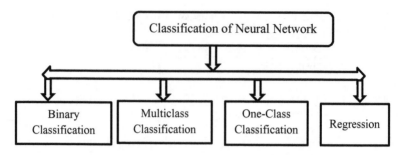

Fig. 1 Exploration areas of neural network for cardiac diseases detection and prediction

based on features of HRV signal have the greatest potential to reduce the burden of heart disease by enabling faster and more efficient diagnostic decision taking [15].

A new fast learning neural classifier for single-hidden-layer feedforward networks (SLFNs) and modeled extreme learning machine (ELM) [16, 17] have recently been investigated to optimize the effectiveness of SLFN. Unlike neural network machine learning (like back-propagation (BP) models), which may experience difficulties in automatically tuning process parameter (learning speeds, having to learn epochs, etc.) and/or local minima, ELM is entirely systematically deployed without recursive tuning, and, in principle, so users do not need to interfere. In fact, ELM's learning speed is incredibly high as compared to other conventional approaches. In the ELM technique, the learning specifications of hidden neurons include input synaptic weights which can be individually allocated randomly as well as the network solved analytically can be mathematically calculated via simple and standardized reverse process. In the training phase, the ELM has the ability of learning fast without time-consuming process of learning with a corrected nonlinear activation function [18]. In addition, the ELM methodology can provide a good result in generalization. Furthermore, the standard ELM's fundamental estimation capability with an additive or RBF activation function [19, 20] has also been established. A neural network classifier can be used in four possible ways, shown in Fig. 1. Online version of the classification problem is needed due to the rapidly growing need of streaming data [21, 22]. For this, online sequential extreme learning machine (OSELM) which is modified version of ELM has been employed to binary classifies the cardiac heart diseases (either healthy or CAD, CHF).

2 Methodology

For detection and classification of CAD and CHF, nine different chaos attributes were extracted from preprocessed and segmented HRV database. The chaos and nonlinear features, namely, correlation dimension (CD), detrended fluctuation analysis (DFA), aApproximate eEntropy (ApEn), the results of the Poincare plot as SD1/SD2 ratio, Hurst exponent(HE), Permutation entropy (PE), improved multiscale permutation entropy (IMPE), and cumulative bi-correlation (CBC) have been extracted from segmented HRV database. Figure 2 shows a proposed adaptive ML model for CAD and CHF detection. All the features are not sensitive to escalation for interpretation and comprehension of healthy and CAD database. Therefore, they were ranked using Fisher score ranking method. The most important top five ranked attributes were applied to attributes space transformation technique as Generalized Discriminant Analysis (GDA). The GDA transfer top ten attributes to a new attribute. The values of new feature were first regularized in the range of -1 to 1, after this, fed to online sequential extreme learning machine (OSELM) having sigmoid, hardlim, RBF, and sine activation function binary classifier. The simulated results show that GDA with Gaussian or RBF kernel function and (OSELM) classifier with sine activation function achieved better accuracy (AC), sensitivity (SE), specificity (SP), and positive prediction value (PPV) as compared to other considered kernel function.

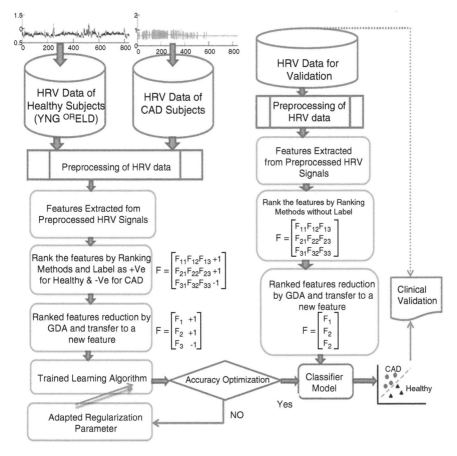

Fig. 2 Framework of the proposed ML for cardiac heart disease detection. The right part of ML has been employed for training and left part for validation of ML

2.1 Fundamentals of ELM

The authors [17, 23] have stated that the fundamentals of ELM can be described in three phases for given training features (X) and class label (T) set defined as $\{X_K, T_K\}_{K=1, 2...., M}$ and $X_K = \{x_{K1}, x_{K2}, ..., x_{Kn}\}^t \in R^n$. Here M, K, and t represent number of samples, number of input features to the n input layer, and transpose of the input features matrix. Notation $T_K \in \{-1, 1\}$ represents output corresponding to sample X_K for binary classification. ELM consist of m number of hidden layers' nodes with activation function G (.) between input and output layer. The construction of ELM is shown in Fig. 3.

Following three phases involved in learning of ELM

1. First take random value of input weights $(W) = \{W_{m1}, W_{m2}, ..., W_{mn}\}^t$ and biases $B = \{B_1, B_2, ...B_m\}$ of hidden nodes (N). This value does not change during learning and validation of ELM.
2. Compute the hidden layer (N) output by using activation function $G(.)$ as $G(W X + B)$:

$$N = \begin{bmatrix} \varnothing(W_1 X_1 + B_1,) & \cdots & \varnothing(W_m X_1 + B_m) \\ \vdots & \cdots & \vdots \\ \varnothing(W_1 X_n + B_1,) & \cdots & \varnothing(W_m X_n + B_m) \end{bmatrix}_{n \times m}$$

3. Compute the output weight $\beta = N^\dagger T$, where $N^\dagger$ represents Moore-Penrose generalized inverse of N and $\beta = \{\beta_1 \beta_2, ... \beta_m\}^t$ weight between hidden layers and output node. Minimize the learning error as well as norm of the output weights by $\|N\beta - T\|^2$ and $\|\beta\|^2$.

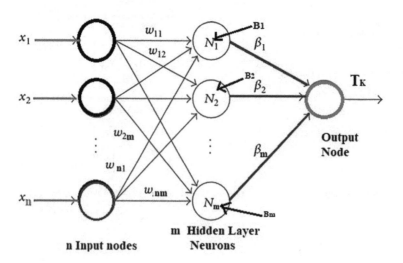

Fig. 3 Represents construction of extreme learning machine. It consists of input nodes, hidden layer neurons and output node

2.2 Analytical Concept of OSELM

The concept of batch learning of ELM originates the analytical derivation of OSELM [23]. The training data can be viewed sequentially, i.e., one or the other by one or block by block of constant or varying duration, and this process can be eliminated for training once training has been completed. It is processed in two stages:

First stage: Firstly set $L = 0$, where L denotes Lth block of data. At first, training data (M_0) should not be less than m. For this training data, output of hidden layer (N_0) is defined as $N_0 = [F(W_i, b_i, X_j)]$, where $i = 1$ to m and $j = 1$ to M_0, F is an activation function, weight between hidden layer and output (β_0) is defined as $\beta_0 = P_0 N_0^{\mathrm{T}} T_0$, where $P_0 = \left(N_0^{\mathrm{T}} N_0 \right)^{-1}$, and T_0 denotes the class level (M_0) [22].

Second stage sequential: In this stage, the output of partial hidden layer neurons (N_{L+1}) is evaluated using Moore-Penrose inverse ($N^\dagger$) same as ELM where $(L + 1)$thth block of new observation ($N)_{L+1}$ denotes number of training data in $(L + 1)$th block. The output weight matrix $\beta^{(L+1)}$ is calculated as follows:

$$\beta^{(L+1)} = \beta^{(L)} + P_{L+1} N_{L+1}^{\mathrm{T}} \left(T_{L+1} - N_{L+1} \beta^L \right)$$

Where $P_{L+1} = P_L - P_L N_{L+1}^{\mathrm{T}} \left(I + N_{L+1} P_L N_{k+1}^{\mathrm{T}} \right)^{-1} N_{L+1} P_L.$

3 Box Plot

The box plot is a graphic approach representing five numerical statistics of a sample group in its conventional form in order to visualize its scattering and skewness [24]. All descriptions are concentrated on the median and refer to the smaller measurement, a first half part of the sample median (first quartile, $Q1$), the median (second quartile, $Q2$), the second half of the sample median (third quartile, $Q3$), and the largest assessment. The range between the first and third quartiles is defined as the interquartile range (IQR) and offers an indicator of data distribution (IQR = $Q3 - Q1$). The IQR refers visually to the display's only box, and it occupies about 50 percent of findings closest to the mean. The highest and the lowest findings are those which are beyond the lines (or whiskers) that link the IQR to a smallest or largest non-outlier value (e.g., within 1.5 IQR). In addition, the conventional box plot may also have a probability distribution of approximately 95% around the median. The labeling and structure of a box plot is shown in Fig. 4.

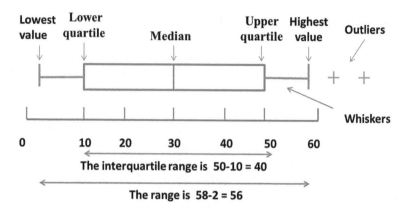

Fig. 4 A brief labeling with interquartile range, outliers median, and structure of a box plot

4 Attributes' Dimension Reduction by Generalized Discriminant Analysis

Dimension reduction relates to the procedure of translating a collection of large-scale data into smaller-dimensional data ensuring it eloquently conveys similar information. Usually these methods are used to solve ML problems in order to achieve better attributes for a classification, detection, and prediction of CDs. The box plot of nine features of NSR-CAD and NSR-CHF are shown in Fig. 5a, b which reveals that some considered attributes convey similar information in the form of median IQ value. In these cases, differentiating between the two classes (group) is a challenge. An attribute's dimension transformation technique would be very useful in these cases [25, 26]. Various methodologies have been applied to minimize the classification size of data attributes [27–29]. In this chapter, Generalized Discriminant Analysis (GDA) has been employed for dimension reduction of attributes. An advantage of this method is that space reduction of the input attribute's dimension and discriminating of features are based on nonlinear kernel function [30].

The formulation of GDA has been explained as follows: assume that given training sample set X has α attribute vectors out of β classes' level, let us assume that X_{ij} signifies the jth HRV attributes vector in the ith class, β_i is the class size of the ith class, and ψ is a nonlinear mapping function to facilitate the features data of X which is plotted into upper dimensional attributes space. $\psi : X_k \in R^f \rightarrow \psi(X_k) \in R^F$, $F \gg f$. The interpretations of $\psi(X_k)$ are assumed to be concentrated in space F. Before defining the projection of the input training sample set X into a new set Y by worth of the GDA, two matrices of the within $-$ class scatter matrix ω and the between class scatter matrix ρ in space F are formulated as

$$\omega = \frac{1}{\alpha} \sum_{\beta}^{i=1} \sum_{\beta_i}^{j=1} \psi\left(X_{ij}\right)\psi^t\left(X_{ij}\right) \tag{1}$$

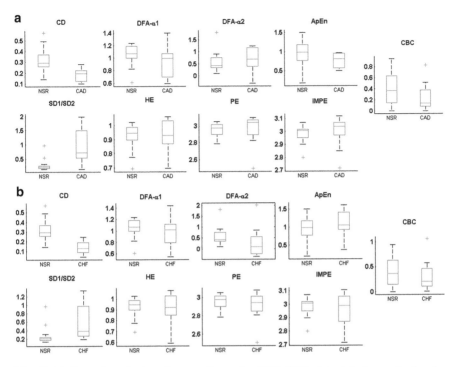

Fig. 5 (**a**) Box plot of nine chaos attributes for NSR-CAD dataset before reduction by GDA. (**b**) Box plot of nine chaos attributes for NSR-CHF dataset before reduction by GDA

$$\rho = \frac{1}{\alpha} \sum_{\beta}^{i=1} \beta_i \left(\sum_{\beta_i}^{j=1} \psi\left(X_{ij}\right) \left(\sum_{\beta_i}^{r=1} \psi\left(X_{ir}\right) \right)^t \right) \tag{2}$$

The GDA's main purpose is to find the projections matrix ∂ so that it can maximize inter-class attrition and reduce intra-class attrition in space F, which is similar to executing the complex Fisher criteria maximizing issue:

$$\partial = \arg\max_{\partial} \left(\frac{\omega^t \rho_\partial}{\omega^t \omega_\partial} \right) \tag{3}$$

The projection vector ∂ is the eigenvector of the matrix $\omega^{-1}\rho$ related with the eigenvalue $\lambda = \omega^t\rho_\partial/\omega^t\omega_\partial$. All solutions of the ∂ lie in the range of (X). As a result, there exist extension coefficients μ_k such that

$$\partial = \sum_{\beta}^{k=1} \mu_k \psi\left(X_k\right) \tag{4}$$

Assume that the kernel function is represented as $K(X_k, X_l) = K_{kl} = \psi(X_k)\psi(X_l)$ and acting the eigen matrix disintegration on the kernel vector as $ED = (K_{kl})_{k, l = 1, 2, ..., ; a}$; hence, α normalized extension coefficient for each projection vector $\mu = \mu / \sqrt{\mu^t K_\mu}$ is calculated. Now, for an attribute matrix X from the test HRV dataset, the projection on the kth eigenvector ∂_k can be computed as

$$Y^k = \partial^{k^t} \psi(X) = \sum_\alpha^{j=1} \partial_j^k \psi(X_j) \psi(X) = \sum_\alpha^{j=1} \partial_j^k K(X_j, X) \tag{5}$$

where ∂_j^k indicates the jth extension factor of the ith eigenvector. For the measurement of the reductions of the function element, $\beta - 1$ eigenvectors vectors connected to the first highest nonzero $\beta - 1$ eigenvalues values are assigned to form the mapping function $(TM)^t = [\partial^1, \partial^2, ..., \partial^{\beta - 1}]$. Therefore, every one HRV feature vector is projected into a new coordinates using the $\beta - 1$ projection vectors [30]. It implies also that optimal solution of eigenvectors for the data is transformed is usually equal to $\beta - 1$. In this chapter, assuming that the class level is 2, i.e., binary class, thus GDA transforms the dimension of nine attribute to a new attribute.

5   Chaos Attributes

5.1   Correlation Dimension

The *correlation dimension* (CD) is a measurement of the fractal dimension of the space taken up by a set of possible points. For M sample points $X(1), X(2), ..., X(M)$, with an embedding space $(m) \in R^m$, the CD is defined as

$$CD = \lim_{r \to 0} \frac{\log(C(r))}{\log(r)} \tag{6}$$

A   correlation   function $C(r)$ is   represented   as

$$C(r) = \frac{1}{M^2} \times \left(\text{number of pairs of } (i,j) \text{ KeywordsIndustry 4.0 with } S(i,j) < r \right),$$

where $S(i, j) = | X_i - X_j |$ in millisecond and $1 \leq i < j \leq M$ [31]. In this work, $m = 10$ and *filtering level* $(r) = \{0.0050...0.1\}$ are taken for the HRV sample analysis. The step to calculate of r value using data extracted from random walker.

5.2   Detrended Fluctuation Analysis

Detrended fluctuation analysis (DFA) is an alteration of root − mean − square (RMS) and based on a random walk which is implemented to assess the chaos of HRV signal. The RMS fluctuation of combined and detrended of N-N time series is called DFA. It is defined as

$$F(n) = \sqrt{\frac{1}{M} \sum_{M}^{k=1} \left[Y(k) - Y_n(k) \right]^2}$$
(7)

Where $Y_n(k)$ is the kth value of integrated $N − N$ time series data of total length k [32]. The α represents the slope of the line relating log $F(n)$ to log (n). Often two particular linear regions on the log − log plot are utilized to represent the short-term α_1, for this $n_1 = 4$, calculated $F(n_1)$ and the long − term scaling α_2, for this $n_2 = 300$ calculated $F(n_2)$.

5.3   Sample Entropy

The application of sample entropy (SampEn) for HRV analysis has been discussed to detect cardiac disease in [33, 34]. For an HRV time series $X(1)$, $X(2)$, ..., $X(M)$, assume $X_m(i)$ denotes the m points $X_i, X_{i+1}, ..., X_{i+m-1}$ which is known as a template and can be reflected a matrix of length m. An example where all the components of the matrix $X_m(j)$ are within a distance r of $X_m(i)$ is known as a template match. Let D_i indicate the number of template matches with $X_m(i)$ and C_i indicate the number of template matches with $X_{m+1}(i)$. The number $P_i = \dfrac{C_i}{D_i}$ is an estimate of the conditional probability that the point X_{j+m} is within r of X'_{i+m-1} given that $X_m(j)$ matches $X_m(i)$. The SampEn is defined for m points:

$$\text{SampEn}(m,r,M) = -\log\left(\sum_{M-m}^{i=1} C_i / \sum_{M-m}^{i=1} D_i \right)$$
(8)

where m is an integer number and r is a positive real number. In this work, standard value $m = 2$ and $r = 0.2 \times$ std. deviation (NN) were used for HRV analysis.

5.4   Poincare Plot as SD1/SD2 Ratio

The Poincare plot investigation is a nonlinear and graphical method to assess the chaos of NN interval (HRV). This plot scatters the graph of present NN intervals and previous NN interval. Two neighboring NN intervals signify a single point in the scattered plot. The first *NN* interval (NN_i) denotes the X-abscissa, and the second interval as NN_{i+1} denotes Y-ordinate. Standard deviation one (SD_1) for short *NN* interval and standard deviation two (SD_2) for long *NN* intervals were calculated for chaos analysis of HRV signal. For calculation of these intervals, we have taken 150 samples for short and 350 samples for long out of 500 *NN* intervals. The value of SD1/SD2 may likewise be listed to describe the relationship between short and long terms [35].

5.5   Hurst Exponent

Hurst exponent (HE) is a method of measuring the smoothness of the data from a fractal time series. It is based on the asymptotic execution of the rescaled observation range:

$$HE = \frac{\log\big(R(n)/S(n)\big)}{\log(T)} \tag{9}$$

Here *n* is the analysis time period (like $n = M$, $M/2$, $M/4$…where 2, 4, 8) which is referred to as blocks size, $R(n)$ is the range of the first *n* values, and $S(n)$ is their standard deviation (S.D). $R(n)/S(n)$ is the respective rescaled range value, and T is the population sample length. *M* is observations of a time series [36].

5.6   Permutation Entropy

Permutation entropy (PE) is a suitable test for exposing the nonlinearity of HRV time series. Due to its easy concept, the PE has also been studied most extensively of physiological signals, based on fewer features, computationally and fairly immune to interference and artifacts. For the data series $\{X(i), i = 1, 2, 3…M\}$, the PE can be represented as the entropy for both the sequences and ordering of the K symbols (O) [37]:

$$H = -\sum_{K}^{L=1} \pi_L \ln\big(\pi_L\big) \tag{10}$$

where $\pi_1 \pi_2 ……\pi_K$ signify the probability distribution of every symbol series [38] and $\sum_{L=1}^{K} \pi_K = 1$. In this work, standard value $O = 4$ and time delay of 1 are chosen for HRV analysis.

5.7   Improved Multiscale Permutation Entropy

The *multiscale permutation entropy* (MPE) method cannot provide a consistent investigation for short HRV time series. An improved MPE (IMPE) has been presented to overcome this problem [39] to define a real-valued time series $\{X(i), i = 1, 2, 3,..., M\}$ of length M for IPEM formulation with such an embedding space $\{(m) \in R^m\}$. Many subsequent coarse-grained versions [40] are set by averaging the sets of data series within equally spaced extending period S frames, which is termed the scale factor. Therefore, in this process chosen, separate time series is $\eta_i^s \mid (i = 1, 2...S)$. For a given scale factor S and embedding *dimension m*, there is a different calculation of the *probability entropy* of each of $\eta_i^s \mid (i = 1, 2...S)$; this then measures the average values of probability entropy. It is defined as

$$\text{IMPE}(X,S,m) = \frac{1}{S}\sum_{S}^{i=1}\text{PE}(\eta_i^s) \qquad (11)$$

For HRV analysis, standard value $m = 4$, *scale (S)* = 4 and time delay of 1 have been used.

5.8   Cumulative Bi-Correlation

The bi-correlation is the joint moment of three $NN(i)$, $NN(i + \tau)$, *and* $NN(i + 2\tau)$ samples and defined as $E[X(i); X(i + \tau); X(i + \tau_0)]$, where E denotes expected value of three samples, τ and τ_0 delays between samples. We have taken $\tau_0 = 2\,\tau$ so that the measurement of joint moment can be function of τ [41]. The bi-correlation is not commonly known for the calculation of HRV signal disorder, but the cumulative bi-correlation (CBC) was introduced for the nonlinearity test, with the constraint that the second delay (τ_0) is double the first delay (τ) [42]. For the definite set of delays, the CBC is a composite function of bi-correlation, and for each interval, the CBC is the summation of the bi-correlation's cumulative values up to the interval delay τ. The delay of 1 is chosen for NN analysis.

6   Parameters Used for Simulation

The detection and classification of CAD and CHF has been performed by 1-NLPELM using sigmoid activation function and multiquadric functional additive node. The multiquadric function was considered for RBF hidden nodes. The sigmoid function and multiquadric function are defined as $\varnothing(A, B, X) = 1/1 + \exp - (A^tX + B)$ and $\varnothing(A,B,X) = \sqrt{(\|X - A\|_2^2 + B^2}$. The optimal values of user-specified parameters like regularization parameter γ for 1-NLPELM were selected using tenfold cross-validation method. Analyzing classifier output for data-sets, the following performance parameters calculated:

$$\text{Accuracy} \left(\text{AC}\right) = \left(\text{TP} + \text{TN}\right) / \left(\text{TP} + \text{TN} + \text{FN} + \text{FP}\right) \tag{12}$$

$$\text{Sensitivity} \left(\text{SE}\right) \text{ or true positive rate} \left(\text{TPR}\right) = \text{TP} / \left(\text{TP} + \text{FN}\right) \tag{13}$$

$$\text{Specificity} \left(\text{SP}\right) \text{ or true negative rate} \left(\text{TNR}\right) = \text{TN} / \left(\text{FP} + \text{TN}\right) \tag{14}$$

$$\text{False positive rate} \left(\text{FPR}\right) = \left(1 - \text{SP}\right) \text{ using confusion matrix.} \tag{15}$$

where TP = true positive, FN = false negative, TN = true negative, and FP = false positive.

7 Results

To understand the reduction capability of GDA using RBF kernel function, the box plots of the chaos attribute for NSR-CAD and NSR-CHF datasets are shown in Fig. 5a, b and after reduction of chaos features by GDA is shown Fig. 6a, b. The box plot patterns of nine chaos features associated with datasets are positioned close to each other (median value indicated by red line in box) before reduction of attributes. After attribute space reduction by GDA method, a new attribute is generated which is well separated within the attribute dimension. So, the new feature not only pro-vides improvements in the detection capability but also makes a suitable tool for good discrimination of NSR-CAD and NSR-CHF dataset. For this reason, GDA

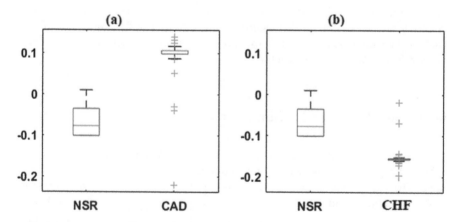

Fig. 6 Box plot, after attributes reduction by GDA with RBF kernel function for (**a**) NSR – CAD dataset (**b**) NSR – CHF dataset

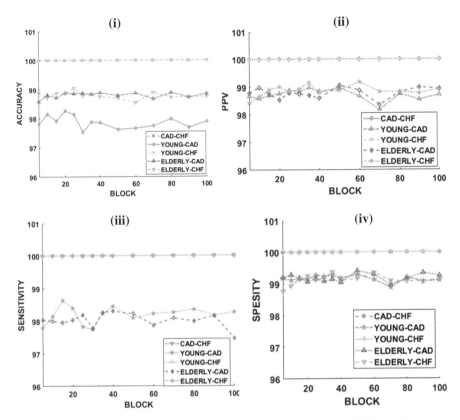

Fig. 7 Variation of classification parameters Vs. Block size when using OSELM with hardlim activation and GDA with Gaussian kernel for parameters (**i**) accuracy (**ii**) PPV (**iii**) sensitivity (**iv**) specificity

reduction scheme is an appropriate tool for better discrimination of NSR-CAD and NSR-CHF dataset.

The variation of classification parameters like PPV, SEN, and SP with respect to block size (5, 10, 15, ..., 100) for OSELM and GDA as feature reduction scheme with different kernel and activation functions is shown in Fig. 7. For evaluation of each parameter, mean of 10 cross validation with 100 times random subjects are selected from datasets for each block. To understand the effect of varying block size on a parameter, the following dataset combination of CAD – CHF, NSR(YNG) – CAD, NSR (YNG) – CHF, and NSR (ELDERLY) – CHF was used. The parameters AC, V, SEN, and SE of different datasets are plotted for OSELM classifier with hardlim activation function and GDA with Gaussian and RBF kernel as feature reduction scheme. It is observed that even after increasing the block size, there is no significant change in value of classification parameters. The simulation graph reveal that less than 40 blocks are appropriate for detection and classification of CHF and CAD subjects. So, the block size is chosen in such a way that optimum

Table 2 Results achieved by OSELM and OSELM combine with GDA

Datasets	Training				Validation			
(Training and validation size)	AC	PPV	SEN	SE	AC	PPV	SE	SP
OS − ELM with hardlim activation function								
NSR − CAD (84 × 1, 47 × 1)	100	100	100	100	81.83	79.12	76.6	87.08
NSR − CHF (80 × 1, 60 × 1)	100	100	100	100	77.07	76.17	69.84	82.65
	OS − ELM with sine activation function							
NSR − CAD (84 × 1, 47 × 1)	100	100	100	100	90.94	91.17	86.72	94.42
NSR − CHF (80 × 1, 60 × 1)	100	100	100	100	81.53	81.22	75.35	87.06
	OS − ELM with sigmoid activation function							
NSR − CAD (84 × 1, 47 × 1)	100	100	100	100	85.11	83.23	82.32	89.26
NSR − CHF (80 × 1, 60 × 1)	100	100	100	100	79.2	80.2	71.98	86.78
GDA with Gaussian Kernel + OS − ELM with sigmoid activation function								
NSR − CAD (84 × 1, 47 × 1)	100	100	100	100	98.26	98.08	97.88	98.81
NSR − CHF (80 × 1, 60 × 1)	100	100	100	100	**100**	**100**	**100**	**100**
GDA with Gaussian Kernel + OS − ELM with sine activation function								
NSR − CAD (84 × 1, 47 × 1)	100	100	100	100	98.23	98.7	97.22	99.17
NSR − CHF (80 × 1, 60 × 1)	100	100	100	100	**100**	**100**	**100**	**100**
GDA with RBF Kernel + OS − ELM with sine activation function								
NSR − CAD (84 × 1, 47 × 1)	100	100	100	100	**99.34**	**99**	**97.38**	**99.32**
NSR − CHF (80 × 1, 60 × 1)	100	100	100	100	97.87	97.41	97.99	97.96

The best classification parameters are signposted by boldface in the table

value of testing and validation parameters is achieved. The parameters for different activations function and kernel are tabulated in Table 2.

In order to determine the classification parameters and validate the performance of proposed method in terms of *AC*, PPV, SE, and SP, simulation analysis has been conducted on the dataset of various subjects. 50 samples for training and 62 samples for validation have been taken for CAD − CHF, 84 and 47 have been taken for NSR − CAD, 80 and 60 for NSR − CHF, 80 and 52 NSR − CAD, and 80 and 60 NSR − CHF datasets have been used for training and validation purpose, respectively. These standard databases have been obtained from PhysioNet website.

The performance parameters achieved by OSELM and OSEL+GDA are listed in Table 2. The numerical simulation results shows that OSELM with hardlim activation function achieved an AC, PPV, SE, and SP of 81.83, 79.12, 76.6, and 87.08, respectively, for NSR − CAD datasets while OSELM with sine activation function attained 90.94, 91.17, 86.72, and 94.42, respectively. When GDA with kernel function is combined with OSELM, the classification performance has significantly increased. For instance, GDA with RBF kernel +OSELM with sine activation function achieved classification performances 98.34, 99, 97.38, and 99.32, respectively, for NSR-CAD group. GDA with Gaussian kernel + OSELM with sine activation function produced 100% classification performances for NSR-CHF dataset. This result reveals that proposed method achieved better results as compared to OSELM + various type of activation function.

8   Discussion

Table 1 revealed that the cardiac heart diseases like CAD and CHF have also been proven to become one of the leading causes of death, which is the major reason why precise heart failure (HF) risk prediction is vitally important for preventing and treating it [43]. A quick and efficient CAD and CHF diagnosis is essential for evading a life-threatening event [44]. In addition to timeliness, AC, PPV, SE, and SP play an incredibly important role in the medical sphere, because it is linked to a person's life. There has been done a terrific and substantial number of works on the diagnosis and detection of cardiac diseases using ML techniques. In contrast, there is yet to be a gap regarding compatibility of methodology or classification algorithm suitable with datasets. However, it is demonstrated that the methodology of selection and reductions of features increased the performance and accuracy of classification models. In addition, it is also evident that classifier ensembles have demonstrated to have enhanced classification AC [45]. There are some factors that could not be ignored in health-related issues, such as time taken to execute the procedure and technical challenge that depends on the number of functions, precision, and sweeping generalization. Several researchers have focused on methodology to avoid the integration of unnecessary traits, as per assessment. Using state-of-the-art methods such as genetic algorithm (GA) in [46–48], LS-SVM in [49], information gain in [50], and F − score in [45] for attribute selection has helped to counteract the question of so many other attributes and thus decrease the processing time and the size of the computing. When an insight assessment of the articles was conducted, it was realized that certain researches have lessened the dimensionality utilizing advanced detection methods. For instance, principal component analysis (PCA) in [49, 51, 52] chaos features in [53], and minimal max significance redundancy in [54] are incredibly effective in reducing dimensions. Many research focused on obtaining the maximum accuracies through implementing methods that are exceptionally efficient and consistent, for example, GA with SVM to accomplish more than 98% AC in [46] PCA and SVM to achieve more than 99% AC in [49], PCA to gain more than overall AC in [52], and a set of bagged decision trees (DT) to obtain approximately 99%. AC in [44], some of those methods, and their prediction accuracy are shown in Table 3. What's troubling is that most of the methods were applied to small database and there's still a desperate need to test them on a broad dataset. The most research haven't addressed whether attribute reduction affects the knowledge of systems or not.

Table 3 Summary of existing methods applied for CAD and CHF disease detection and classification

Reference	Detection of subjects	Proposed scheme	Database	Accuracy (in %)
[46]	CHF	GA with SVM	CHF2DB and NSR	98.79
[49]	CAD	PCA and SVM	Long – term HRV	99.2
[51]	CAD	GA and neural network	Z-Alizadeh Sani Database	93.85
[55]	CHF and CAD	DT	A dataset of 2346 patients' records	94
[56]	Paroxysmal atrial fibrillation (AF)	SVM	AF database	87.7
[57]	CHF risk factor	Rules-based classifier.	Cleveland	86.7
[58]	CAD	Rules and fuzzy experts approach.	Advanced Medical Research Institute	84.2
[44]	CHF	Ensemble of bagged DT	PhysioNet database	98.8
[59]	sudden cardiac deaths (SCD)	t-test for feature ranking and DT, kNN, and SVM	MIT-BIH and NSR	94.7
[60]	CHF and CAD	Multilayer perceptron NN	NSR and long-term ST	97.83
[54]	CHF	DTC wavelet transform	MIT – BIH NSR, Fantasia, and BIDMC CHF	99.86
[61]	Chronic heart failure diagnosis	Least-square SVM	A dataset of 152 heart sound	95.39
[62]	HF patients' mortality	Random forest	Intelligent monitoring in ICU	82.1
[63]	Heart failure risk	Neural Networks and Long Short – term Memory network.	–	66.55
[64]	CAD	Random Forest, C5.0, and fuzzy modeling.	UCI	90.50
[65]	Heart disease (CAD,CHF,MI)	Fuzzy rules – based	Personal health record	69.22
	This paper CHF and CAD	GDA with RBF, Gaussian kernel and OSELM with sine activation	PhysioNet database	100 for CHF and 98.34 CAD

9 Conclusion

In this chapter, a new approach has been discussed for classification of coronary heart diseases such as CAD and CHF. For this, nine nonlinear features have been extracted from HRV signal. In order to enhance the detection capability of proposed model, the dimension of nine features were reduced using GDA technique. The results of the comparative study have indicated that the GDA with OSELM binary classifier outperforms as compared to other existing techniques. The GDA with Gaussian kernel + OSELM with sine activation function achieved classification performances of 100% for NSR-CHF datasets. The GDA with RBF kernel + OSELM with sine activation function attained an AC of 99.34%, PPV of 99%, and SP of 99.32% for NSR-CAD. Hence, this proposed scheme can be employed for online coronary diseases monitoring and diagnosis of CAD and CHF subjects.

References

1. B. L. Dake and C. L. Oltman, "Cardiovascular, metabolic, and coronary dysfunction in high-Fat-Fed obesity-resistant/prone rats," *Obesity*, vol. 23, no. 3, pp. 623–629, 2015, doi: https://doi.org/10.1002/oby.21009.
2. World Health Organization, "Noncommunicable Diseases. Country Perfil 2011," *World Health Organization*, 2011. http://www.who.int/nmh/publications/ncd_profiles2011/en/.
3. S. Yusuf *et al.*, "Cardiovascular Risk and Events in 17 Low-, Middle-, and High-Income Countries," *N. Engl. J. Med.*, vol. 371, no. 9, pp. 818–827, 2014, doi: https://doi.org/10.1056/NEJMoa1311890.
4. D. Prabhakaran *et al.*, "Two-year outcomes in patients admitted with non-ST elevation acute coronary syndrome: results of the OASIS registry 1 and 2." *Indian Heart J.*, vol. 57, no. 3, pp. 217–25, 2005, [Online]. Available: http://www.ncbi.nlm.nih.gov/pubmed/16196178.
5. A. Bayés De Luna, "Nueva terminología de las paredes del corazón y nueva clasificación electrocardiográfica de los infartos con onda Q basada en la correlación con la resonancia magnética," *Revista Espanola de Cardiologia*, vol. 60, no. 7, pp. 683–689, 2007.
6. S. Mendis *et al.*, "World Health Organization definition of myocardial infarction: 2008-09 revision," *Int. J. Epidemiol.*, vol. 40, no. 1, pp. 139–146, 2011, doi: https://doi.org/10.1093/ije/dyq165.
7. "Institute of Health Metrics and Evaluation. GBD Profile: India," *http://www.healthdata.org/sites/default/files/files/country_profiles/GBD/ihme_gbd_country_report_india.pdf. Accessed April 30, 2014.*
8. U. Rajendra Acharya, O. Faust, N. Adib Kadri, J. S. Suri, and W. Yu, "Automated identification of normal and diabetes heart rate signals using nonlinear measures," *Comput. Biol. Med.*, vol. 43, no. 10, pp. 1523–1529, 2013, doi: https://doi.org/10.1016/j.compbiomed.2013.05.024.
9. Y. Mobssite, B. B. Samir, and A. F. B. Mohamad Hani, "Signal and image processing for early detection of coronary artery diseases: A review," in *AIP Conference Proceedings*, 2012, vol. 1482, pp. 712–723, doi: https://doi.org/10.1063/1.4757564.
10. D. M. Salerno *et al.*, "Exercise seismocardiography for detection of coronary artery disease," *Am. J. Noninvasive Cardiol.*, vol. 6, no. 5, pp. 321–330, 1992, doi: https://doi.org/10.1159/000470383.
11. A. Cassar, D. R. Holmes, C. S. Rihal, and B. J. Gersh, "Chronic coronary artery disease: Diagnosis and management," in *Mayo Clinic Proceedings*, 2009, vol. 84, no. 12, pp. 1130–1146, doi: https://doi.org/10.4065/mcp.2009.0391.
12. M. R. Patel *et al.*, "Low diagnostic yield of elective coronary angiography," *N. Engl. J. Med.*, vol. 362, no. 10, pp. 886–895, 2010, doi: https://doi.org/10.1056/NEJMoa0907272.
13. C. Martin-Isla *et al.*, "Image-Based Cardiac Diagnosis With Machine Learning: A Review," *Frontiers in Cardiovascular Medicine*, vol. 7. pp. 1–10, 2020, doi: https://doi.org/10.3389/fcvm.2020.00001.
14. A. Moreno, J. Rodriguez, and F. Martínez, "Regional Multiscale Motion Representation for Cardiac Disease Prediction," in *2019 22nd Symposium on Image, Signal Processing and*

Artificial Vision, STSIVA 2019 – Conference Proceedings, 2019, pp. 1–15, doi: https://doi. org/10.1109/STSIVA.2019.8730231.

15. H. Bagher-Ebadian, H. Soltanian-Zadeh, S. Setayeshi, and S. T. Smith, "Neural network and fuzzy clustering approach for automatic diagnosis of coronary artery disease in nuclear medicine," *IEEE Trans. Nucl. Sci.*, vol. 51, no. 1 I, pp. 184–192, 2004, doi: https://doi.org/10.1109/ TNS.2003.823047.

16. G. Bin Huang, Q. Y. Zhu, and C. K. Siew, "Extreme learning machine: A new learning scheme of feedforward neural networks," in *IEEE International Conference on Neural Networks - Conference Proceedings*, 2004, vol. 2, pp. 985–990, doi: https://doi.org/10.1109/ IJCNN.2004.1380068.

17. G.-B. Huang *et al.*, "Extreme learning machine: Theory and applications," *Neurocomputing*, vol. 70, no. 1–3, pp. 489–501, 2006, doi: https://doi.org/10.1016/j.neucom.2005.12.126.

18. S. Ding, H. Zhao, Y. Zhang, X. Xu, and R. Nie, "Extreme learning machine: algorithm, theory and applications," *Artif. Intell. Rev.*, vol. 44, no. 1, pp. 103–115, 2015, doi: https://doi. org/10.1007/s10462-013-9405-z.

19. G. Bin Huang, L. Chen, and C. K. Siew, "Universal approximation using incremental constructive feedforward networks with random hidden nodes," *IEEE Trans. Neural Networks*, vol. 17, no. 4, pp. 879–892, 2006, doi: https://doi.org/10.1109/TNN.2006.875977.

20. G. Bin Huang, D. H. Wang, and Y. Lan, "Extreme learning machines: A survey," *Int. J. Mach. Learn. Cybern.*, vol. 2, no. 2, pp. 107–122, 2011, doi: https://doi.org/10.1007/ s13042-011-0019-y.

21. Q. Leng, H. Qi, J. Miao, W. Zhu, and G. Su, "One-Class Classification with Extreme Learning Machine," *Math. Probl. Eng.*, vol. 6, no. 2, pp. 447–461, 2015, doi: https://doi. org/10.1155/2015/412957.

22. C. Gautam, A. Tiwari, and Q. Leng, "On the construction of extreme learning machine for online and offline one-class classification—An expanded toolbox," *Neurocomputing*, vol. 261, pp. 126–143, 2017, doi: https://doi.org/10.1016/j.neucom.2016.04.070.

23. Guang-Bin Huang, Hongming Zhou, Xiaojian Ding, and Rui Zhang, "Extreme Learning Machine for Regression and Multiclass Classification," *IEEE Trans. Syst. Man, Cybern. Part B*, vol. 42, no. 2, pp. 513–529, 2011, doi: https://doi.org/10.1109/tsmcb.2011.2168604.

24. F. Marmolejo-Ramos and T. Siva Tian, "The shifting boxplot. A boxplot based on essential summary statistics around the mean," *Int. J. Psychol. Res.*, vol. 3, no. 1, pp. 37–45, 2010, doi: https://doi.org/10.21500/20112084.823.

25. A. Kampouraki, G. Manis, and C. Nikou, "Heartbeat time series classification with support vector machines," in *IEEE Transactions on Information Technology in Biomedicine*, 2009, vol. 13, no. 4, pp. 512–518, doi: https://doi.org/10.1109/TITB.2008.2003323.

26. B. COY, "Dimension Reduction for Analysis of Unstable Periodic Orbits Using Locally Linear Embedding," *Int. J. Bifurc. Chaos*, vol. 22, no. 01, p. 1230001, 2012, doi: https://doi. org/10.1142/s0218127412300017.

27. S. Dua, X. Du, S. Vinitha Sree, and V. I. Thajudin Ahamed, "Novel classification of coronary artery disease using heart rate variability analysis," *J. Mech. Med. Biol.*, vol. 12, no. 4, p. 1240017, 2012, doi: https://doi.org/10.1142/S0219519412400179.

28. I. Babaoğlu, O. Fındık, and M. Bayrak, "Effects of principle component analysis on assessment of coronary artery diseases using support vector machine," *Expert Syst. Appl.*, vol. 37, no. 3, pp. 2182–2185, 2010, doi: https://doi.org/10.1016/j.eswa.2009.07.055.

29. D. Giri *et al.*, "Automated diagnosis of Coronary Artery Disease affected patients using LDA, PCA, ICA and Discrete Wavelet Transform," *Knowledge-Based Syst.*, vol. 37, pp. 274–282, 2013, doi: https://doi.org/10.1016/j.knosys.2012.08.011.

30. B. M. Asl, S. K. Setarehdan, and M. Mohebbi, "Support vector machine-based arrhythmia classification using reduced features of heart rate variability signal," *Artif. Intell. Med.*, vol. 44, no. 1, pp. 51–64, 2008, doi: https://doi.org/10.1016/j.artmed.2008.04.007.

31. P. Grassberger and I. Procaccia, "Measuring the strangeness of strange attractors," *Phys. D Nonlinear Phenom.*, vol. 9, no. 1–2, pp. 189–208, 1983, doi: https://doi. org/10.1016/0167-2789(83)90298-1.

32. H. V. Huikuri, T. H. Mäkikallio, C. K. Peng, A. L. Goldberger, U. Hintze, and M. Møller, "Fractal correlation properties of R-R interval dynamics and mortality in patients with depressed left ventricular function after an acute myocardial infarction.," *Circulation*, vol. 101, no. 1, pp. 47–53, 2000, doi: https://doi.org/10.1161/01.CIR.101.1.47.

33. J. S. Richman and J. R. Moorman, "Physiological time-series analysis using approximate entropy and sample entropy.," *Am. J. Physiol. Heart Circ. Physiol.*, vol. 278, no. 6, pp. H2039–H2049, 2000, doi: https://doi.org/10.1103/physreva.29.975.

34. M. Vollmer, "A robust, simple and reliable measure of heart rate variability using relative RR intervals," *Comput. Cardiol. (2010).*, vol. 42, no. 6, pp. 609–612, 2016, doi: https://doi.org/10.1109/CIC.2015.7410984.

35. P. W. Kamen, H. Krum, and A. M. Tonkin, "Poincaré plot of heart rate variability allows quantitative display of parasympathetic nervous activity in humans.," *Clin. Sci. (Lond).*, vol. 91, no. 2, pp. 201–8, 1996, doi: https://doi.org/10.1042/cs0910201.

36. R. Acharya, U. N. Kannathal, and S. M. Krishnan, "Comprehensive analysis of cardiac health using heart rate signals," *Physiol. Meas.*, vol. 25, no. 5, pp. 1139–1151, 2004, doi: https://doi.org/10.1088/0967-3334/25/5/005.

37. S. M. Pincus, "Approximate entropy as a measure of system complexity," *Proc. Natl. Acad. Sci. U. S. A.*, vol. 88, no. 6, pp. 2297–2301, 1991, doi: https://doi.org/10.1073/pnas.88.6.2297.

38. R. Yan, Y. Liu, and R. X. Gao, "Permutation entropy: A nonlinear statistical measure for status characterization of rotary machines," in *Mechanical Systems and Signal Processing*, 2012, vol. 29, pp. 474–484, doi: https://doi.org/10.1016/j.ymssp.2011.11.022.

39. G. Manis, M. Aktaruzzaman, and R. Sassi, "Bubble entropy: An entropy almost free of parameters," *IEEE Trans. Biomed. Eng.*, vol. 64, no. 11, pp. 2711–2718, 2017, doi: https://doi.org/10.1109/TBME.2017.2664105.

40. R. Yan, Q. Zheng, and W. Peng, "Multi-scale entropy and Renyi cross entropy based traffic anomaly detection," in *2008 11th IEEE Singapore International Conference on Communication Systems, ICCS 2008*, 2008, pp. 554–558, doi: https://doi.org/10.1109/ICCS.2008.4737245.

41. D. Kugiumtzis and A. Tsimpiris, "Measures of Analysis of Time Series (MATS)," *J. Stat. Softw.*, vol. 33, no. 5, 2010.

42. R. Kalpana, M. Chitra, and G. Ratna-Sagari, "A Case Study Analysis of EEG Signals under Conditions of Cognition," *Asian J. Med. Sci.*, vol. 7, no. 4, pp. 41–49, 2015, [Online]. Available: http://www.airitilibrary.com/Publication/alDetailedMesh?docid=20408773-201510-201512080004-201512080004-41-49.

43. O. W. Samuel, G. M. Asogbon, A. K. Sangaiah, P. Fang, and G. Li, "An integrated decision support system based on ANN and Fuzzy_AHP for heart failure risk prediction," *Expert Syst. Appl.*, vol. 68, no. 2, pp. 163–172, 2017, doi: https://doi.org/10.1016/j.eswa.2016.10.020.

44. R. Mahajan, T. Viangteeravat, and O. Akbilgic, "Improved detection of congestive heart failure via probabilistic symbolic pattern recognition and heart rate variability metrics," *Int. J. Med. Inform.*, vol. 108, no. 1, pp. 55–63, 2017, doi: https://doi.org/10.1016/j.ijmedinf.2017.09.006.

45. S. Bashir, U. Qamar, and F. H. Khan, "IntelliHealth: A medical decision support application using a novel weighted multi-layer classifier ensemble framework," *J. Biomed. Inform.*, vol. 59, no. 1, pp. 185–200, 2016, doi: https://doi.org/10.1016/j.jbi.2015.12.001.

46. S. N. Yu and M. Y. Lee, "Bispectral analysis and genetic algorithm for congestive heart failure recognition based on heart rate variability," *Comput. Biol. Med.*, vol. 42, no. 8, pp. 816–825, 2012, doi: https://doi.org/10.1016/j.compbiomed.2012.06.005.

47. D. Tay, C. L. Poh, and R. I. Kitney, "A novel neural-inspired learning algorithm with application to clinical risk prediction," *J. Biomed. Inform.*, vol. 54, pp. 305–314, 2015, doi: https://doi.org/10.1016/j.jbi.2014.12.014.

48. P. Pławiak, "Novel methodology of cardiac health recognition based on ECG signals and evolutionary-neural system," *Expert Syst. Appl.*, vol. 92, no. 2, pp. 334–349, 2018, doi: https://doi.org/10.1016/j.eswa.2017.09.022.

49. A. Davari Dolatabadi, S. E. Z. Khadem, and B. M. Asl, "Automated diagnosis of coronary artery disease (CAD) patients using optimized SVM," *Comput. Methods Programs Biomed.*, vol. 138, no. 2, pp. 117–126, 2017, doi: https://doi.org/10.1016/j.cmpb.2016.10.011.

50. A. Mustaqeem, S. M. Anwar, A. R. Khan, and M. Majid, "A statistical analysis based recommender model for heart disease patients," *Int. J. Med. Inform.*, vol. 108, no. 2, pp. 134–145, 2017, doi: https://doi.org/10.1016/j.ijmedinf.2017.10.008.

51. Z. Arabasadi, R. Alizadehsani, M. Roshanzamir, H. Moosaei, and A. A. Yarifard, "Computer aided decision making for heart disease detection using hybrid neural network-Genetic algorithm," *Comput. Methods Programs Biomed.*, vol. 141, no. 2, pp. 19–26, 2017, doi: https://doi.org/10.1016/j.cmpb.2017.01.004.

52. R. J. Martis, U. R. Acharya, K. M. Mandana, A. K. Ray, and C. Chakraborty, "Application of principal component analysis to ECG signals for automated diagnosis of cardiac health," *Expert Syst. Appl.*, vol. 39, no. 14, pp. 11792–11800, 2012, doi: https://doi.org/10.1016/j.eswa.2012.04.072.

53. N. C. Long, P. Meesad, and H. Unger, "A highly accurate firefly based algorithm for heart disease prediction," *Expert Syst. Appl.*, vol. 42, no. 21, pp. 8221–8231, 2015, doi: https://doi.org/10.1016/j.eswa.2015.06.024.

54. V. K. Sudarshan *et al.*, "Automated diagnosis of congestive heart failure using dual tree complex wavelet transform and statistical features extracted from 2 s of ECG signals," *Comput. Biol. Med.*, vol. 83, no. 1, pp. 48–58, 2017, doi: https://doi.org/10.1016/j.compbiomed.2017.01.019.

55. M. Tayefi *et al.*, "hs-CRP is strongly associated with coronary heart disease (CHD): A data mining approach using decision tree algorithm," *Comput. Methods Programs Biomed.*, vol. 141, pp. 105–109, 2017, doi: https://doi.org/10.1016/j.cmpb.2017.02.001.

56. K. H. Boon, M. Khalil-Hani, and M. B. Malarvili, "Paroxysmal atrial fibrillation prediction based on HRV analysis and non-dominated sorting genetic algorithm III," *Comput. Methods Programs Biomed.*, vol. 153, pp. 171–184, 2018, doi: https://doi.org/10.1016/j.cmpb.2017.10.012.

57. Purushottam, K. Saxena, and R. Sharma, "Efficient Heart Disease Prediction System," in *Procedia Computer Science*, 2016, vol. 85, pp. 962–969, doi: https://doi.org/10.1016/j.procs.2016.05.288.

58. D. Pal, K. M. Mandana, S. Pal, D. Sarkar, and C. Chakraborty, "Fuzzy expert system approach for coronary artery disease screening using clinical parameters," *Knowledge-Based Syst.*, vol. 36, no. 2, pp. 162–174, 2012, doi: https://doi.org/10.1016/j.knosys.2012.06.013.

59. H. Fujita *et al.*, "Sudden cardiac death (SCD) prediction based on nonlinear heart rate variability features and SCD index," *Appl. Soft Comput. J.*, vol. 43, pp. 510–519, 2016, doi: https://doi.org/10.1016/j.asoc.2016.02.049.

60. G. Altan, Y. Kutlu, and N. Allahverdi, "A new approach to early diagnosis of congestive heart failure disease by using Hilbert–Huang transform," *Comput. Methods Programs Biomed.*, vol. 137, pp. 23–34, 2016, doi: https://doi.org/10.1016/j.cmpb.2016.09.003.

61. Y. Zheng, X. Guo, J. Qin, and S. Xiao, "Computer-assisted diagnosis for chronic heart failure by the analysis of their cardiac reserve and heart sound characteristics," *Comput. Methods Programs Biomed.*, vol. 122, no. 3, pp. 372–383, 2015, doi: https://doi.org/10.1016/j.cmpb.2015.09.001.

62. F. Miao, Y. P. Cai, Y. X. Zhang, X. M. Fan, and Y. Li, "Predictive modeling of hospital mortality for patients with heart failure by using an improved random survival forest," *IEEE Access*, vol. 6, no. 1, pp. 7244–7253, 2018, doi: https://doi.org/10.1109/ACCESS.2018.2789898.

63. B. Jin, C. Che, Z. Liu, S. Zhang, X. Yin, and X. Wei, "Predicting the Risk of Heart Failure with EHR Sequential Data Modeling," *IEEE Access*, vol. 6, no. 2, pp. 9256–9261, 2018, doi: https://doi.org/10.1109/ACCESS.2017.2789324.

64. S. A. Mokeddem, "A fuzzy classification model for myocardial infarction risk assessment," *Appl. Intell.*, vol. 48, no. 5, pp. 1233–1250, 2018, doi: https://doi.org/10.1007/s10489-017-1102-1.

65. J. K. Kim, J. S. Lee, D. K. Park, Y. S. Lim, Y. H. Lee, and E. Y. Jung, "Adaptive mining prediction model for content recommendation to coronary heart disease patients," *Cluster Comput.*, vol. 17, no. 3, pp. 881–891, 2014, doi: https://doi.org/10.1007/s10586-013-0308-1.

Interference Reduction in ECG Signal Using IIR Digital Filter Based on GA and Its Simulation

Ranjit Singh Chauhan

Abstract Electrocardiogram (ECG) signal carries most important information in the cardiology. Care should be taken to avoid interference in the ECG. This chapter discusses ECG signals with the help of infinite-impulse-response (IIR) digital filter. To avoid too many computations, IIR digital filters have fewer coefficients and potential of sharp roll-offs, which is acceptable for real-time processing. In this chapter, an attempt has been made to generate ECG waveforms with the help of a suitable MATLAB model. Coefficients of IIR digital filter are worked out with genetic algorithm (GA). Using designed filter, the ECG signal was de-noised by removing the interference. Results clearly indicate that there is noise reduction in the ECG signal.

Keywords Electrocardiogram signal · Infinite-impulse-response · Digital filters · Interference · Genetic algorithms

1 Introduction

1.1 Electrocardiogram Signal

Electrocardiogram (ECG) signal is the information or recording of the activity/ action of the heart in the form of graph. ECG is the most important signal to cardio-vascular disease. ECG signal contains lots of information about heart. This record-ing of the activity (particularly electrical action) in the form of signal helps the doctor for the diagnosis of patient. The various time intervals in a basic ECG signal are shown below in Fig. 1.

Generally, ECG signal has frequency range of 0.05–100 Hz and 1–10 mV is its dynamic range. There are normally five types of peaks and other valleys in ECG signal which are normally written off as by the different types of letter, i.e., P, Q, R,

R. S. Chauhan (✉)
JMIETI Radaur, Radaur, Haryana, India

© The Author(s), under exclusive license to Springer
Nature Switzerland AG 2021
A. K. Manocha et al. (eds.), *Computational Intelligence in Healthcare*, Health
Information Science, https://doi.org/10.1007/978-3-030-68723-6_12

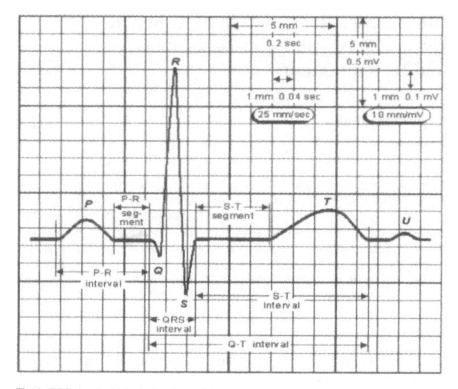

Fig. 1 ECG signal with basic time interval

S, and T. There remains few percent cases in which there is one more peak, which is termed as letter U. Mainly, the accurate, precise, and consistent detection of the labeled QRS signal/complex gives the performance of ECG analyzing system. Now doubt P and T waves are also helpful in the analysis of ECG signal. The various types of cardiac disorders are indicated by the doctor, comparing the results or deviations with normal electrical patterns.

On the basis of precise and accurate ECG signal, the doctor gives correct diagnosis of cardiac vascular diseases. But, in the case of ECG signal, as like other analog signals, ECG also has much of interference, often coming from electricity, environment, and so on, which made it complicated to diagnose the patient and give the proper treatment. Wherever the interference comes from, we should filter it. Hence, interference rejection is one of the most essential and critical problems in the benefit of human beings. With more recent technology, digital filters are now capable of being implemented.

1.2 Digital Filters

In digital signal processing (DSP), digital filtration is the utmost important process and powerful tool. No doubt its amazing performance and consistent results are among the unique and major reasons that DSP has become a great standard. The main and popular advantages of digital filters over analog filters are:

- *Accuracy and precise*: Digital filters are more *accurate and precise*. An analog filter cannot be very accurate and precise for its operation.
- *Programmability*: Digital filters are *programmable*. The function or working of digital filter can be resolute by a program which remains identical as per conditions.
- *Designing*: Digital filters are easy to *design*, and on a general-purpose computer or workstation, it can be easily *tested* and *implemented*.
- *Stability*: Digital filters are more *stable* than analog filters particularly with respect to both time and temperature, while the features or characteristics of an analog filter (having active components or circuitry) change with time.
- *Frequency range*: Digital filters can be used with *low frequency* range of signals more precisely and accurately while their counterpart's, i.e., analog filters cannot. True phase response can be achieved with the help of digital filters.
- *Versatility*: In the capability to process signal in a diversity of methods, digital filter is much more *versatile* and adaptable than analog types of filter. The digital filters have the capability to change the characteristics of the signal.
- *Hardware requirement*: The hardware requirements of digital filters are relatively *modest*, *optimize*, and *compact* in association with the corresponding analog filters.

Consider low-pass-type filter with gain of value 1.0 ± 0.0001 from D.C. to 500 Hz (hertz) and gain smaller than 0.0001 intended for frequencies greater than 501 Hz. The whole conversion takes place within single 1 Hz which is not predictable from an operational amplifier (analog type) circuit. In such case, the digital types of filters can easily achieve *thousands* times improved performance. This builds a strong difference in the filtering approaches. In some cases, it is extremely difficult and not possible to meet specified performances digital filters are capable to achieve. Further, the digital filter can easily modify the characteristics under software control.

The several stages for the design of digital type of filters have been mentioned in the process diagram as presented above in the Fig. 2. This whole process for the design of digital types of filters can be conveniently broken down into five main stages as follows:

Stage 1: Performance specifications
It includes:

(a) *Type of filters:* Digital filters are classified mainly in to four types on the basis of their frequency response. These filters are termed as low-pass (LP), high-

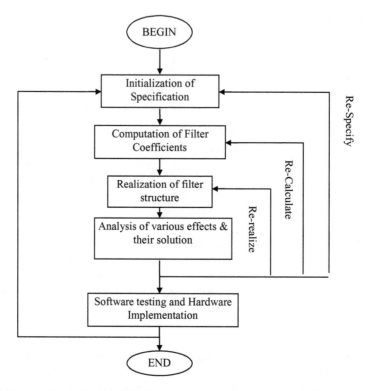

Fig. 2 Process diagram for digital filter

pass (HP), band-pass (BP), and band-reject or band-stop (BS). In this proposed
chapter, low-pass filter has been considered for applying the algorithms.

(b) *Frequency/phase response specifications:* After deciding on the type of filter to
be used, the specifications of the frequency response characteristics are decided.

   • High-pass filter is one which passes frequencies from cutoff frequency
   $\omega_{p1} = \omega_p$ or $f_{c,l}$ to $\omega_{p2} = \pi$ with a unity gain.
   • Band-stop or band-reject filter is one which stops frequencies in the chosen
   range from $\omega_{s1} = f_{c,l}$ to $\omega_{s2} = f_{c,h}$.
   • Band-pass filter is one which allows or passes frequencies in the chosen
   range from $\omega_{p1} = f_{c,l}$ to $\omega_{p2} = f_{c,h}$.
   • Magnitude response, phase response, impulse response, and pole-zero
   response is stated for the design of filter.
   • In few types of applications, the magnitude response or phase response
   shows more interest and progress of attainable estimate to a specified
   condition.
   • By cascading the filter with an all pass section, phase response can be
   corrected.

The frequency response of a filter is also specified in the form of magnitude
response, which is described in brief in the following section:

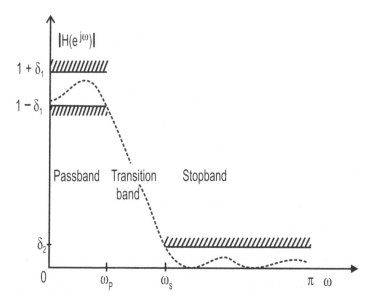

Fig. 3 Magnitude response of low-pass filter

(c) *Magnitude response:* The practical possible solution is being found out by having some relaxation in desired performance, like the following:

- Few acceptable tolerances can be considered in the magnitude response keeping the specifications of digital filter in the pass-band and stop-band.
- A transition band is always stated among the pass-band and stop-band.

Figure 3 indicates the magnitude response of a low-pass type of digital filter. The various specifications for IIR digital filter are:

ω_p – frequency of pass-band edge
ω_s – frequency of stop-band edge
δ_1 or δ_p – pass-band ripple value
δ_2 or δ_s – stop-band ripple value
$H(j\omega)$ – frequency response
$|H(j\omega)|$ – magnitude response

The various filter conditions are specified for the range of frequency between $0 \leq \omega \leq \pi$.

Stage 2: Calculation of coefficients
The focus of this step is to find out the filter coefficients which are obtained by calculating the pulse transfer function which is labeled as $H(z)$, satisfying or approximating the various specifications of a given frequency response for the design of digital type filter. The pulse transfer function denoted as $H(z)$ should be a causal transfer function and rational function. The pulse transfer function for FIR is given by $H(z) = \sum_{x=0}^{M-1} b_x z^{-x}$

The pulse transfer function for infinite-impulse-response type of digital filter is given below in Eq. 1.

$$H(z) = \frac{B(z)}{A(z)} = \frac{\sum_{x=0}^{M-1} b_x z^{-x}}{1 + \sum_{x=1}^{N-1} a_x z^{-x}} \tag{1}$$

where $A(z)$ is the z-transform of input value given as $x(n)$ and $B(z)$ is z-transform of output given by $y(n)$ of the filter, while a_x and b_x are the filter coefficients.

Stage 3: Structure realization

The objective of this stage is to realize the pulse transfer function into an appropriate filter structure or filter network. The main fundamental aspect of image or signal processing is filtering. This involves the operation of the spectrum of a signal by allowing or rejecting certain portions, according to the frequency of that portion. This also depends on the kind of application and manipulation of the signal. The implementation of digital filters is done through the three major fundamental building blocks, i.e., adder, multiplier, and a delay or advance element.

- Adder is having two inputs and one output, and its function is to add the two inputs together.
- Multiplier is a gain element, and its purpose is to multiply the input signal by some constant value.
- Delay or advance element delays or advances the incoming signal by one sample.

The realization of digital filters can be done using either a signal flow graph or a block diagram. Figure 4 depicts signal flow graph, and Fig. 5 shows the three major basic elements in block diagram.

A second-order system is represented by difference equation as given:

$$y(n) = b_0 x(n) + b_1 x(n-1) + b_2 x(n-2) - a_1 y(n-1) - a_1 y(n-2) \tag{2}$$

and the corresponding block diagram representation is given below in Fig. 6.

Few typical structures for FIR are direct form structure, cascade form, frequency-sampling form, lattice type, etc. Similarly, for IIR are direct form, lattice form, parallel form, cascade form etc.

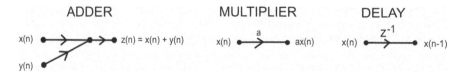

Fig. 4 Signal flow graph of basic elements

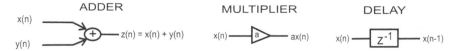

Fig. 5 Block diagram of basic elements

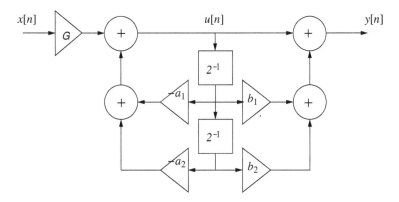

Fig. 6 Second-order system

Stage 4: Analysis of finite word length

In this step, the various effects due to finite word length (quantized, rounded off, etc.) are analyzed on filtering operation and filter performance. The main effects of this finite word length are quantization error, round-off error (least significant bits lost), and overflow error (most significant bits lost).

The coefficient quantization, round-off error, and overflow error behavior can vary from one filter structure to another. It is very important to find the coefficients and select a realization that is not sensitive to finite word length effect. If the solution does not meet the specifications, then we have to re-realize, recalculate, or re-specify.

Stage 5: Hardware and software implementation

This involves implementing software code or hardware circuit which performs actual filtering, and the process testing involves:

- Verifying the performance of filter
- Modeling the truncation for assessing round-off error
- Looking the peaks in frequency response calculate overflow situations

On the basis of unit pulse response of a discrete system, we can divide digital filters into two parts. First is called FIR type filters, i.e., finite duration of the unit pulse response of a system. Second is known as IIR-type filters, which give the infinite (unlimited or vast) duration of unit pulse response. As clear from the name, this suggests that the impulse response in infinite duration of the unit pulse response system is of vast duration. Suppose, in a digital type of filter, the present output $y(n)$ is considered exclusively from the present and previous input values denoted as

$(x(n), x(n-1), x(n-2)...)$, then filter is assumed to be non-recursive filters. The recursive filter can be defined as one in which along with the input values, we use previous output values as well. These input values, just like the old ones, are kept in the memory of the processor. The dictionary meaning of the word recursive is running back, and therefore it clearly indicates and mentions to the circumstances that the formerly considered output values will run back into the consideration of the new outputs. Therefore the expression for a recursive type of filter contains not only the terms involving the input values like $(x(n), x(n-1), x(n-2)...)$; on the other hand, also relation is having the output value may be like $(y(n-1), y(n-2), ...)$. In another term a *non-recursive* type of the filter is commonly referred as a finite impulse response digital filter, and a *recursive* type of the filter is stated to as an infinite impulse response digital filter.

The above referred definitions point to the different "impulse responses" which are classified in two types of filters. When a *unit impulse* is applied at the input of system, then the impulse response of digital type of filter is the output sequence received from the said filters. (A unit impulse is nothing else but a very modest input sequence containing a single value, i.e., 1 at initial time $t = 0$, which is trailed by zeros at all successive sampling times). Now, the FIR type filter as the name clearly indicates is the one which have finite duration impulse response. To explain further, whenever an impulse is applied as input to a FIR type of filter, the output will always consist of a finite duration sequence. The unique traits of FIR type of digital filters are that they are characterized by transfer function which is not a rational function, as given by Eq. 3:

$$H(z) = \sum_{k=0}^{M-1} b_k z^{-k} \tag{3}$$

In contrast, an IIR type of digital filter can be characterized by the one system whose impulse response supposedly remains for eternity as the recursive, i.e., the prior output, relation feedback energy into the filter input, and makes it go on forever continuously. But the term IIR cannot be considered to be appropriate or up to the mark as the real impulse responses of almost all IIR type of filters diminish practically to zero in a finite interval of time. Yet, the abovementioned two terms are the most often and commonly used terms in the application of signal and image processing.

The discrete difference equation for IIR type of digital filter can be given in the following way, as exposed below in Eq. 4:

$$\sum_{m=0}^{m=N} a_m y(n-m) = \sum_{k=0}^{k=M} b_k x(n-k) \tag{4}$$

To denote a_m and b_k, respectively, the coefficients of digital filter correlated to the feedback and the feed-forward part of the realized digital IIR filter are used. The filter input is denoted as, $x(n)$, where n is the total number of the specified sample; in the same manner, $y(n)$ symbolizes the output equivalent to the mentioned sample

n. As shown in the data given above, the ranges of M and N are termed as either the filter word length or the order of the digital filter. The right-hand side of equation explains at length the feed forward in the function of digital filter. And the left-hand side elaborately explains the feedback in the mentioned digital filter function. Either or both sides of the difference equation may constitute a filter function. Supposedly, if only the one side (right-hand side) of the difference equation is being used, then the filter is a FIR type of digital filter ($M \neq 0$ and $N = 0$). In case if we are using the both sides of the difference equation, then filter is an IIR type of filter ($M \neq 0$ and $N \neq 0$). The unique or uncharacteristic instance is when only the one side (left side) of the differential equation is used ($M = 0$ and $N \neq 0$). In this unique scenario, the filter is referred as "all-pole" filter. Basically, the all pole for the filter is an IIR-type filter, as all filters which involve the feedback process have an infinite impulse response.

Digital filters are commonly described by the z-domain. Equation 5 shows the z-transform of Eq. 4:

$$Y(z) \sum_{m=0}^{m=N} a_m z^{-m} = X(z) \sum_{k=0}^{k=M} b_k z^{-k} \tag{5}$$

The main motive of providing the z-transform of the difference equation is that the features of the any type of digital filters are defined by their pulse transfer function labeled as $H(z)$, in the form of z domain. The overall purpose of the pulse transfer function of any filter (or any discrete system) is to describe the relationship among the input value and output value of the filter (or system) as represented in Fig. 7:

The overall relationship between the input of filter $X(z)$ and the output of the filter $Y(z)$, i.e., the pulse transfer function of the filter $H(z)$, is given by Eq. 6 mentioned as below:

$$H(z) = \frac{B(z)}{A(z)} = \frac{\sum_{x=0}^{M-1} b_x z^{-x}}{1 + \sum_{x=1}^{N-1} a_x z^{-x}} \tag{6}$$

The numerator of the above function describes the feed forward part of the digital filter function, and the value of the denominator describes the feedback part of the filter function in z-domain.

The following are the advantages of IIR type of digital filters over FIR digital type filters:

- They are steadier and can be realized competently in hardware.
- This type of filters utilizes both a feed forward part or polynomial (as the roots are zeros) and a feedback polynomial (as the roots are poles), so it has immensely sharp transition trait for a given order of filter.

Fig. 7 Block diagram
representation of transfer
function of a filter

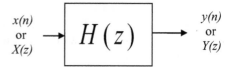

$$x(n) \text{ or } X(z) \quad \longrightarrow \quad H(z) \quad \longrightarrow \quad y(n) \text{ or } Y(z)$$

- As in the case of analog type filters with poles, an IIR digital filter normally has nonlinear phase with true features.
- Signal feedback occurs and IIR digital filters both fall in the recursive type of system.
- Conversion from analog filter to digital filter is very easy and accurate. IIR digital filters are typically more effectual designed in the terms of memory condition and computation period.

As the error surface of infinite-impulse-response (IIR) of digital filters are usually multimodal and nonlinear, so there is requirement or scope of global optimization methods in order to escape local minima, precise due to lack of instrumentation, thus offering a great advantage over analog implementation.

1.3   Genetic Algorithm

In the early seventies, Holland suggested that genetic algorithms are the computer algorithms or programs that replicate the natural processes of the evolution. Further, De-Jong expanded the GAs for optimization of functions, and an elaborated scientific model of GA was brought forward by Goldberg in the year of 1970. Genetic algorithms (GAs) are random exploration approaches that can be applied to find an optimal result to the progression function of an optimization problem. The basic function of GAs is to operate/handle population of the distinct in each set of generation. The population of an individual in each iteration (*generation*) where each distinct term, which is considered as the *chromosome*. This will represent the unique candidate solution to the optimization problem. As per Darwin's theory, fit individuals survive and represent a solution to the minor problems. Further, the individual survived within the population reproduces and recombines their genetic ingredients which help us to produce the new individuals which are termed as *offspring*. The genetic ingredients are demonstrated by some data arrangement, utmost a finite word length of the attribute. By means of nature, *selection* offers the essential driving mechanism for the better solutions and optimal values to survive. The value of each solution is associated with a *fitness* value that reflects with other random solutions. The process of recombination is activated through a *crossover* principle that includes the interactions or portions of data strings among the identical chromosomes. The new ingredients of genetics are also familiarized through *mutation* that is responsible for the strings random alterations. The chances or frequency of occurrence of these all above genetic operations is measured or controlled by the certain probabilities (values of the crossover probability and mutation probability). In the projected algorithm, an effort has been made to increase the convergence rate of the optimization problem in which the genetic algorithm constraints are described below:

Size of population   The population size covers all candidate solutions for supplementary processing. During the initialization of the search, size of the population must have maximum value. There will be miscellaneous random solutions. But as there is progress in the search of solution, the worth of the solutions in the population should get improved until the optimum solution is found. The complete population size converges to this better or optimal solution. The size of the population is one of the very important factors of GAs. The larger the value of the initial population, the more possibility to get the best solution for any problem. This best solution will be closer to optimal solution of the problem. No doubt this will increase the execution time of the algorithm.

Selection operator   The selection operation helps us to choose the initial solution to be used for crossover operator. The fitness of the solution is the recognizing factor for this decision. Often the superiority of the solution depends on the value of fitness function and is applied for the selection by relating it to the different individuals in the population. To get the better and optimal solution particularly in terms of specific optimization objectives, the better is the significance of fitness function, and the best will be preferred for recombination. But different types of the selection schemes have been established over the last few years. Most important and significant are roulette wheel selection, linear rank selection, tournament selection, etc. A straightforward and most commonly used selection model is the roulette-wheel-selection which is shown in Fig. 8. Their proportional fitness helps us to select the solutions. In our chapter and simulation results, stochastic universal sampling (SUS) has been used for selection function. SUS is type of single-type phase sampling algorithm with zero bias and minimum spread. As an alternative of the single pointer active in roulette wheel approaches, SUS also uses N equally spread out pointer, where the value of N is the required number of selections. The value of population size is scuffled arbitrarily, and a unique value of the random number is generated, i.e., ptr which exists in the range 0–N. Then N individuals are selected by creating the N pointers space out by one, $[ptr, ptr + 1, ptr + 2, \ldots, ptr + (N - 1)]$, and choosing the individuals for the pointer. Thus an individual is very carefully chosen to a least expected numbers of the trails ($et(i)$) times, thus attaining minimum number of spread. While accumulation, as an individual is nominated exclusively on their locus in the population, i.e. stochastic universal sampling type selection has nil bias.

Crossover operation   The method of combining properties of genes of designated solutions to profit a novel value of solution is known as crossover. Overall idea behind is if the "right (R)" portions of the two respectable solutions are joint together into a novel solution, the superiority of this new value of solution must be superior to the parent solution of the problem. A single child is produced by breeding of two parents. That child inherits the properties from both the parents, and as per fitness functions, the child may be inferior or better than either parent solution. Partially

Fig. 8 Model of roulette
wheel selection

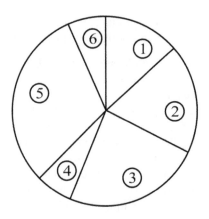

matched crossover (PMX), order crossover (OX), cycle crossover (CX), and single-point crossover (SPX) are some of the crossovers used in generic algorithm in past. Single-point crossover is illustrated as shown in Fig. 9.

In two point crossover, two points are chosen, and bits in between them are exchanged as shown in Fig. 10.

Mutation operator The existence of mutation operator is just because crossover classically uses the properties of existing solution, and it cannot give solutions with new evidence. Mutation arises due to slight random agitation of the solution candidate. However there are small probabilities to mutate a separate population. The mutation operator aims at regaining data which was misplaced during the search operation, i.e., prevention of population from early concurrence. In an old-fashioned way, it is less or more a secondary operator which is achieved only with low value of probability. Though an effective search technique is the one in which crossover and mutation mechanism and probabilities counterpart. Reciprocal exchange, inversion, etc. are some of the mutation functions. Mutation is illustrated as shown in Fig. 11.

Fitness function Another problem-dependent function is the fitness function, representing the degree of quality of any assumed result. The function must somehow generate a total ordering in the space of solution. The visibility of minor improvements in the result to the procedure is vital. The inverse of the error produced by program output defines fitness.

The initial use of digital filter for ECG has been reported. The results were inferior, as the digital filters were very much at their early stages at the time. As the digital filter has become extra mature, this work has gained more attention over past few years. The defects reported formerly have now almost been corrected. Mitov (2004) described the interferences in ECG. Chavan and Uplan (2008) by using rectangular window presented a new approach of FIR filters.

The chapter is systematized as follows: Section 2 presents the model to generate ECG signal. Section 3 introduces the basics of IIR digital filter and designing of IIR digital filter using GA. The performance of the novel technique is considered on the

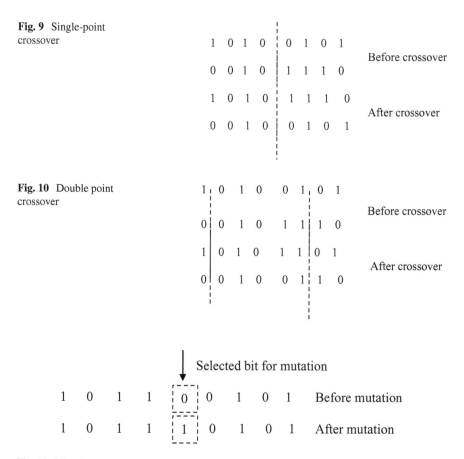

Fig. 9 Single-point crossover

Fig. 10 Double point crossover

Fig. 11 Mutation

real ECG signal exaggerated by power line interference and baseline wander in the fourth section. Finally, attention on conclusion has been drawn in the last section of this chapter.

2 Model Used to Generate ECG Signal

MATLAB software is used for analysis of ECG signal. Many technical computing problems are solved by a high-performance interactive system called MATLAB. The algorithm is designed to give the data in workspace. The inputs are given to the model to get the final results. In the model the time scope indicates the output used as real-time application as shown in Figs. 12 and 13.

It is observed that there is some nôise in the signal. In the last 10 years, several methods of eliminating the artifacts in the ECG signals were suggested. These

Fig. 12 Model of ECG
signal

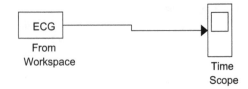

Fig. 13 ECG signal in time scope

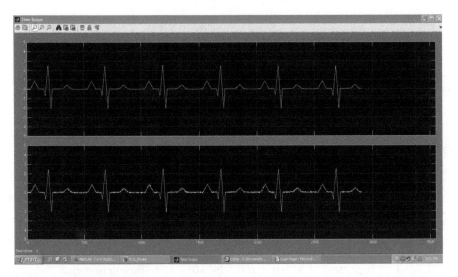

methods are of two types, i.e., nonadaptive and adaptive filtering. The nonadaptive
filtering method includes FIR filter, IIR filter, and notch-type filter. The low-pass
type of filter with cutoff frequency equal to 0.5 Hz can be helpful to eliminate the
intrusion of baseline, which can filter out the signal element with frequency less
than 0.5 Hz, whereas the frequency more than 0.5 Hz is conserved; the digital filter
can be realized non-recursively and recursively types (FIR and IIR digital type of
filters). This chapter presents the IIR digital filter to remove level of noise.

3   Design of IIR Digital Filters Based on GA

Suppose the IIR type of digital filter with the input and output relationship directed as

$$y(n) + \sum_{i=1}^{M} b_i y(n-i) = \sum_{i=0}^{L} a_i x(n-i) \tag{7}$$

whereas $x(n)$ and $y(n)$ are the filter's input and output value, respectively, and M ($\geq L$) is denoted as the order of the filter. The pulse transfer function of the above IIR type of digital filter can be rewritten as given below:

$$H(z) = \frac{A(z)}{B(z)} = \frac{\sum_{i=0}^{L} a_i z^{-i}}{1 + \sum_{i=1}^{M} b_i z^{-i}} \tag{8}$$

A significant and difficult task for the scientist/researchers is to find out the optimal values of coefficients a_i and b_i such that the frequency response of the desired filter approaches a preferred characteristic while maintaining the stability of the intended filter.

The width of various frequencies bands, i.e., pass-band, stop-band, values of ripples for pass-band, and stop-band, are accepted design specifications that are to be fulfilled during the design of digital various filters.

Objective or goal of filter designing is optimization of digital filter design with an arbitrary magnitude response. Thus, the fitness function must be based on the magnitude/phase response of the filter undergoing evaluation and the desired magnitude response. The design of IIR type of digital filter can be reflected as an combinational optimization problem of the function called as cost function specified as $J(f)$ which must be

$$\min J(f) \tag{9}$$

In above function, w is filter coefficient vector written as $[a_0, a_1, \ldots, a_L, b_1, \ldots, b_M]$. The overall purpose is to optimize or minimize/reduce the cost function $J(f)$ by adjusting the value of w. The value of cost function (in this case the time-averaged cost function) is typically stated as

$$J(f) = \frac{1}{N} \sum_{n=1}^{N} \left(d(n) - y(n) \right)^2 \tag{10}$$

where the preferred and actual responses of the digital filter are respectively denoted as $d(n)$ and $y(n)$. The number of various samples required for the control of cost function is given by N. The fitness value of the optimal solution i in the size of population is resolute by using fitness formula given by

$$fit(x) = \frac{1}{p + J(f)x} \tag{11}$$

where $J(f)$ is the value of cost function computed for x and p is the number of poles lies outside the circle (with unity radius).

```
Process GA
    Parameters;
    Start check conditions
            Compute fitness function for each individual
            Selection mechanism
            Crossover operation
            Mutation method
        Stop loop
    Stop process
```

Fig. 14 Basic pseudo code of GA

The selection, crossover, and mutation operators as demonstrated in the last section establish the basic pseudo code of GA which is presented in Fig. 14. The mentioned code is repetitive until some predetermined conditions are satisfied. This process helps us to generate the successively better and better individuals of the species.

The overall flow chart for the design of infinite impulse response digital type filter through GA is displayed below in Fig. 15.

The procedure for implementing GA is as follows:

- Initialize the desired frequency specifications of the filter, generate the population, chromosome, etc.
- Obtain the fitness function based on stability, performance function, etc.
- Use reproduction method to choose chromosome based on relative fitness function.
- Identify the coefficients after the crossover operation and mutation.
- Each calculated coefficient is verified upon preferred format. Compute frequency response and write final coefficient set.
- Otherwise go to the step number 2, until condition is satisfied, generally extreme number of the iterations (termination) or a satisfactorily response.

The GA-based IIR (GAIIR) filter produces optimal coefficients of filter that assure frequency template, i.e., both magnitude response and phase response. Figure 16 shows model for filtering ECG signal using GA-based IIR digital filter.

4 Simulation Results

The simulated ECG signal has been considered in this section. The range of frequency of this signal is from 0.05 Hz to about 15 Hz.

In this case, GAs has been run for simulation results. The various types of parameters set for analysis with the help of GAs is shown in Table 1 given below.

The IIR filter is designed using the genetic algorithm with the parameters shown above. The values of coefficients obtained using GA for first example is tabulated in

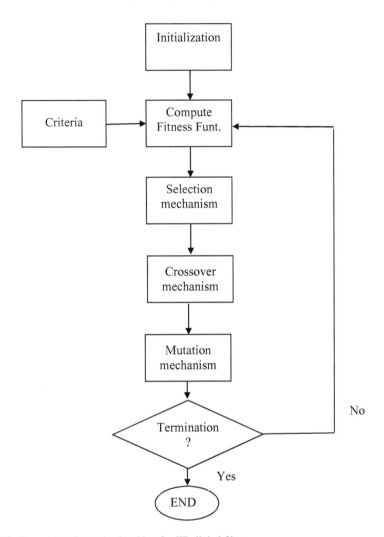

Fig. 15 Flow chart of genetic algorithm for IIR digital filter

Table 2. It is also observed that the optimal values of coefficients can be calculated with the help of simulated annealing. It is also observed that the above calculated optimal values of coefficients give least value of MSE (mean square error) equal to 0.3275 and MSD (mean standard deviation) equal to 0.3105.

With the help of calculated optimal coefficients, the frequency response of designed filter can be seen in Fig. 17.

Through the optimal coefficients, the magnitude response of IIR digital low-pass-type filter with respect to normalized frequency using GA is illustrated in Fig. 17(a). It is shown between gain varying 0 to −60 dB and normalized frequency ranging from 0 to 1 (×π radian/sample). The zoom in curve of magnitude response

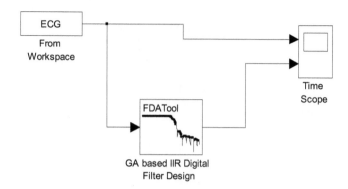

Fig. 16 Model used to remove Interference

Table 1 Parameters for GA technique

Classes	Values
Population size	50
Generation size	500
Crossover probability	0.80
Mutation probability	0.02
Selection operation	*Stochastic universal sampling*
Cross over operation	*Double point*
Mutation operation	*Reciprocal exchange*

Table 2 Values of Coefficients Designed Using GA

Coefficients	Proposed method
a_0	0.3739
a_1	0.7459
a_2	0.3739
b_1	1.0000
b_2	0.3116
b_3	0.1789

for transition band is highlighted in Fig. 17(a). It is plotted between gain through the calculated coefficient and normalized frequency. It is observed that for normalized frequency that increases from 0.90 to 0.95 ($\times\pi$ radian/sample), the response decreases sharply from −27 dB to −37 dB. This effect in magnitude response provides us better transition band than general.

Figure 17(b) shows the phase response of low-pass type of IIR digital filter using GA. It is displayed between angle ranging between 0 and −3 radian and normalized frequency varying from 0 to 1 ($\times\pi$ radian/sample). It is evidently seen that specifications are satisfactory.

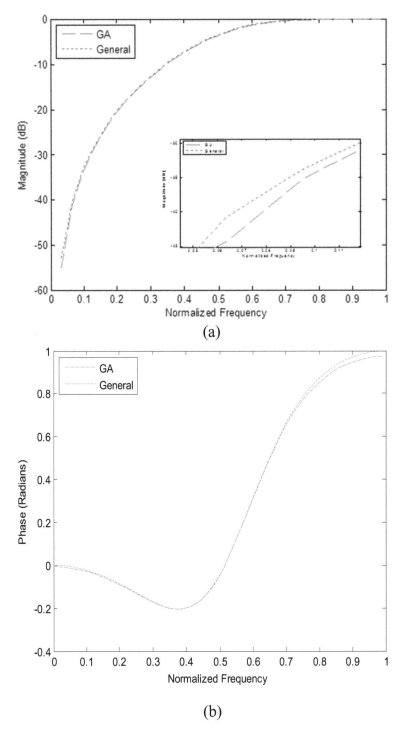

Fig. 17 Response of designed filter: (**a**) magnitude response; (**b**) phase response

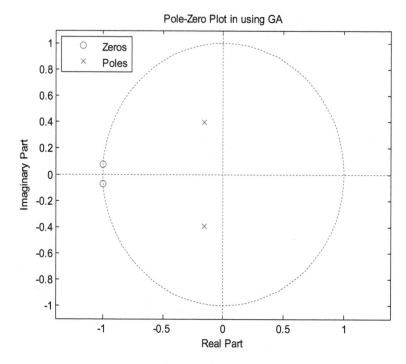

Fig. 18 Pole and zero behavior of designed filter using GA

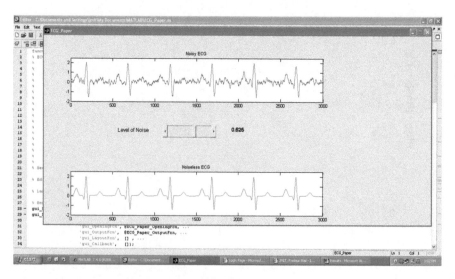

Fig. 19 Noisy and noiseless ECG signal

The resulting pole are at $-0.1558 \pm 0.3932i$ and zero are at $-0.9975 \pm 0.0712i$. It can be realized that the pole-zero position of considered filter lies inside a unit sphere. It expresses that the considered filter is also stable with the projected method. Figure 18 demonstrates the location of pole and zero of the IIR low-pass-type digital filter intended with the help of heuristic algorithm with factors given in the table for GA algorithm.

The designed filter is applied to noisy ECG which reduces the level of noise. The noisy and noise less ECG response is depicted in Fig. 19.

5 Conclusion

In this chapter, the GA technique is discussed to create a novel set of digital type IIR filters. The proposed digital IIR-type filter possesses true magnitude response, phase response, and pole-zero plot. A model is discussed to run the ECG signal, and another model is used to remove the noise. The result of the simulations verifies that, using the projected GAIIR filter, both the selectivity and transient duration of proposed filter are at satisfactory level. As an illustration, GA-based digital low-pass IIR type of filter has been used to eradicate the level of interference from the noisy ECG signal to make noiseless signal for better treatment.

Bibliography

1. David E. Goldberg, Genetic Algorithm in search, optimization and machine Learning. Pearson Education Edition, Delhi, 2005.
2. J. G. Proakis and D. G. Manolakis, Digital Signal Processing: Principles, Algorithms, and Applications. 4th Edition, Pearson Education, Inc., New Delhi, 2007.
3. Joelle Skaf and P. Boyd Stephen, "Filter Design with Low Complexity Coefficients," IEEE Trans. on Signal Processing, vol. 56, no. 7, pp. 3162–3170, July 2008.
4. K.D. Abdesselam, "Design of Stable, causal, perfect reconstruction, IIR Uniform DFT Filters," IEEE Trans. on Signal Processing, vol. 48, no. 4, pp. 1110–1117, 2000.
5. C.C. Tseng and S.C. Pei, "Stable IIR Notch Filter design with optimal pole placement, IEEE Trans. on Signal Processing, vol. 49, no. 11, pp. 2673–2681, 2001.
6. Li Liang, Majid Ahmadi, Maher Ahmed, and Konrarh Wallus, "Design of Canonical signed digital filters using Genetic Algorithms," IEEE Trans. on Signal Processing, vol. 3, no. 1, pp. 2043–2047, 2003.
7. Sabbir U. Ahmad and Andreas Antoniou, "Design of Digital filters using Genetic Algorithms," IEEE Trans. on Signal Processing, vol. 1, no. 1, pp. 1–9, 2006.
8. J.E. Cousseau, Stefan Werner, and P.D. Donate, "Factorized All-Pass Based IIR Adaptive Notch Filters" IEEE Trans. on Signal Processing, vol. 55, no. 11, pp. 5225–5236, 2007.
9. H.A. Oliveira, Antonio Petraglia, and M.R. Petraglia, "Frequency Domain FIR Filter Design Using Fuzzy Adaptive Simulated Annealing" in IEEE International Symposium on Signal Processing and Information Technology, 2007, pp. 884–888.
10. B.W. Jung, H.J. Yang, and J. Chun, "Finite Wordlength Digital Filter Design Using Simulated Annealing," IEEE Trans. on Signal Processing, pp.546-550, 2008.

11. Chaohua Dai, Weirong Chen, and Yunfang Zhu, "Seeker Optimization Algorithm for Digital IIR Filter Design," IEEE Trans. On Evolutionary Computation, vol. 57, no. 5, pp. 1710–1718, 2010.
12. R.S. Chauhan and Sandeep K. Arya, "IIR digital filter design through Genetic Algorithm", Elixir Advn. Engg. Info., vol. 30, no. 1, pp. 1796-1799, 2011.
13. M. Lagerholm, "Clustering ECG complexes using hermite functions and self-organizing maps," IEEE Transactions on Biomedical Engg., vol. 47, 2000.
14. M.S. Chavan, R.A. Aggarwal and M.D. Uplana, "Interference Reduction in ECG using Digital filtering," WSEAS Trans. on Signal processing, vol. 4, no. 5, pp. 340–349, 2008.
15. A. K. Ziarani and A. Konrad, "A nonlinear adaptive method of elimination of power line interference in ECG signals," IEEE Trans. Biomed. Eng., vol. 49, no. 6, pp. 540–547, Jun. 2002.
16. Jacek Piskorowski, "Digital Q-Varying Notch IIR Filter with Transient Suppression", IEEE Trans. on Instrumentation and Measurement, vol. 59, no. 4, pp. 866–873, April 2010.
17. He Qi, Zhi Guo Feng, Ka Fai Cedric Yiu and Sven Nordholm, "Optimal Design of IIR filters via the Partial Fraction Decomposition Method" IEEE Trans. on Circuits and Systems II, vol. 66, no. 8, pp. 1461–1467, Nov. 2018.
18. Anastasia Volkova, Matei Istoan, Florent De Dinechin and Thibault Hilaire, "Towards Hardware IIR filters Computing Just Right: Direct Form I Case Study" IEEE Trans. on Computers, vol. 68, no. 4, pp. 597–608, April 2019.
19. Hsien-Ju Ko and Jeffrey J. P. Tsai, "Robust and Computationally efficient digital IIR filter Synthesis and Stability Analysis Under Finite Precision Implementations" IEEE Trans. on Signal Processing, vol. 68, no. 4, pp. 1807–1822, March 2020.

Contactless Measurement of Heart Rate from Live Video and Comparison with Standard Method

A. N. Nithyaa, S. Sakthivel, K. Santhosh Kumar, and P. Pradeep Raj

Abstract Heart rate (HR) is one of the essential physiological parameters and acts as an indicator of person's physiological condition. This work deals with the noncontact measurement of human HR from live video. It is a real-time application using a camera. The algorithm for face detection is used to recognize human faces, and HR information is extracted from the color variation in facial skin caused by blood circulation. The variation in the blood circulation causes changes in the pixel intensity of the live video recorded. The extraction of the specific frequency is achieved by band-pass filtering, and the pixel intensity average is calculated. Finally, HR of the subject is measured using frequency domain method. The measured HR from the proposed contactless procedure is compared to the standard method using the patient monitoring system, and experimental accuracy is determined in terms of differences in the beats per minute. This method of noncontact measurement of heart rate from live face video can able to give a high range of accuracies under well-controlled environmental conditions. The accuracy can be improvised by using high-quality cameras and by increasing the pixel intensity. This approach provides benefits for medical and computing applications.

Keywords Heart rate · Face detection · Band-pass filter · Pixel intensity

1 Introduction

Heart rate is the measurement of the number of heart beats per minute [22]. The HR depends on the number of ventricular contractions, which is the lower chamber of the human heart. The abnormality in the HR is specified by two terms: tachycardia (too fast) and bradycardia (too slow). The human HR can differ according to the person's age and physical needs [4], while a normal HR does not guarantee that a

---

A. N. Nithyaa (✉) · S. Sakthivel · K. Santhosh Kumar · P. Pradeep Raj
Rajalakshmi Engineering College, Chennai, India
e-mail: nithyaa.an@rajalakshmi.edu.in; sakthivel.s.2016.bme@rajalakshmi.edu.in

© The Author(s), under exclusive license to Springer
Nature Switzerland AG 2021
A. K. Manocha et al. (eds.), *Computational Intelligence in Healthcare*, Health
Information Science, https://doi.org/10.1007/978-3-030-68723-6_13

257

subject is free of health problems. It is a useful benchmark for identifying the range of person's health issues.

As the society becoming more conscious on health issues, various contactless health monitoring systems are developed [11]. In most of the situations, continuous HR monitoring is necessary, but the problem is with the skin contact, and it will be uncomfortable to the patient to be continuously connected to a monitoring device. So the contactless heart rate monitoring is an essential tool.

This work deals with a new approach to a contactless method for monitoring HR using continuous live video stream [5]. The human cardiovascular system allows circulation of blood throughout the parts of the human body which is mediated by the heart that continuously pumps the blood. It is possible to extract heart rate from facial skin color variations as for every heartbeat the heart pumps the blood to every body part including facial area [21].

In order to record the HR in real-time applications, the proposed method uses OpenCv, and it is implemented using Python, which is a programming language [1]. This approach can be used in day-to-day applications like driver monitoring.

2   Experimental Method

The proposed method consists of three major steps such as (1) preprocessing, (2) signal extraction, and (3) post-processing (Figs. 3 and 4).

2.1   Preprocessing

2.1.1   Face Detection

Human face detection is one of the computing technologies used in various human face recognition applications in the form of digital images [10]. It can be known as a specialized case of object class detection. These detection techniques can be used to identify the sizes and locations of the objects in the given image which is of the given class [18].

The first object detection frame is the Viola-Jones method which gives the rate of competitive object detection in the real time [15]. It was primarily done to overcome the problem of human face detection.

2.1.2   ROI Detection/Tracking

A region of interest (ROI) is a subset of an image. ROI is labelled in the facial region that are used for analysis. The forehead is the most suitable body part as it provides detailed skin color variations in the face

Fig. 1 Haar Features for face detection

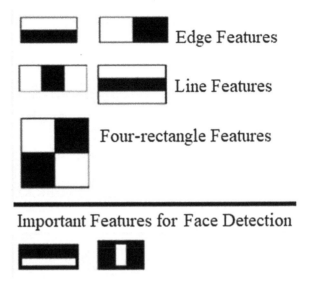

Edge Features

Line Features

Four-rectangle Features

Important Features for Face Detection

Two rules followed to find the ROI: first is to exclude the region of the eye because blinking of an eye can interfere with estimated heart rate frequency. Second is to isolate the ROI boundary region; otherwise in the detection process non-facial pixels might be included from the background [7].

Paul Viola and Michael Jones presented an effective method using Haar cascades to detect the human face, which is trained by machine learning principles [1]. A set of both positive images (facial pictures) and negative images (non-facial pictures) are used for training. The Viola-Jones detection method has the following key features which are used to detect the human face easily [1]:

(a) Converts the pixel intensity values into an integral image
(b) Haar features: Identify rectangular shaped objects, shown in Fig. 1
(c) AdaBoost Learning Algorithm: Used to select the best features from the entire set
(d) Cascade filtering: Used to discard the negative window and aimed only on the positive window (Fig. 2)

2.2 Signal Extraction

2.2.1 Applying Band-Pass Filtering

A device or a process that removes some unnecessary feature or component of a signal is called as a filter [6].

A band-pass (BP) filter is a filtering device that passes a certain range of frequencies and eliminates the frequencies outside of the given range [3]. The difference

Fig. 2 Face Detection
with OpenCV – Computer
Vision

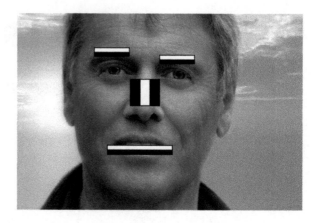

between upper cutoff frequencies and the lower cutoff frequencies is called as the bandwidth of the filter [20].

Here, we apply a band-pass filter with FL = 0.8 Hz and FH = 3 Hz, which are 48 bpm and 180 bpm, respectively.

2.2.2   Averaging Pixel Intensity

A small block which represents the amount of grayscale intensity of the given image is called a pixel [19]. Integers 0 (black)–255 (white) is the range of the pixel values for most of the images [9]. Average color value in ROI in each frame is calculated pushed to a data buffer which is 150 in length.

2.3   Post-processing

2.3.1   Measuring the Heart Rate

Fast Fourier transform (FFT) is applied to the positive window formed by the last 200 frames of signal [1]. Since the normal HR is between 35 and 195 BPM, frequency domain filtering can be used to correct the false reading. The HR obtained from the frequencies between 0.5 Hz and 3 Hz [12].

There are few chances of interferences from power line frequencies. The spectrum, which is close to the HR, is influenced by continuous component. During which the summing frequency takes effects on spectral density, the detection algorithm will run on webcam frequencies [13].

First, the zero hertz component detected is avoided. The maximum heart rate frequencies is a ratio which is the calculation between median and maximum of the spectrum (Fig. 3).

Fig. 3 Block diagram of the proposed method

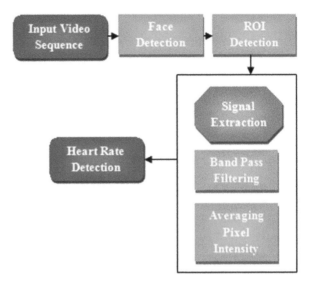

To ensure the accuracy of the measurement, parallel heart rate test was done using patient monitoring system (Fig. 4).

3 Flow Chart Explanation

3.1 Importing Python Modules

The import keyword allows the user to import predefined modules in the Python program, to make use of the functions available under the modules.

An import statement is written with "import" keyword followed by the name of the module. In a Python program, this will be declared first, under any shebang line or general comment. So, in the Python file, main.py import is used to import Python modules. When importing a module, it will be available in the current program as a separate namespace. It will refer to the functions in dot notations, as in module function.

3.2 Helper Methods (Defining Methods in Python)

A helper method is a term used to describe some method that is reused often by other methods or parts of a program. Helper methods are typically not too complex and help shorten code for frequently used minor tasks. Using helper methods can also help to reduce error in code by having the logic in one place.

Fig. 4 Flow chart to detect
heart rate

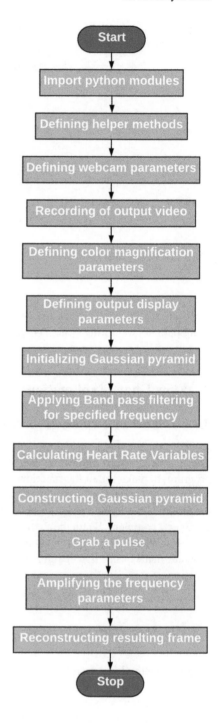

3.3   Webcam Parameters

It is used to build interesting applications using live face video stream from the computer's webcam. OpenCV platform provides as a video capture object which handles opening and closing of the webcam [2]. Creating the object can be used to keep reading frames. The code will first open the webcam, capture the frame, down-scale them by a factor of 2, and display in a window. The OpenCV's video capture function is creating the video capture object [8]. Once the object is created, it starts an infinite loop and keeps on reading the frames from the Webcam until a keyboard interrupt is encountered.

3.4   Output Video

It is the video that is displayed in the monitor that captures the facial skin color changes, and it can be recorded and saved as a separate file.

3.5   Color Magnification Parameters

Eulerian Video Magnification for Python is a Python implementation for revealing subtle changes. The goal is to identify temporal variation in the given video [16]. The input for the proposed method is the standard live video. One of the inputs is obtained; spatial decompositions and temporal filtering are applied to the frames. The hidden information can be identified by amplifying the obtained signal. The technique is used to visualize facial blood flow and also identify small motion. This method can be used to run-in real-time applications. The code defines the variables that are used for color magnification

3.6   Output Display Parameters

The display parameters determine the text location in the output frame. The font color can be defined using the RGB color scale [8]. The output box color can also be defined using the RGB color scale.

3.7   Initialize Gaussian Pyramid

Gaussian pyramids are used to work with images of different resolutions [23]. In some situations, it is essential to deal with images of differing resolutions of the same image while dealing with image in which we are not sure about the object size that the image contains in it, for example, facial image/video. In those cases, it is in necessary to construct a set of images with different resolutions, and objects can be searched in all the images. These set of images with the different resolutions are called as image pyramids

3.8   Band-pass Filter for Specified Frequencies

It used to allow specific information from the face that is selected from region of interest

3.9   Grab a Pulse

FFT is a tool used for analysis of frequency [14]. FFT usually converts the time domain into frequency domain of a signal. FFT is a faster version of the DFT (Discrete Fourier Transform), which can be applied when the no. of samples in the given signal is a power of 2 [17]. The N point DFT can be computed by using

$$x_n = \frac{1}{N} \sum_{N-1}^{k=0} X_k \cdot e^{i2\pi kn/N}, \quad n \in \mathbb{Z}$$

where x_n is the discrete time signal with a period of N. In order to determine the frequency, FFT was computed and then analyzed. Once the signal's frequency was obtained from the spectrum, the HR was recorded from heart rate (HR) = 60 * frequency [17].

3.10   Reconstruct Resulting Frame

The resulting frame of the output video is constructed with the desired height and width. When the live video gets started, it will show notification as "Calculating HR…" If the face is detected, it will start calculating the heart rate and show results as "Heart Rate: (Desired Heart rate value)." Press "e" on keyboard to terminate the live video and stop the execution of the program.

4   Result and Discussion

The outputs obtained are the heart rate of the subjects by recording live face video. The chosen subjects are in good health at the time of detecting the heart rate. The HR is measured at two conditions: (a) resting condition and (b) after 5 minutes of physical exercise (Table 1).

The subjects are listed with their heart rate obtained from the video recording. First the heart rate of the subjects is measured in their resting condition and after doing physical exercise from remote HR measurement technique. Meanwhile, to check the accuracy of the resultant heart rate, subject's heart rates are measured from standard heart rate measurement method using patient monitoring system. The difference in the heart rate obtained from proposed method and standard method is tabulated as the error in the below Table 2. The measurement from the proposed method is quite accurate from the standard heart rate measurement (Figs. 5, 6, 7, 8, 9, and 10).

Table 1 Heart rate obtained from the proposed method and standard method (patient monitoring system)

Subject	Age	Gender	Heart rate (resting condition)	Heart rate (after physical exercise)	Standard heart rate (resting condition)	Standard heart rate (after physical exercise)
1	55	M	84	90	82	89
2	21	M	72	88	75	90
3	10	F	69	83	70	80
4	8	M	72	81	73	84
5	25	F	78	82	75	86
6	48	F	79	80	76	82
7	30	F	76	82	74	82
8	34	M	79	87	79	88
9	61	M	80	85	81	84
10	56	F	77	83	77	84
11	9	M	74	80	71	83
12	62	M	82	89	80	88
13	52	F	72	81	75	81
14	29	M	73	82	75	84
15	51	F	78	86	77	83
16	26	F	77	85	73	82
17	46	M	72	79	72	82
18	41	F	73	80	70	79
19	17	M	71	82	73	85
20	16	M	76	81	74	80
21	33	F	69	78	70	80

Table 2 Experimental accuracy

Subjects	Error (resting condition)	Error (after physical exercise)
1	2	1
2	3	2
3	1	3
4	1	3
5	3	4
6	3	2
7	2	0
8	0	1
9	1	1
10	0	1
11	3	3
12	2	1
13	3	0
14	2	2
15	1	3
16	4	3
17	0	3
18	3	1
19	2	3
20	2	1
21	1	2

Fig. 5 Comparison of standard HR and HR obtained from the proposed method at resting condition

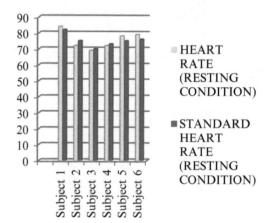

5 Conclusion

Heart rate (HR) measurement is an essential diagnostic parameter, as any unusual changes in the HR are directly related to the cardiovascular system functional changes which in turn useful in day-to-day life applications. The proposed method is used to monitor the heart rate of multiple subjects quickly and makes sure there is feasibility to implement mobile applications

Fig. 6 Comparison of standard HR and HR obtained from the proposed method after physical exercise

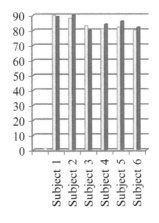

HEART RATE (PHYSICAL EXERCISE)

STANDARD HEART RATE (AFTER PHYSICAL EXERCISE)

Fig. 7 Sub 2 heart rate at resting condition

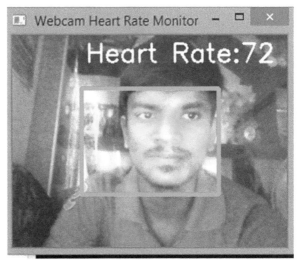

Fig. 8 Sub 2 heart rate after physical exercise

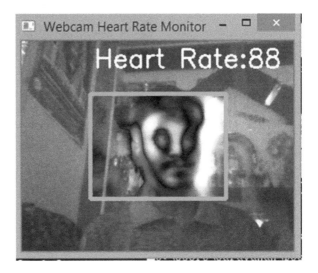

Fig. 9 Sub 6 heart rate at
resting condition

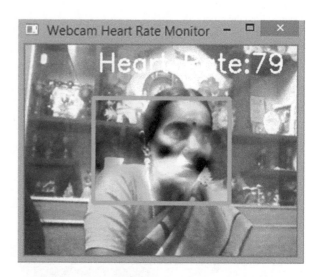

Fig. 10 Sub 6 heart rate
after physical exercise

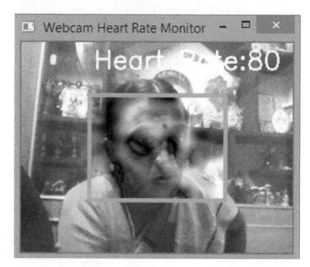

This method of contactless heart rate measurement from live video can be able
to give accurate results under well-controlled environmental conditions, but there is
a degradation in performance when variations in environmental illumination and
subjects motions. The accuracy can be improvised by using high-quality cameras
and by increasing the pixel intensity.

In the near future, we intend to study the camera quality's importance, no. of
human faces that can be recognized at a single moment, and the maximum distance
between subjected person and the camera. Also, we envision to enforce the heart
rate monitoring algorithm on various platforms.

References

1. Carmen Nadrag, Vlad Poenaru, George Suciu *"Heart rate measurement using face detection in video"*, IEEE 2018.
2. C. G. Scully, J. Lee, J. Meyer, A. M. Gorbach, D. Granquist-Fraser, Y. Mendelson, and K. H. Chon, *"Physiological parameter monitoring from optical recordings with a mobile phone,"* IEEE transactions on bio-medical engineering, vol. 59, Feb. 2012.
3. Chen Wang, Thierry Pun, Guillaume Chanel *"A Comparative survey of methods for Remote Heart rate detection from frontal face detection",* Frontiers in Bioengineering and Biotechnology, Volume 6, Article 33, May 2018.
4. D. Grimaldi, Y. Kurylyak, F. Lamonaca, and A. Nastro, *"Photoplethysmography detection by smartphone's videocamera,"* in 2011 IEEE 6th International Conference on Intelligent Data Acquisition and Advanced Computing Systems (IDAACS), vol. 1, 2011.
5. F. Lamonaca, Y. Kurylyak, D. Grimaldi, and V. Spagnuolo, *"Reliable pulse rate evaluation by smartphone,"* in 2012 IEEE International symposium on Medical Measurements and Applications Proceedings(MeMeA), 2012.
6. Guha Balakrishnan, Fredo Durand, John Guttag *"Detecting Pulse from head motion in video"*, IEEE conference on computer vision and pattern recognition, CVPR.2013.440, IEEE 2013.
7. H. Rahman, Hamidur, M. Ahmed, S. Begum, and P. Funk: *"Real time heart rate monitoring from facial RGB color video using webcam,"* 9th Annual Workshop of the Swedish Artificial Intelligence Society, 2016.
8. Isabel Bush *"Measuring Heart rate from video"*, Standard computer science, CA 94305, 2014.
9. Jean Pierre Lomaliza and Hanhoon park *"Improved heart rate measurement from mobile face videos"*, Electronics 2019,8,663, June 2019.
10. Jing Wei, Hong Luo, Si J. Wu, Paul P. Zheng, Genyue Fu and Kang Lee *"Transdermal optical imaging reveal basal stress via Heart rate variability Analysis- A Novel methodology comparable to Electrocardiography"*, Frontiers in Bioengineering and Biotechnology, Volume 9, Article 98, Feb 2018.
11. Kumar, M., Veeraraghavan, A., and Sabharwal, A, *"DistancePPG: robust non-contact vital signs monitoring using a camera"*, Biomed. Opt. Exp. 6, 1565–1588. doi:https://doi.org/10.1364/BOE.6.001565, 2015
12. L.K. Mestha, S. Kyal, B. Xu, and H.J. Madhu, *"Video-based estimation of heart rate variability,"* US8977347, 2015.
13. M. Garbey et al. *"Contact-free measurement of cardiac pulse based on the analysis of thermal imagery"*, IEEE Trnas Biomed Eng, 2007.
14. M. Lewandowska, J. Rumiński, T. Kocejko and J. Nowak, *"Measuring pulse rate with a webcam — A non-contact method for evaluating cardiac activity,"* Federated Conference on Computer Science and Information Systems, Szczecin, 2011.
15. M. Lunawat, A. Momin, V. Nirantar, and A. Deshmukh, *"Heart pulse monitoring: The smart phone way,"* Journal of Engineering Research and Applications, vol. 2, 2012.
16. M.-Z. Poh, D. McDuff, and R. Picard *"Non-contact, auto-mated cardiac pulse measurements using video imaging and blind source separation"*, Optical Society of America, 2010.
17. N. H. Mohd Sani, W. Mansor, Khuan Y. Lee, N. Ahmad Zainudin, S. A. Mahrim, *"Determination of Heart Rate from Photoplethysmogram using Fast Fourier Transform"*, International Conference on Bio Signal Analysis, Processing and Systems (ICBAPS), IEEE 2015
18. P. Viola and M. Jones, *"Rapid object detection using a boosted cascade of simple features",* In CVPR, 2001.
19. R. B. Lagido, J. Lobo, S. Leite, C. Sousa, L. Ferreira, J. Silva-Cardoso *"Using the smartphone camera to monitor heart rate and rhythm in heart failure patient"*, IEEE 2014.
20. S. Kwon, H. Kim, and K. S. Park, *"Validation of heart rate extraction using video imaging on a built-in camera system of a smartphone"*, In *EMBS*, 2012.

21. Xiaobai Li, Jie Chen, Guoying Zhao, Matti Pietikainen *"Remote Heart rate measurement from face videos under realistic situations"*, IEEE conference on computer vision and pattern recognition, CVPR.2014.543, IEEE 2014.
22. Xiao-Rong Ding, Yuan-Ting Zhang, Jing Liu, Wen-Xuan Dai, Hon Ki Tsang *"Continuous Cuffless blood pressure estimation using pulse transit time and photoplethysmogram intensity ratio"*, IEEE Transactions on Biomedical Engineering, 2015.
23. W. Verkruysse, L. O. Svaasand, and J. S. Nelson, *"Remote plethysmographic imaging using ambient light"*, Optics express, 2008.

Automatic Melanoma Diagnosis and Classification on Dermoscopic Images

Bethanney Janney. J, S. Emalda Roslin, and J. Premkumar

Abstract Automatic identification of skin carcinoma is significant. The dangerous types of cancer found in humans are skin cancer. Melanoma is the deadlier type of skin cancer. Healing can be beneficial on early diagnosis of melanoma. This paper aims to propose a skin cancer diagnosis algorithm that can automatically classify lesions as malignant or benign. Segmentation is done in the initial phase after choosing the finest image development methods accomplished by applying and comparing various noise removal filters on images. A perfect optimized segmentation methodology relies on thresholding, watershed algorithms are implemented on dermoscopy images, and the differentiated object is derived for GLCM attributes and qualitative techniques. To identify malignant or benign samples, the attributes are therefore supplied in to the support vector machine as a source. As perceived by experimental findings, SVM classification system with watershed segmentation has the potential to distinguish benign and malignant melanoma with a higher overall categorization efficiency.

Keywords Dermoscopic skin lesions · Image enhancement · Watershed segmentation · Feature extraction · SVM classifier

1 Introduction

Of most of the recognized forms of cancer, skin cancer, is considered as well established. It is frequently seen in the Caucasian white people. Melanoma, basal skin cancer (BSC), and squamous skin cancer (SSC) are predominant forms of skin cancer. Between these three, both basal and squamous are termed non-melanocytic skin cancer (NMSC) unlike the other skin conditions [11]. Melanoma seems to be the

Bethanney Janney. J (✉) · J. Premkumar
Department of Biomedical Engineering, Sathyabama Institute of Science and Technology, Chennai, India

S. Emalda Roslin
Department of Electronics and Communication Engineering, Sathyabama Institute of Science and Technology, Chennai, India

© The Author(s), under exclusive license to Springer Nature Switzerland AG 2021
A. K. Manocha et al. (eds.), *Computational Intelligence in Healthcare*, Health Information Science, https://doi.org/10.1007/978-3-030-68723-6_14

most severe growth in the skin often occurring in specific people with reduced mela-nin pigment [21]. It is reported that the absorption of ultraviolet radiation from the sun stimulates more remarkable than 90% of skin cancer occurrences. The infected individual's recovery rate is dropping, and certain infections appear black or brown in appearance [8]. Earlier time identification as well as skin malignancy diagnosis will prevent it from expanding or being dangerous. Utilization of microscopic approaches in melanoma cancer determined from pathologist is a very dull proce-dure. It also suffers from the variance of inter and intra-observer. The methods for instance biopsy is intrusive and so aching and dangerous. Dermatoscopy has been one of the methods for scanning used in melanoma detection. Dermatoscopy is indeed a nonintrusive type of scanning [13]. The very essential part for melanoma detection acts as precise classification and defining set of melanoma. They are cat-egorized as benign and malignant. Dermoscopic image has enhanced recognition efficiency by 50%, and perfect correctness of skin cancer diagnosis with dermos-copy lies between 75% and 84%. This suggests the essential of computer-based analysis platforms [5, 16]. This paper work aims at developing a computer-based skin cancer detection system and an accurate classification between benign and malignant melanoma that can improve the diagnosis rate of melanoma.

2   Related Works

Aljanabi et al. [1] proposed artificial bee colony algorithm for segmentation of the lesions. For each image a binomial image was obtained, and then the quantitative value of precision, sensitivity, specificity, dice coefficient, and Jaccard index was contrasted with ground truth (GT). Accuracy showed the segmentation evaluation significant connection with the aggregate pixel.

Arezoo Zakeri and Alireza Hokmabadi [2] presented a computer-assisted diag-nostic scheme to enhance the computational capability of standard ABCD assess-ment. The features obtained from local analysis of lesion intensity characterize melanin production and surface (PDT) attributes. The findings suggest that PDT structures are optimistic characteristics that can increase the identification efficiency of pigmented skin lesions in conjunction with standard ABCD features.

Jaisakthi et al. [10] used the GrabCut and k-means statistical models to imple-ment a skin carcinoma process. The process includes of two different phases: pre-processing with filtering methods to eradicate ambient noise or pels. The GrabCut neural network is utilized for optimization of the lesion from normal skin. To improve the boundary, the second phase utilizes the k-mean clustering algorithm with shade attributes in the lesion. The current proposal acquired better Dice coef-ficient values for PH2 and ISIC.

Riaz Farhan et al. [7] implemented method for predicting melanoma by. The borders of the lesion look distorted in this technique, like stripes and color patterns rather than regular streaks with normal borders, to separate the lesion and isolate the area of importance from the remainder of the picture through the use of an active contour approach supported by Kullback Leibler's difference within skin and tumor; attributes are derived from Local Binary Patterns (LBP) which often take the entire attributes of skin cancer. Throughout the current scheme, findings obtained on both PH2 and ISIC databases are more accurate with KNN and SVM.

Seeja and Suresh [23] presented a U-net algorithm based on the convolutional neural network (CNN) used for segmentation operations. The shade, pattern, and structure characteristics were then derived from its differentiated picture, and all the attributes derived from those same approaches have been incorporated into the classifier SVM System, Naïve Bayes, random forest, and K-nearest neighbor to identify surface picture which is neither carcinoma nor harmless lesion. The findings indicate the efficiency of the proposed solution. For image segmentation, the Dice efficiency rate of 77.5% is attained, and the SVM classification system provided 85.19% precision.

Muniba Ashfaq et al. [17] described a Smart Melanoma Prediction Method. In that way, the method involves isolating the textural properties of the skin infection including the characteristics of shade. In multilayer feed-forward, the identified attributes can be used to learn artificial neural models. The trained network for test specimen categorization is evaluated. This research involves three frames of simulations, which include 50%, 70%, and 90% of the information for use in training, whereas the existing 50%, 30%, and 10% were the test frames. The attributes measure the proportion between size and shape. The need for modified sample size in conjunction with ABCD functionality actually increases their detection of skin cancer.

3   Materials and Methods

The approach for determining classification pertaining to skin lesion via SVM classifier is provided in detail. Initially dermoscopic picture is subjected toward grayscale imaging and it's preprocessed for expulsion of clamor, for example, hairs and air pockets. The preprocessing acts as an essential step which helps in accurate diagnosis of varied skin lesion types. Many techniques were developed for noise reduction; here we use four different filtering techniques for example, median, Laplacian, mean and Gaussian filter. Then enhanced image is further segmented via thresholding and watershed segmentation algorithm. Besides, the segmented form of image is further then extracted on the basis of GLCM features and using fundamental form of statistical approach. The features are then fed directly as input for SVM and are used for distinguishing the unique features from that of malignant and benign forms of skin sores. The group of data is then distributed as training as well as test data for accounting, which is followed by examining the net accuracy of system performance. A conceptual illustration in the form of schematic diagram is depicted in Fig. 1.

Fig. 1 Schematic diagram
of skin lesion classification
using SVM classifier

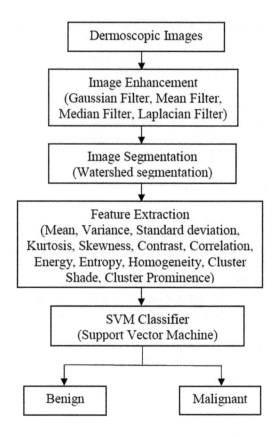

3.1 Image Enhancement

The very first step is image acquiring. Picked up image type is employed for preprocessing. Preprocessing is the step for enhancing an image. The enhancement stage
is employed for filtering noises along with image brightening. Using this process
fur, air pockets, and clamor artifacts are eliminated [20]. It is essential to eliminate
these artifacts before segmentation. Therefore preprocessing poses a prominent
impact in segmentation technique. Our proposed work imparts Gaussian, mean,
Laplacian, and median filter for preprocessing, and comparative results are
obtained [3].

3.2 Watershed Segmentation

Segmentation splits an image into its respective sections or objects. Accurate segmented outcomes are beneficial for evaluation, prediction, and treatment [24].
Watershed segmentation is a picture segmentation process based on geometry. The

watershed conversion for picture segmentation was proposed by Hanzheng Wang et al. [9] in grayscale computational morphology. To separate contacting objects in a picture, watershed division is utilized. The transformation of the watershed is often beneficial to this task. It discovers in a picture watershed slope lines and catchment bowls by treating it as a layer with high light pels and low dark pels. Watershed transforms function perfectly if you can identify or tag items in the forefront and backgrounds.

3.3 Feature Extraction

Precise and reliable extraction of the attribute is important as it influences the quality of the identification of skin lesions. For texture attribute measurements, the output of the GLCM is used to provide a quantity of intensity variance at the pixel of significance. Ordinarily, in light of two parameters, the co-event matrix is determined. These are the relative separation among pixel pair d estimated in pixel number and their relative direction. It is typically quantized in four angles (e.g., $0°$, $45°$, $90°$, and $135°$) [25]. A GLCM is a vector attributing the amount of columns and rows in the image to the volume of gray, G. The array vector $P(i, j \mid \Delta_x, \Delta_y)$ is the proportional wavelength subdivided via a sequence of pixels $(\Delta_x \Delta_y)$. GLCM is also represented as $P(i, j \mid d, \theta)$ comprising the quadratic statistical likelihood values for gray level i and j varies at a certain distance inclination specific attributes are derived through this approach, G is the total of the gray scales chosen, where μ seems to be the average, P, μ_x, μ_y, σ_x and σ_y are indeed the means and periodic deviations of P_x and P_y [14]. GLCM operates on gray level picture matrix to derive most common attributes like mean, variance, standard deviation, skewness, kurtosis, entropy, energy, contrast, cluster shade, correlation, cluster prominence, and homogeneity [4].

3.4 Skin Lesion Classification

Support vector machines (SVM) are supervised processing configurations. Such learning models are correlated with processing algorithms prone to distinguish information and to recognize characteristics of data provided. Similar strategies are given for grouping activities. SVM can be utilized if the data has exactly two categories. The classifier picks the right hyperplane to distinguish one class data points from the other category. Since it is important to define two categories, the two characteristics are taken as f_1 and f_2. In this work, the linear SVM classifier can be used to write the general equation as:

$$f_1 w_1 + f_2 w_2 + \text{bias} = 0 \tag{1}$$

where

f_1 - source 1 (attribute1)
f_2 - source 2 (attribute 2)
w_1 is the weight initialized to the first input
w_2 is the weight initialized to the second input

The value of one of the attributes can be determined by means of the expression below:

$$f_2 = -\frac{f1w1}{w2} - \frac{b}{w2} \tag{2}$$

where interrupts $b/w2$ and gradient is the proportion of weights ($w1/w2$). Thus support arrays are discovered through figuring the range among arrays and serializing the support arrays as two points. Then the weights and bias constraints are computed employing orthonormal formulae that would be used to categorize the data [22].

4 Experimental Analysis

This segment addresses the findings of automated skin lesion categorization as cancerous or harmless on images collected from the dermoscopy technique database. It is found that the result obtained due to the application of above SVM classifier is much more accurate than the other methods. For research and benchmarking purposes, the PH2 dataset was developed to simplify relative trainings on dermoscopic image segmentation and organization algorithms. PH2 is a dermoscopic image database developed from Pedro Hispano Hospital, Matosinhos, Portugal's Dermatology Service [15]. Preprocessing is further then carried out using five filters, viz., Gaussian, median, mean, and finally Laplacian filter. Figure 2 shows the resultant images rendered from various filters which (a) serve as the source image, (b) represent output for Gaussian filter, (c) indicate result for mean filtering, (d) indicate result for median filtering, and (e) indicate result for Laplacian filtering, respectively.

Comparative representation indicated four filtered images which appeared clear over the fact that the net output for median filter proved as best for removing noise. In determining the best approach, each kernel method is validated with three error metrics expressed as peak signal-to-noise ratio (PSNR), mean squared error (MSE), and structural similarity index (SSIM) [18]. The average squared deviation between the normalized picture and the real picture is the total square error.

From the experimental results, lower the value of MSE indicates lesser error, whereas PSNR is specified as proportion underlying quality measurement to that of actual picture to normalized picture. PSNR is found to be inversely proportional with MSE. For better reconstructed image the PSNR value is high. Mathematical

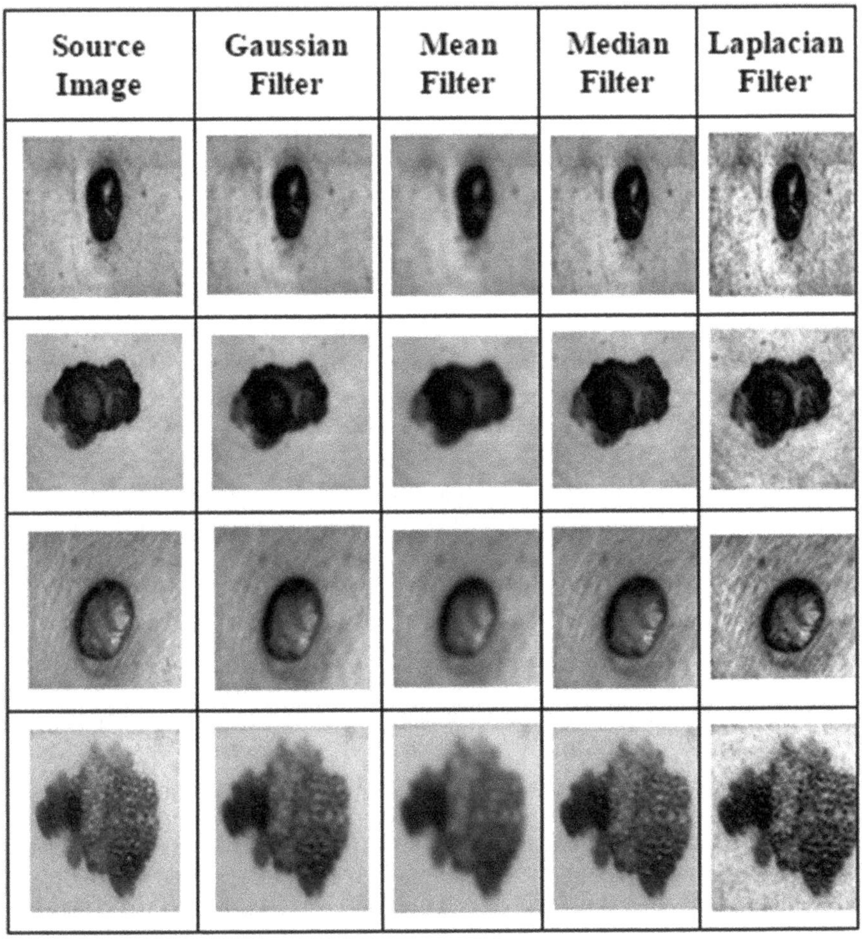

Source Image	Gaussian Filter	Mean Filter	Median Filter	Laplacian Filter

Fig. 2 Results of different filters: (**a**) source image, (**b**) Gaussian, (**c**) mean, (**d**) median, and (**e**) Laplacian filtering

equation from the findings rendered in the form of MSE and PSNR is denoted below as:

$$\text{MSE} = \frac{1}{MN} \sum_{i=1}^{M} \sum_{j=1}^{N} \left(f_1(i,j) - f_2(i,j) \right)^2 \tag{3}$$

where

f_1 - source picture
f_2 - output picture

$$\text{PSNR} = 10\log\left[\frac{(255)^2}{\text{mse}}\right] \tag{4}$$

Structural similarity index measure SSIM is evaluated for measuring image quality and quantifying parameter. SSIM is utilized to determine the comparison among original and compressed images. It is specified in Eq. (5)

$$\text{SSIM}(x,y) = \frac{\left(2\mu_x\mu_y + C_1\right)\left(2\sigma_{xy} + C_2\right)}{\left(\mu_x^2 + \mu_y^2 + C_1\right)\left(\sigma_x^2 + \sigma_y^2 + C_2\right)} \tag{5}$$

from which representations of x and y are comparable pictures. The average pixel quantities are μ_x and μ_y, while the standard deviations at patches x and y are σ_x and σ_y. Where c_1, c_2 is added as constants which prevent instabilities when $\sigma_x \sigma_y$ is close to zero. The numerical values lie between -1 and 1 for ssIm index. For same images arithmetic value is constantly 1.The quantitative metrics are computed.

Analyses are completed for 200 data and formulation is completed for 50 data result. In the proposed work, PH2 database is used [12]. It comprises an array of 200 dermoscopic pictures and their Boolean kernel. The following Table 1 displays the evaluated parameters.

Table 1 clearly demonstrates that mse level is small and that the psnr level for median filters is high. For dermoscopic images, median filter is desired to reduce noise. Figures 3, 4, and 5 display a pictorial evidence of three assessing parameters, viz., PSNR, MSE, and SSIM for four filters showing median filter efficiency is higher than other three filters.

The proposed technique of watershed segmentation provides better result on segmentation of skin lesion. The segmented sample images are seen in Fig. 6. Methods of extraction of features are utilized to remove shape, color, and texture from the separate regions of the lesions. Extracted, those texture attributes by GLCM are shown in Tables 2 and 3.

In the proposed system, SVM classifier is tested on a dataset containing 200 images that includes benign and malignant kinds of skin lesions. The database is organized equally for training set (benign 40, malignant 40) and testing set (benign 50, malignant 50). Specificity, sensitivity, and precision are the parameters utilized to identify the efficiency of classifiers. Figure 7 displays SVM performance evaluation classifier, and parameter validated for the classifier is shown in above Table 4. These parameters can be evaluated using the formula given below [6].

$$\text{Specificity} = \left[\text{TN} \times 100 / (\text{TN} + \text{FP})\right] \tag{6}$$

$$\text{Sensitivity} = \left[\text{TP} \times \frac{100}{(\text{TP} + \text{FN})}\right] \tag{7}$$

Table 1 PSNR, MSE, and SSIM performance evaluation of various filters

Input image	Gaussian filter			Mean filter			Laplacian filter			Median filter		
	PSNR	MSE	SSIM	PSNR	MSE	SSIM	PSNR	MSE	SSIM	PSNR	MSE	SSIM
1.	39.534	25.756	0.5862	35.356	28.031	0.5561	45.871	30.301	0.7610	69.534	21.946	0.8486
2.	37.213	26.981	0.6532	36.821	28.567	0.4453	49.544	31.515	0.7070	67.213	23.039	0.8143
3.	37.012	25.941	0.6700	35.702	29.578	0.4586	56.231	30.284	0.7347	67.012	22.751	0.8182
4.	39.032	25.497	0.5829	35.231	29.031	0.5893	55.324	33.596	0.7452	69.032	22.236	0.8125
5.	32.451	25.032	0.6916	35.003	29.320	0.5241	46.894	31.180	0.7552	72.451	23.096	0.8621
6.	38.421	23.302	0.5844	33.534	29.003	0.6521	47.563	34.271	0.7721	68.421	23.081	0.8098
7.	39.570	26.013	0.5789	36.432	27.412	0.5294	49.863	32.152	0.7231	69.570	21.569	0.8654
8.	37.403	25.781	0.5962	35.022	27.610	0.4561	52.687	32.331	0.7778	67.403	21.563	0.8234
9.	36.804	26.541	0.6358	36.423	28.040	0.4783	53.612	31.564	0.7465	66.804	22.636	0.8147
10.	38.324	27.035	0.6583	37.044	29.006	0.5234	52.314	30.562	0.7120	68.324	22.521	0.8045
11.	30.562	26.587	0.6725	36.528	28.451	0.5412	51.035	31.898	0.7621	70.562	21.036	0.7985
12.	30.245	26.031	0.6851	36.541	29.059	0.5874	50.896	32.549	0.7013	70.245	21.784	0.8014
13.	31.856	25.142	0.6654	35.122	29.009	0.5652	52.764	37.324	0.7450	71.856	22.458	0.7991
14.	39.310	25.001	0.5921	35.030	28.064	0.5231	51.234	38.787	0.7865	69.310	22.684	0.8561
15.	38.501	26.358	0.5968	36.458	27.333	0.4912	52.894	30.987	0.7102	68.501	23.895	0.8452
16.	39.711	27.560	0.6210	37.543	27.491	0.4875	49.321	30.569	0.7560	69.711	22.348	0.8012
17.	39.023	26.980	0.6541	36.345	27.587	0.4520	48.712	31.879	0.7210	69.023	20.998	0.7968
18.	38.251	25.001	0.6998	35.468	28.008	0.4421	47.235	38.345	0.7342	68.251	21.365	0.8128
19.	37.659	27.451	0.6740	37.212	28.145	0.4568	48.210	30.724	0.7124	67.659	23.120	0.8079
20.	37.002	26.314	0.6547	36.377	27.634	0.5161	45.871	31.591	0.7014	67.002	22.001	0.8251

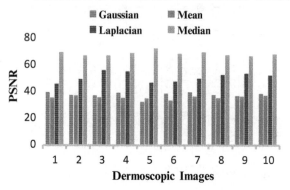

Fig. 3 Relation of Gaussian, standard, and Laplacian filters PSNR values

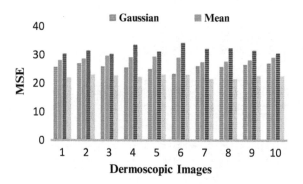

Fig. 4 Relation of Gaussian, standard, and Laplacian filters MSE values

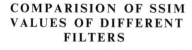

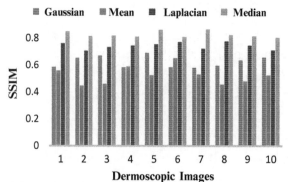

Fig. 5 Relation of Gaussian, standard, and Laplacian filters SSIM values

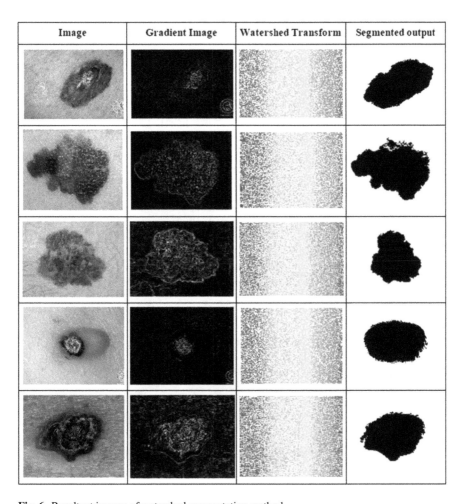

Fig. 6 Resultant images of watershed segmentation method

Table 2 Extracted features of benign images

Attributes	Img 1	Img 2	Img 3	Img 4	Img 5
Mean	7.025121	7.042754	7.293105	7.941474	7.375152
Variance	2.472146	2.614041	2.251743	1.994152	2.572131
Standard deviation	1.621475	1.589923	1.692841	1.794025	1.678453
Kurtosis	7.206723	7.021086	7.321148	7.406741	7.134352
Skewness	−2.256542	−2.157045	−2.271325	−2.282014	−2.187145
Contrast	1.841602	2.218624	2.245513	2.364673	2.192044
Correlation	7.399340	7.942075	7.923140	8.435146	7.849735
Energy	3.278201	3.197956	3.345715	3.297153	3.264012
Entropy	6.317930	5.921883	6.247511	6.587102	6.408211
Homogeneity	8.381254	8.641372	8.701357	8.492154	8.633342
Cluster shade	43.261019	45.836114	49.143015	52.59613	53.921045
Cluster prominence	2381.1427	2393.1748	2482.1024	2581.1327	2701.1075

Table 3 Extracted features of malignant images

Attributes	Img 1	Img 2	Img 3	Img 4	Img 5
Mean	6.748145	7.238214	6.923145	6.856143	6.892377
Variance	1.734125	1.899044	1.672371	1.757133	1.789245
Standard deviation	2.641153	1.862130	1.971011	1.812377	2.378711
Kurtosis	3.072164	4.047254	4.721334	4.831754	4.925763
Skewness	−1.276524	−1.263137	−1.38217	−1.492398	−1.492347
Contrast	2.821764	2.743218	3.027167	3.147542	2.897476
Correlation	9.375712	9.562977	9.576434	8.972148	8.994271
Energy	2.179021	2.194284	2.202177	2.186758	2.214724
Entropy	7.076433	7.261247	6.934564	6.891324	7.012545
Homogeneity	9.210755	9.133881	8.986151	9.142844	8.990231
Cluster shade	99.724066	93.24157	97.87124	84.13574	87.12784
Cluster prominence	3271.1086	3148.2014	3189.124	3012.725	3167.197

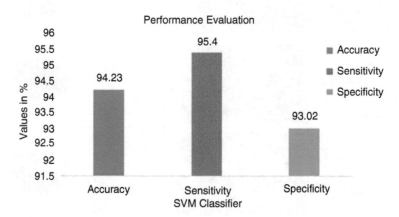

Fig. 7 Performance evaluation of SVM classifier

$$\text{Precision} = \left[\left(TP + TN \right) \times 100 / \left(TP + TN + FP + FN \right) \right] \qquad (8)$$

Where

- False positive (FP): benign picture being wrongly assessed as malignant
- False negative (FN): malignant picture being wrongly assessed as benign
- True positive (TP): malignant picture being assessed accurately as malignant
- True negative (TN): benign picture being assessed accurately as benign

4.1   Discussion

From the experimental findings watershed segmentation is provided to address the challenges of automated dermoscopic image identification of benign and malignant. The automatic skin cancer identification including dermoscopic images is effectively tested to determine the features of skin lesions in a noninvasive way. The suggested method was examined for benign and malignant lesions on 200 images from the PH2 dataset. This database provided ground-truth images which assisted to compare our technique's results with radiologist's manual evaluation. As far as Table 2 is regarded, median filter is preferred for dermoscopic images to minimize noise which clearly shows that for median filters, the mse level is small and that the psnr level is large. Median filtering and watershed segmentation algorithm assisted in precisely segmenting the lesion area. Then we extract array of texture features from the segmented images employing GLCM technique. Tables 2 and 3 display the characteristics derived from the benign and malignant images. Figure 7 and Table 4 show the SVM Classifier's performance analysis with 94.23% accuracy. While the supporting vector machine approach and U-net algorithm are used for identification in the analysis by Seeja and Suresh [23], the classification accuracy rate is 85.19%. Based on its precision, specificity, and sensitivity, the output result of the proposed SVM classifier system provides better results relative to many other classifications [19].

5   Conclusion

The target of this work is to classify melanoma as healthy and cancerous based on watershed segmentation, method of extraction of GLCM features, and classifier of SVM. In the whole study, the efficiency of five preprocessing filters used in skin lesion images for noise removal was discussed and compared. Median filter is observed to be more appropriate in dermoscopic images for noise removal. The use of gradient magnitude with watershed segmentation in our technique provides the highest outcomes and prevents overlapping between the lesion and healthy skin. The segmentation outcome was then used by the GLCM feature extraction technique, which makes it possible to analyze the melanoma spot analysis and guides

Table 4 Parameters validated for the SVM classifier

Metrics	SVM classifier
True positive	83
True negative	80
False positive	06
False negative	04
Accuracy	94.23
Sensitivity	95.40
Specificity	93.02

for the cancer spread direction. The SVM algorithm is used to identify a skin abrasion as healthy and carcinogenic. However, performance of SVM classifier might be enhanced by increasing number of features that can very well classify the skin images based on the parameters proposed.

Acknowledgments We, the authors, would like to thank Sathyabama Institute of Science and Technology, Department of Biomedical Engineering for providing facilities for carrying on and executing the research work.
Compliance with Ethical StandardsConflict of interest: Authors declare that they have no conflict of interest.

References

1. Aljanabi M, Ozok Y, Rahebi J, Abdullah A (2018) Skin Lesion Segmentation Method for Dermoscopy Images using Artificial Bee Colony Algorithm. Symmetry 10(8):347–357
2. Arezoo Zakeri, Alireza Hokmabadi (2018) Improvement in the diagnosis of melanoma and dysplastic lesions by introducing ABCD-PDT features and a hybrid classifier. Biocybernetics and Biomedical Engineering 38(3):456–466
3. Azadeh Noori Hoshyar, Adel Al-Jumailya, Afsaneh Noori Hoshyar (2014) Comparing the Performance of Various Filters on Skin Cancer Images. Procedia Computer Science, Elsevier 42:32–37
4. Bethanney Janney J and Emalda Roslin S (2018) Classification of melanoma from dermoscopic data using machine learning techniques. Multimedia tools and applications, Springer 79:3713–3728
5. Cheng Lu, Mrinal Mandal (2015) Automated analysis and diagnosis of skin melanoma on whole slide histopathological images. Pattern Recognition 48:2738–275
6. Ebtihal Almansour, Arfan Jaffar M (2016) Classification of Dermoscopic Skin Cancer Images using Color and Hybrid Texture. International Journal of Computer Science and Network Security 16(4):135–139
7. Farhan Riaz, Sidra Naeem, Raheel Nawaz, Miguel Coimbra (2018) Active Contours Based Segmentation and Lesion Periphery Analysis for Characterization of Skin Lesions in Dermoscopy Images. IEEE Journal of Biomedical and Health Informatics 23(2):489–500
8. Guerra Rosas E, Álvarez Borrego J (2015) Methodology for diagnosing of skin cancer on images of dermatologic spots by spectral analysis. Biomedical Optics Express 6(10):3876–3891
9. Hanzheng Wang, Xiaohe Chen, Randy H. Moss, Joe Stanley (2010) Watershed segmentation of dermoscopy images using a watershed technique. Skin Research and Technology 16:378–384
10. Jaisakthi S M, Mirunalini P, Aravindan C (2018) Automated skin lesion segmentation of dermoscopy images using GrabCut and k-means algorithms. IET Computer Vision 12(8):1088–1095
11. Jeffrey E. Gershenwald, Richard A. Scolyer, Kenneth R. Hess (2017) Melanoma Staging: Evidence-Based Changes in the American Joint Committee on Cancer Eighth Edition Cancer Staging Manual. CA: Cancer Journal for Clinicians 67(6):474–492
12. Khalid Eltayef, Yongmin Li, Xiaohui Liu (2017) Detection of Melanoma Skin Cancer in dermoscopy images. IOP Conf. Series: Journal of Physics. doi: https://doi.org/10.1088/1742659 6/787/1/012034
13. Maglogiannis I, Doukas C N (2009) Overview of advanced computer vision systems for skin lesions characterization. IEEE Transactions on Information Technology in Biomedicine 13(5):721–733

14. Md. Al-Amin, Md. Badrul Alam Miah, Md. Ronju Mia (2015) Detection of Cancerous and Non-cancerous Skin by using GLCM Matrix and Neural Network Classifier. International Journal of Computer Applications 132(8):44–49
15. Mendonca T, Ferreira P M, Marques J S, Marcal A R, Rozeira J (2013) PH2 - A dermoscopic image database for research and benchmarking. 35th Annual International Conference of the IEEE EMBS 5437–5440
16. Monisha M., Suresh A, Bapu B T, Rashmi M R (2018) Classification of malignant melanoma and benign skin lesion by using back propagation neural network and ABCD rule. Cluster Computing: 1–11
17. Muniba Ashfaq, Nasru Minallah, Zahid Ullah, Arbab Masood Ahmad, Aamir Saeed, Abdul Hafeez (2019) Performance Analysis of Low-Level and High-Level Intuitive Features for Melanoma Detection. Electronics 8:672–682
18. Nurwahidah Mamat, Wan Eny Zarina Wan Abdul Rahman, Shaharuddin Soh, Rozi Mahmud (2016) Evaluation of Performance for Different Filtering Methods in CT Brain Images. AIP Conference Proceedings. https://doi.org/10.1063/1.5055479
19. Odeh S M, Baareh A M (2016) A comparison of classification methods as diagnostic system: A case study on skin lesions. Computer Methods and Programs in Biomedicine 137:311–319
20. Ramya Ravi R, Vinod Kumar R S, Shanila N (2018) Artifacts Removal in Melanoma using Various Preprocessing Filters. International Journal of Engineering and Technology 7(3.27):104–107
21. Rebecca L. Siegel, Kimberly D. Miller, Ahmedin Jemal (2019) Cancer Statistics 2019. CA: Cancer Journal for Clinicians 69:7–34
22. Samy Bakheet (2017) An SVM Framework for Malignant Melanoma Detection Based on Optimized HOG Features. Computation 5(4):1–13
23. Seeja R D, Suresh A (2019) Deep Learning Based Skin Lesion Segmentation and Classification of Melanoma using Support Vector Machine. Asian Pac J Cancer Prev 20(5):1555–1561
24. Sumithra R, Suhil M, Guru D S (2015) Segmentation and classification of skin lesions for disease diagnosis. Procedia Computer Science 45:76–85
25. Wei L S, Gan Q, Ji T (2018) Skin Disease Recognition Method Based on Image Color and Texture Features. Computational and Mathematical Methods in Medicine 8145713:1–10

GI Cloud Design: Issues and Perspectives

V. Lakshmi Narasimhan, A. K. Sala, and Anne Shergill

Abstract Gastroenterology is a field of medicine that has its roots deeply embedded in the technological revolution of the twenty-first century. It emerges as a specialty dominated by ever-evolving imaging and diagnostic modalities that have surpassed archaic means of diagnosing and treating various gastroenterological disorders. This article highlights advancement in Cloud-computing technology that has the potential to change the way healthcare professionals in gastrointestinal (GI) work in the inpatient and outpatient setting. Cloud-based technology for storing, retrieving, and manipulating patient-specific data will set to transcend from being used in government or corporate organizations to outpatient and inpatient GI services across the nation. For example, various gastroenterological procedures, including esophagogastroduodenoscopy, colonoscopy, and endoscopic retrograde cholangiopancreatography, are reported in the electronic medical record system as a PDF file. This PDF file can range between 200 and 500 kilobytes in memory size with approximately five to ten pictures in each PDF file on an average. Such files are retrieved – on average – two to three times (in hospital) and two to three times during follow-up visits. Further, in an academic institution and particularly tertiary care facilities, with GI fellows working across multiple subdivisions of GI – namely, hepatology, pancreatobiliary, and advanced endoscopy – the number of average procedures in a day can range between 15 and 20. In the outpatient setting comprising primarily of private GI practices, this number can range between 10 and 15. In addition, the number of GI specialist can vary based on the hospital size and is often different for various programs. However for a tertiary care facility, this number can average around three to five attending physicians and five to six GI fellows at any given time. As a consequence, GI the services are likely to expand with limitless potential to grow in terms of practicing physicians, training physicians, and patient

---

An earlier version of the paper appeared in the American Journal of Gastroenterology, 2019 [22].

V. L. Narasimhan (✉)
Department of Computer Science, University of Botswana, Gaborone, Botswana

A. K. Sala
Smaragdine Technologies Pvt. Ltd., Hyderabad, India

A. Shergill
Banner University Medical Center, Tucson, AZ, USA

population being served. The amount of data that needs to be stored, categorized, analyzed, and retrieved would be enormous. Further, context-based searching and retrieving are also required. Further a plethora of services are needed, and future services should be relatively easily added, besides maintaining existing services properly. All these issues besides others can be addressed thru proper design of the GI Cloud. This chapter describes the architecture of the GI Cloud, besides addressing various issues therein, including possible vendor lock-in and Cloud interoperability standards. The performance of the GI Cloud has been evaluated using parametric modelling technique, and the results indicate that GI Cloud can successfully enhance the performance of the medicos involved in this field; the details are also provided in this chapter.

Keywords Gastroenterology · Cloud computing · Data services · Software services · Privacy and security services · Portability and interoperability services · HIPPA compliance service · Human computing service · Universal access and reliability service · Total quality of service (TQoS) · Parametric performance modelling

1 Introduction

Modern technology is catapulting the way medicine is practiced today and, while every technological enhancement betters patient care and experience, they also bring along shortcomings that need to be overcome on a continual basis. In the past decade, GI has successfully ventured toward electronic documentation and record keeping, but the only thing certain about future is further change in our infrastructure to accommodate the growing patient population, patient-specific database, and healthcare provider-driven management of the same. Practicing medicine today in the inpatient or outpatient setting is centered on patient satisfaction, which in turn serves as a parameter for quality of healthcare being delivered. Healthcare professionals dedicatedly strive to provide a wholesome experience that begins with the initial patient encounter and continues throughout the course of outpatient followup or hospital course, entailing various diagnostic and therapeutic interventions. It is therefore the need of the hour to identify how innovative technology can aid in this task to better patient care experience at large. A cohesive approach systematically works with the ever-expanding patient database and procedural reporting of effective reproduction and recall of this dataset. And this necessity gave rise to one of the most current and talked about technological advancements in medicine relating to data storage, analyses, retrieval, and value-adding, called "The Cloud."

GI is a specialty fueled by procedural expertise and viewing and analyzing large amount of data. It encompasses a wide array of procedures, ranging from esophagogastroduodenoscopy, colonoscopy, and endoscopic ultrasound to endoscopic retrograde cholangiopancreatography. Each procedure is reported and documented electronically, while procedure reports comprise of detailed description of the procedure along with pictorial illustration. The challenges to be addressed include the need to accommodate ever-expanding patient database with a plethora of quality of service factors, such as information security, privacy, portability reliability, and interoperability of datasets. Considering this scenario, Cloud-based technology emerges as the single most vied advancement to address this, as the Cloud offers a viable, yet cheaper alternative.

This chapter deals with the design of a comprehensive GI Cloud and its associated services therein, besides addressing various practical technical issues. The rest of the chapter is organized as follows: Section 2 outlines the problem statement, while Sect. 3 describes a typical Cloud environment. Section 4 details the services architecture of the GI Cloud, and Sect. 5 discusses other issues of the GI Cloud. A parametric performance evaluation model for the GI Cloud is presented in Sect. 6, while the conclusion summarizes the chapter and offers pointers for further work in this arena.

2 Problem Statement

A widely used definition of Cloud computing developed by the US National Institute of Standards and Technology's (NIST) states [5]: "Cloud computing is a model for enabling ubiquitous, convenient, on-demand network access to a shared pool of configurable computing resources (e.g., networks, servers, storage, applications, and services) that can be rapidly provisioned and released with minimal management effort or service provider interaction." The model consists of five essential characteristics, namely, self-service on demand, ubiquitous network access, metered use, elasticity, and resource pooling; three service models, namely, infrastructure as a service, platform as a service, and software as a service; and four deployment models, namely, public Cloud, private Cloud, community Cloud, and hybrid Cloud. Further, the National e-Governance Plan (NeGP) has led to the creation of common ICT infrastructure, such as State Wide Area Networks (SWANs), state data centers (SDCs), and Common Service Centers (CSCs), as well as the development of guidelines and standards to ensure interoperability, standardization, and integration of various services to provide a unified face of the government to the people. The progress of NeGP and other national initiatives [2, 3], such as National Data Centers (NDCs), NICNET, National Knowledge Network (NKN), and National Optical Fiber Network (NoFN), highlight the fact that core ICT infrastructure has been rolled out and there is considerable reach in terms of connectivity both at the national and state level [23].

Such groundbreaking advancements always stem from the absolute need to bring about a change in the existing methodology and approach in GI. While outlining the need to adopt Cloud-based technology, it is prudent to recognize why this change is essential. There is a huge disparity between the ever-increasing volume of patient-specific data and the corresponding lack of suitable infrastructure to hold and work with the dataset. The need for deployment of automatic features that facilitate patient-specific data storage, search, retrieval, and processing are critically felt. These are met by Cloud-based technology, for data handling and processing in GI. Being content with the status quo invariably results in stagnation and regression in any field. But this is particularly true for a dynamic field like GI, where modern concepts continually challenge the existing ones. Cloud computing offers efficient solution to several of the problems and issues encountered in GI. Indeed, experiences at few GI practices [1, 2] indicate that this is the technological way forward in the field GI.

The GI Cloud architecture presented in this chapter is to be seeded initially on national and state data center assets (adapted for the Cloud through virtualization) and connected through existing network infrastructure such as the Internet, SWANs, and NKN; the services of private Cloud providers [23] may also be inducted depending on the demand. The GI Cloud will provide services to government departments, citizens, and businesses through the Internet as well as mobile connectivity. Furthermore, the Cloud will provide accelerated delivery of e-services to citizens and businesses and support a number of other objectives, including increased standardization, interoperability, and integration.

3   Overview of the Cloud Environment

Cloud computing refers to making best use of resources on remote servers made available at national and state data centers and accessed via the Internet for storing and processing of a wide variety of datasets (see Fig. 1). Cloud has transformed the way legacy IT infrastructure is managed, and its adoption has resulted in improved innovation and cost efficiency, quicker product deployment, time to market, and the ability to automatically scale up or scale down the applications that are on demand [15, 17]. Over a period of time, Cloud has emerged in scope, and applications are growing rapidly from conceptual models to reality. There are many more aspects, such as economical, contractual, legal, and security that are still to be explored in depth and maturity [9].

The advantages of the Cloud environment include the following [8, 9, 11, 12]: (i) reduced overall costs, (ii) round-the-clock and round-the-year availability, (iii) capacity flexibility, (iv) access from anywhere, (v) automatic updates on supporting software, (vi) minimum migration time, (vii) low carbon footprint, (viii) security, (ix) HIPPA compliance, and (x) simplicity of overall use.

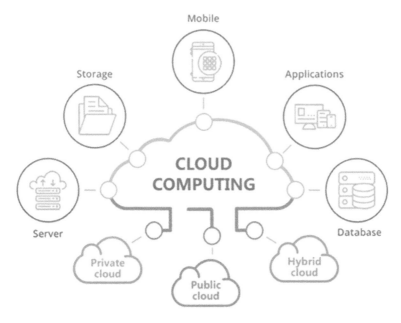

Fig. 1 A Typical Cloud environment

4 Services Architecture of the GI Cloud

The US National Institute of Standards and Technology's (NIST) definition of Cloud computing [5] is the most widely adopted one and has been adopted by various governments and establishments including hospitals. The GI Cloud is envisaged to be established initially on national and state data center assets (adapted for the Cloud through virtualization) and connected through existing network infrastructure. A hospital may also engage the services of private Cloud providers to address security-related considerations. The GI Cloud will provide services to various patients and businesses through the Internet as well as mobile connectivity. The hospital's Cloud-based service delivery platform will also support a number of other objectives including increased standardization, interoperability, integration, a move toward an OPEX model, the pooling of scarce, under-utilized resources, and the spread of best practices [23]. It will also support ongoing cost-effectiveness and manageability. Cloud computing also facilitates speeding up the development and roll out of e-hospital applications, thereby enhancing agility in customizing and deploying ICT to meet specific business needs, while at the same time increasing government ICT efficiency (through reuse and economies of scale). As a consequence, a well-defined adoption strategy and roadmap are critical for realizing this vision and to establish the envisaged Cloud-computing platform. Our GI Cloud provided in Fig. 2a and b is further elaborated below:

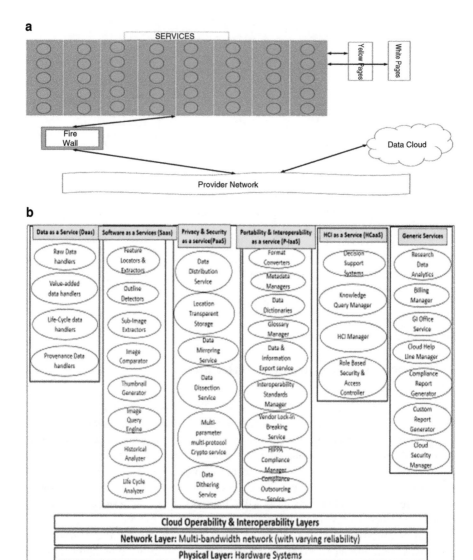

Fig. 2 (**a**) Information architecture of the GI Cloud. (**b**) Detailed information services architecture of the GI Cloud

4.1 Data as a Service (DaaS)

Data as a Service (DaaS) – Datasets available in different forms (text, audio, video, images, and animations) can be made available to customers across continents, countries, and regions, giving them a feel that the data is locally available, provided users have network connectivity [13]. The service is offered at varying costs to the end-user, while most times the data storage on these infrastructure remains free of cost to those who maintain very low volumes of data. For application developers who are looking to host applications offered by different vendors for different models, they can be set at varying price tags. The services are offered at much cheaper costs based on the volume application developer choses to have and different types of data storage technologies that are available at a very cheaper cost. Application developers need only to strike a balance between the cost and the data access speeds. The nature of services in in our GI Cloud's DaaS includes, but not limited to, the following four services:

- *Raw data handlers*: Raw data that gets generated and stored cannot be used in the form as received; one needs a variety of analytical tools that are made available in the Cloud. Raw data types include text, images, audio, video, telemetry, and geospatial data. Application developers need to go through the SLAs (service-level agreements) and NDAs (nondisclosure agreements) with DaaS service providers to meet the QoS (quality of service) offered and promised by the vendors. In cases where application developers want the servers not to be exposed to public, there is always a chance to have the DaaS service provider host their services either on private Cloud or on localized server environments which are caged in Cloud infrastructure environment, and only the clients and no one else are given access to very sensitive information on the designated systems.
- *Value-added data handlers* – Value-added data handler handles data from multiple raw sources so that one can get type of data that is available from more than one source and the format in which the user wants.
- *Life cycle data handlers* – Life cycle data handlers deals with data of a single entity or a person but over a life cycle or set of entity or person over their entire life cycle. So this data is deeper data on a particular entity or a person.
- *Provenance data handlers* - Provenance[1] data handler relates to both data and provenance-related information, i.e., how the data originally was collected, namely, the model of the instrument, resolution, and accuracy.

4.2   Software as a Service (SaaS)

Software as a Service (SaaS) [14] is a distribution model of the complete software required from a third-party providers to host applications that are available to all customers round the clock and 365 days a year, with little or no impact to the business [18, 19]. SaaS works in tandem with infrastructure as a service (IaaS) and

---

[1]Provenance relates to the collection and maintenance of all metadata along with the actual collected data. For example, a particular dataset might have been collected using a particular model and made of a meter; then not only these details but also their accuracy and resolution would also be recorded so that when people try to use the datasets later, they would understand as to how the original data was actually collected. In many real-world scenario, such provenance information is critically important in managing/controlling the overall system.

platform as a service (PaaS) – the three main categories of Cloud computing. SaaS is a hosted application management model, where providers host customers' software, which become the main link to delivery. The source of application is one and the same for all the customers and in situations like new feature inclusions, functionalities, updates, etc. can be rolled out with a push of a button. This service is also in line with policies framed in SLA. The end customer can make best use of the application programming interface (API) provided by SaaS provider and go hand in hand taking their complete benefits. Email, financial management, customer relationship management, sales management, business intelligence tool, ticketing systems, and customer and technical support systems are many such fundamental business applications that are available over multiple SaaS models. SaaS services in our GI Cloud work with a variety of images, such as, optical, ultrasound, and X-ray. SaaS services are mainly image processing services, which include the following eight services:

- *Feature Locators and Extractors* – feature extractors and locators is a service which can locate the relevant features and extract those features from a given image. They call for a variety of image processing algorithms to be employed and where decisions cannot be made by a single algorithm confidently then majority voting mechanism can be used.
- *Outline Detectors* – outline detector basically detects the outline of an entity that is of interest in a given image using multiple outline detection algorithms.
- *Sub-image extractors* – sub-image extractor will extract the sub-images from the image once the entity has been identified. An Image extractor algorithm will be used to extract sub-images there are in. A variety of algorithms needs to be used based on whether it is ultrasound image, optical image, or X-ray image.
- *Image Comparators* – image comparator will compare two or more images or sub-images using a variety of algorithms and then give a scale how well the images compare. This includes intensity comparison as well, and, therefore, images need to be intensity codified as well.
- *Thumbnail Generators* – thumbnail generator simply refers to algorithm that will generate the thumbnail of a given ultrasound or optical image. This service is useful for quick browsing needs.
- *Image-based Query Engine* – image-based query engine is an engine in which one can give a present image or a sub-image, and a query can be made on the retrieval of images in the database which are similar in nature, and one can give percentile comparison using more than one similarity metric.
- *Historical Data Analyzers* – historical data analyzer will do image-based analysis of the history of that entity or an individual.
- *Life Cycle Analyzers* – life cycle analyzer extracts all the comparable data and gives user the race- and gender-specific life cycle analyses.

4.3   Privacy and Security as a Service (P-SaaS)

Privacy and Security as a Service (PaaS) relates to offering privacy and security to each individual dataset [6, 10]. A given patient's dataset is cut into several pieces and held at several locations using several cryptographic protocols. The underlying algorithms are generated at run time, and only the system knows where an actual user's datasets are stored and how they can be retrieved and rebuilt for any use. P-SaaS consist of six services as described below:

- *Data Distribution Service* – data distribution service relates to distribution of a given patient data across multiple destinations so that even if one part of the dataset is compromised, one needs the entire data to know the details about the individual. This does a hash-based distribution, and that hash function is known only to the computer. We have a collection of hash functions and which one is taken for an individual is random and is only known to the system.
- *Location Transparent Storage* – location transparent storage refers to the location of the part data storage is transparent.
- *Data Mirroring Service* – data mirroring service provides replication of data, and the location of the mirrored data is not known to the user but only known to the algorithm.
- *Data Dissection Service* – data dissection service relates to dividing the dataset of an individual combining with other individual datasets and storing it in multiple locations. The dissection process is also algorithmically controlled.
- *Multiparameter multi-protocol Crypto Service* – Multi-parameter multi-protocol Crypto Service offers multiple encryption algorithms with multiple bits. The choice of algorithm and number of bits used is left to the user or the system.
- *Data Dithering Service* – data dithering service relates to dithering the data so that only approved users get actual data all other users will get only ranged data.

4.4   Portability and Interoperability as a Service (P-IaaS)

Portability and Interoperability as a Services (P-IaaS) provides mechanisms for porting datasets across Clouds and also interoperability between various datasets and also between various Clouds [11, 16]. This service got nine different sub-services as detailed below:

- *Format Converters* – Format converters have the ability to convert raw data from one format to another format, or user-given format is also allowed.
- *Metadata Managers* – Metadata managers store the data about the data.[2]

---

[2]An example in the C programming language "int" refers to integer but stored only using 2 bytes, whereas in java "int" also refers to integers but use 4 bytes to store.

- *Data Dictionaries* – Data dictionaries refer how data from one source can be made equivalent to data from another source. It is the mechanism by which one can understand the semantics of the data.
- *Glossary Manager* – Glossary manager provides the glossary of terms used in various data sources so that one can glean an idea about the real technical meaning (not the common English term meaning) of a given term.
- *Data and Information Export Service* – Data and information exporting service provides the ability to export data in multiple formats,[3] including variants of XML.
- *Cloud Interoperability Standards Manager* – Cloud interoperability standards manager is about Cloud interoperability, namely, facilitate data movement from one Cloud to another.[4]
- *Vendor Lock-in Breaking Service* – "Vendor lock-in" breaking service refers to the fact that Cloud is genetically tied to a particular vendor; so if a user wants to make more data to another Cloud, one must then need to break the service from the original vendor. This mechanism provides a way to break the service and port the data to another Cloud in a seamless manner.
- *HIPPA Compliance Manager* – HIPPA (Health Information Privacy and Portability Act of the USA) relates to protecting and making the medical data of users portable across a variety of systems and/or platforms. HIPPA is made mandatory in USA medical data arena. We intend to provide HIPPA compliance for privacy and portability verification service.
- *Compliance Outsourcing Service* – HIPPA compliance need not be the core part of a medical practice; instead, the tedious task of HIPPA compliance can be outsourced to a company. This management compliance company has the responsibility of training and monitoring doctors and staff for compliance, including conducting periodic test for compliance and reporting thereof. Also improve compliance as and when issues occur.

4.5   Human Computing as a Service (HCaaS)

Software is used by various users, namely, medical practitioners, specialist, and staff working in the medical practice as well as common people, as evidenced in the application described in [7]. So a variety of services are needed for their support. We provide four services as detailed below:

- *Decision Support System/s* – Decision support system/s refers to the system which present results based on the type of users. For common users results will

---

[3] One can use variants of XML maybe one need to develop GI-specific XML using medical image formats – for example, using Digital Imaging and Communications in Medicine (DICOM).

[4] Cloud interoperability has been proposed by www.omg.org (object management group) and W3C consortium, but practical issues linger for a viable solution.

be sanitized variably but for a specialist results will be presented in detail, along with, if required, past cases of successes and failures.

- *Knowledge-Related Query Manager (KQM)* – The knowledge-related query manager is where domain-specific knowledge-based query can be posed and managed. This will also be tied to the level of user type.
- *Human Computer Interface Manager* – Human computer interface management is for managing HCI for various types of users and/or their roles.
- *Role Based Security and Access Controller* – Based on the role, security and access protocols to both patients and patient data can be managed, transmitted, and stored.

4.6 Generic Services

Generic services offer a wide variety of provisions, and we provide seven services as detailed below:

- *Research Data Analytic Service* – Research data analytic service is limited to medical practitioners and specialist. Current research data comparative analyses of patient with current research prospects can also be provided as a suggestion/recommendation.
- *Billing Management Service* – Billing Management Service relates to the provision of automatic billing.
- *GI-Office Service* – GI-office service is for handling emails, word processing, presentations, etc. This service will automatically correct such things as spelling and grammatical errors using GI-specific data dictionary.
- *Cloud Help Line Manager* – Cloud Help Line Manager provides the single interface in case there is help needed with an issue. This will comprise of chat, telephone, and an APP to provide help.
- *Compliance Report Generator* – For compliance purposes, this provides periodic reporting of compliance and need-based reporting of compliance.
- *A Variety of Customized Report Generators* – These report generators take into consideration the role and nature of service offered and provide tailored reports.
- *Cloud Security Manager* – Cloud Security: Security impacts data at rest, in motion, or in use. It is necessary therefore to address security issues and challenges which impact the Cloud technology adoption. Threats due to improper security policies by Cloud providers earlier have proved to be fatal, and many have reported severe impact to their business operations due to these unrecoverable losses. Over a period of time, Cloud technologies have become more mature, and it is now that they are providing highest levels of security allowing customers to have their very sensitive and confidential information (including those related to intellectual property) stored with very minimal or little chance either for inappropriate or unauthorized access. A Government of India Recommendation [3, 4] "Department of Electronics and IT (DeitY)" set the standards for

interoperability, integration, portability, contract management, data security, operational aspects, etc., for the Cloud. Architecture Management Office (AMO) is an important component of GI Cloud institutional setup and is also responsible for defining guidelines on security and how we address various risks and challenges.

There is a need for a dedicated security team that will constitute AMO toward setting up guidelines and standards to address areas within security. The guidelines and standards will evolve over a period of time. The process of storing the data and moving it to various Cloud models depends on how the application developer wants to securely transmit the sensitive information considering relevant privacy and security guidelines (including regulatory and legal framework of the hosting jurisdiction). Cloud providers will ensure and adhere to the prescribed security guidelines and standards. Security audit agencies will also play an important role ensuring the adherence to all compliances, allowing all stakeholders build a complete ecosystem. Capacity-building exercises is only possible by spreading awareness and enhance knowledge of all security related amongst Cloud users as well as providers.

5   Discussions on the GI Cloud

Key drivers and potential benefits of GI Cloud-computing environment for GI applications include, but not limited to, the following: (i) optimal usage of existing IT infrastructure, (ii) deployment and reusability, (iii) manageability and maintainability, (iv) scalability, (v) agile and efficient service delivery, (vi) security, (vii) cost reduction, (vii) IT solutions deployment for the first time, (viii) reduced effort in managing technology, (ix) increased user mobility, (x) and standardization. These advantages of the GI Cloud would lead to the following runoff benefits to a typical GI Cloud medical practice:

- *Increasing volume of patient-specific data*: GI practices are inundated with sheer volume of patient-specific data, and Cloud-based technology offers a way to handle multiple databases across regions, nations, and continents.
- *Patient information security*: Patient data confidentiality and information security are critical in the medical domain, and Cloud-based storage provides good security features. Cloud is reliable on the counts of both protecting sensitive patient information and restricting access to only approved users.
- *Ease of installation and transference*: Unlike most medical record management systems, Cloud technology offers a seamless transition from the existing patient database with very minimal to no downtime.
- *Easy interoperability*: Interoperability of datasets in the Cloud domain eases investigation of similar cases with peculiar clinical or imaging findings and simultaneously accessing outpatient and inpatient records.
- *Cost-effectiveness*: When the total cost is compared over an extended period, Cloud technology has been proven to be cost effective.

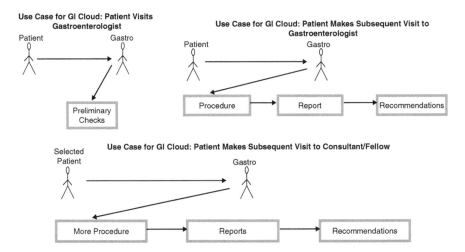

Fig. 3 Three use cases in GI Cloud

Three use cases in the GI Cloud are provided in Fig. 3.

6 Parametric Performance Evaluation of the GI Cloud

A parametric model-based evaluation of the GI Cloud system has been carried out. Table 1 provides typical parameters used for the evaluation of the GI Cloud, which have been obtained after discussions with several experts. Table 2 provides a list of performance indicators and their values, wherein the values are calculated using relative cost unit (RCU) so that depending on the actual cost of individual companies, a suitable multiplier can be employed to calculate the corrected values of various performance indices. It is hoped that these indicators will provide the way forward for the advancement of such systems in various marine sensor network R&D centers around the world.

7 Summary and Conclusions

The architecture of a comprehensive GI Cloud, its needs, and their functionalities are detailed in this chapter. The GI Cloud would enhance many aspects of a typical GI environment which include, but not limited to:

• Enhanced Collaboration: The Cloud technology enhances collaboration and ready exchange information thru shared storage, thereby leading to improved customer service and product development besides reducing time to market.

Table 1 Parameters for evaluating GI Cloud information systems architecture

S. no.	Explanation	Symbol	Average value	Max.
1.	Size of PDF file	a	0.5 MB	1 MB
2.	Number of retrievals per patient per day	b	3	5
3.	Number of patients per day	c	20	35
4.	Number of follow-up visits per patient	d	3	5
5.	Number of tertiary care physicians retrievals per day	e	5	7
6.	Number of tertiary care GI fellow retrievals per day	f	5	7
7.	Number of sub-specialties in GI weightage	g	4	6
8.	Number of maintenance calls per day	h	4	6
9.	Number of images per patient	i	5	7
10.	Number of upgrade requirements per day	j	4	6
11.	Number of internal low-end service calls per day	k	10	18
12.	Number of internal medium-end service calls per day	l	5	8
13.	Number of internal high-end service calls per day	m	3	5
14.	Number of reports to be generated per day	n	40	60
15.	Number of knowledge query management per day	p	50	70
16.	Number of help line management – simple call per day	q	20	30
17.	Number of help line management – medium call per day	r	10	15
18.	Number of help line management – complex call per day	s	5	8
19.	Number of compliance requirements per day	t	1	3
20.	Average viewing time per image	u	4 min	7 min

S.No.	Explanation	Symbol	Relative cost units (RCU)
1.	Data storage cost per GB per month	C1	25
2.	Data access cost per GB	C2	2
3.	Internal low-end service cost per service call	C3	1
4.	Internal medium-end service cost per service call	C4	3
5.	Internal high-end service cost per service call	C5	8
6.	Maintenance cost per service call	C6	15
7.	Upgrade cost per service call	C7	10
8.	Encryption cost per file (0.5 MB)	C8	5
9.	Decryption cost per file (0.5 MB)	C9	5
10.	Air conditioning costs per day	C10	200
11.	Average downtown costs for services upgrade per day	C11	400
12.	Compliance management costs per compliance requirement	C12	500
13.	Average report generation cost per report	C13	10
14.	Average knowledge query management cost per query	C14	2
15.	Help line management per simple call	C15	1
16.	Help line management per medium call	C16	5
17.	Help line management per complex call	C17	10

Table 2 GI Cloud performance indicators

S.No.	Metric name	Symbol	Formula	Typical average value	Metric name
1.	Average execution time on patient data per patient	PI-1	$(a * b + d * e * g) * h*i$	1800	44,100
2.	Average bandwidth used per day	PI-2	$a * b * c * i$	150	1225
3.	Average downtime management per patient	PI-3	$C11/ (b * c)$	6.667	2.2857
4.	Average cost of security per patient	PI-4	$(C8 + C9) * b * e * d$	450	1750
5.	Average ease of use per patient = average execution time on patient data per patient + weighted average service call time + weighted average help call time	PI-5	$\{(a * b + d * e * g) * h*I\} + \{C3 * k + C4 * l + C5 * m\} + \{C15 * q + C16 * r + C17 *s\}$	1419	10,320
6.	Average report generation cost per day	PI-6	$C13 * n$	400	600
7.	Average compliance requirement cost per day	PI-7	$C12 * t$	500	1500
8.	Average network usage cost = patient cost + visit cost + specialty-related cost + InfoSec cost + data access and storage cost	PI-8	$(a * b * c) + (d * f) + (g * i) + (C8 + C9) * i + (C1 + C2) * b * c * i$	8215	33,397
9.	Average GI Cloud usage cost = PI-18 + knowledge query cost + upgrade cost + maintenance cost + aircon cost	PI-9	$PI-8 + (C14 * p) + (C7 *j) + (C6 * h) + C10$	8615	33,887
10.	Average cost of ownership per patient	PI-10	$PI-9/c$	430.75	968.2

- Control on Documents: Cloud allows document control – be they in various formats, titles, and versions, besides offering central file storage and multi-editing facility.
- Easy Management: The existence of SLA (service-level agreement), central resource administration, and managed infrastructure enhances Cloud computing's overall prowess. As a consequence, one gets to enjoy a basic user interface without any requirement for installation of the entire software system. Furthermore, guaranteed and timely management, maintenance, and delivery of the underlying IT services give a typical GI practice considerable advantages over other GI practices.

Such a GI Cloud system is now the order of the day, and already many medical practices are installing and benefitting from a subset of our GI Cloud model. The performance of the GI Cloud has been evaluated using parametric modelling technique, and the results indicate that GI Cloud system can successfully enhance the performance of the scientists and technical people involved in this field; the details are also provided in this chapter. Pointers for further research in this arena include (i) developing cost-benefit model for Cloud migration [21], (ii) developing a simple model for Cloud acceptance, (iii) developing policies for Cloud-based HIPPA compliance, (iv) develop policies for third-party data safety, and (v) making a move toward an OPEX model, the pooling of scarce, underutilized resources, and the spread of best practices [20]. This will also support ongoing cost-effectiveness and manageability. The performance of the GI Cloud has been evaluated using parametric modelling technique, and the results indicate that GI Cloud can successfully enhance the performance of the medicos involved in this field; the details are also provided in this chapter.

References

1. L. Dyrda, "Moving GI Data to the Cloud in the era of Healthcare Consolidation", https://www. beckersasc.com/gastroenterology-and-endoscopy/moving-gi-data-to-the-cloud-in-the-era-of-healthcare-consolidation.html (17th Aug 2019)
2. "Discussions on The GI-Cloud", https://www.meity.gov.in/writereaddata/files/GI-Cloud%20 Strategic%20Direction%20Report%281%29_0.pdf (5th June 2019)
3. India's Department of Electronics and Information Technology (DeitY), www.deity.gov.in (14th Sept 2019).
4. India's Ministry of Electronics and Information Technology Initiative (MeitY), www.meity. gov.in (14th Sept 2019).
5. "NIST Definition of Cloud Computing", https://csrc.nist.gov/publications/detail/sp/800-145/ final (14th Sept 2019).
6. "NIST Cloud Computing Security Reference Architecture", https://csrc.nist.gov/publications/ detail/book/2016/cloud-computing-security-essentials-and-architecture, (14th Sept 2019).
7. V. Lakshmi Narasimhan, "Botswana's Lab-In-A-Briefcase – A Position Paper", ACM Press Proceedings of the Australasian Computer Science Week (ACSW 2019), Sydney, Australia, 29-31 January2019.
8. V. Lakshmi Narasimhan and V.S. Jithin, "Time-Cost Effective Algorithms for Cloud Workflow Scheduling - Extension of An Earlier Work", Proc. of IST Africa Intl. Conf., Gaborone, Botswana, 9-11 May 2018. IEEE Xplore:
9. V. Lakshmi Narasimhan, "Research issues and challenges in Cloud Computing- A Critical Perspective", National Seminar on Computational Intelligence (NSCI '13), SRM University, Kattangalattur, India, Jan. 21–22, 2013.
10. V. Lakshmi Narasimhan, "Cloud Computing – Some Unusual Applications", Proceedings of the ICETT First International Conference on Emerging Technologies in Cloud Computing (INCET-2011)", Sasthamcotta, Quilon, Kerala, India, Mar. 25–26, 2011.
11. D. De, "Mobile Cloud Computing: Architectures, Algorithms and Applications", CRC Press, 2016.
12. Ministry of Electronics and Telecommunications, India, https://www.meity.gov.in/writeread-data/files/GI-Cloud%20Strategic%20Direction%20Report%281%29_0.pdf (5th June 2019)
13. Data As a Service: https://searchdatamanagement.techtarget.com/definition/data-as-a-service (5th June 2019)
14. Software As a Service: https://searchcloudcomputing.techtarget.com/definition/Software-as-a-Service (5th June 2019)
15. Intel Cloud Computing: Transform IT for a Hyper Connected World – Intel Cloud Computing https://www.intel.com/content/www/us/en/cloud-computing/overview.html (17th Sept 2019)

16. Infrastructure as a Service – Tech Target Infrastructure as a Service – Tech Target https://searchcloudcomputing.techtarget.com/definition/Infrastructure-as-a-Service-IaaS (17th Sept 2019)

17. Benefits of Cloud Computing in Business https://www.eukhost.com/blog/webhosting/10-benefits-of-cloud-computing-for-businesses/ (17th Sept 2019)

18. Software as a Service – Tech Target https://searchcloudcomputing.techtarget.com/definition/Software-as-a-Service (17th Sept 2019)

19. IaaS vs DaaS vs PaaS vs SaaS – Which should you choose? – ESDS Blog https://www.esds.co.in/blog/iaas-vs-daas-vs-paas-vs-saas-which-should-you-choose/ (17th Sept 2019)

20. D. De, "Mobile Cloud Computing: Architectures, Algorithms and Applications", CRC Press, 2016. (Chap 4 & 14)

21. D. De, "Mobile Cloud Computing: Architectures, Algorithms and Applications", CRC Press, 2016. (Chap 12)

22. Annie Shergill, V. Lakshmi Narasimhan, Deepti Garg, Amruth K. Sala. "2891 Designing the GI Cloud", American Journal of Gastroenterology, 2019.

23. www.deity.gov.in

A Hybrid Method for Detection of Coronavirus Through X-rays Using Convolutional Neural Networks and Support Vector Machine

P. Srinivasa Rao

Abstract A coronavirus is a group of infectious diseases that were caused by similar viruses called coronaviruses. In human beings, the seriousness of the disease can vary from mild to lethal causing serious illness in old people and with those who are having health issues like cardiovascular disease, diabetes, chronic respiratory, and cancer. There are a limited number of test kits that are available in the hospitals as the number of positive cases increases daily. Hence an automated COVID-19 detection system has to be implemented as an alternative diagnostic method to pause COVID-19 spread in the population. This paper proposes a hybrid deep learning model using a convolutional neural network combined with a support vector machine to detect coronavirus with chest X-ray radiographs. On observing the results that were evaluated based on different evaluation metrics such as precision, recall, F score, rmse, mse, and accuracy, it is seen that the accuracy of the proposed hybrid model using CNN and SVM is 98.07%.

Keywords COVID-19 · Coronavirus · Convolutional neural network · Support vector machine · Chest X-ray radiographs

1 Introduction

In Wuhan, China (2019), coronavirus also called COVID-19 appeared which has become a major health problem [1] in the world. The name severe acute respiratory syndrome coronavirus 2 (SARS-CoV-2) [2, 3] is given to the virus which caused COVID-19, which was recognized as a pandemic by WHO [4]. According to the World Health Organization, coronavirus is an infectious disease transferred from animals (dromedary) close to MERS-CoV virus [5, 6] and SARS-CoV [7] from bats; the COVID-19 can otherwise be termed as a zoonotic disease. The regular

P. Srinivasa Rao (✉)
MVGR College of Engineering, Vizianagaram, Andhra Pradesh, India

© The Author(s), under exclusive license to Springer
Nature Switzerland AG 2021
A. K. Manocha et al. (eds.), *Computational Intelligence in Healthcare*, Health
Information Science, https://doi.org/10.1007/978-3-030-68723-6_16

symptoms that are mostly observed in COVID-19 patients are fever, tiredness, head-ache, and dry cough. In some serious conditions, the signs can be multiple organ failure, severe acute respiratory syndrome, and pneumonia, and it may even cause the death of the person. In COVID-19 infected-people, it is observed that men are more affected than women and the respiratory rates of COVID-19-infected people are more compared to a normal healthy person. According to [8], there are 7,013,972 active cases and 902,315 deaths in the world as of 9 September 2020. Currently, real-time-polymerase chain reaction (RT-PCR) is being used for COVID-19 detection by detecting nucleic acids in blood samples. As compared to COVID-19 cases that are occurring, the RT-PCR test kits available are minimum. An automatic detection system implementation that acts as an alternative method [9] to diagnose the prevention of coronavirus among people is necessary [10–12]. In this scenario, chest X-ray and computed tomography are some of the alternative methods for the detection of COVID-19. The X-ray imaging takes less time when compared to CT imaging which has some drawbacks, and its availability is less. Hence, detection of coronavirus through chest X-rays is a better choice as it is easier, cheaper, and faster. In this paper, we are proposing a methodology using a convolutional neural network combined with a support vector machine for the classification of COVID-19 patients with chest X-rays.

The remainder of the paper is organized as follows: Section 2 discusses literature work, Section 3 presents the methodology, Section 4 describes the environmental setup, Section 5 deals with evaluation metrics and results, and Sect. 6 explains the conclusion and future work.

2 Literature Work

A few studies that were reported by the researchers for the prediction of COVID-19 are, A serious acute respiratory distress syndrome that can be caused to older men having comorbidities are more prone to be affected with coronavirus is observed by analyzing 99 patients tested laboratory data with pneumonia and 2019-nCoV by Nanshan Chen et al. [13]. During close contacts, it is more likely seen that the transmission of coronavirus from human to human has occurred by analyzing transmission dynamics of coronavirus with novel coronavirus-infected pneumonia patient's laboratory-tested data (Quin Li et al.) [14]. A comparison of pre-trained models of the convolutional neural network such as Inception-ResNetV2, InceptionV3, and ResNet50 using chest X-ray images for coronavirus detection in patients has showcased that ResNet50 has obtained better performance than other two methods and state-of-the-art methodologies (Ali Narin et al.) [15]. An experiment with chest CT to detect COVID-19 with 1014 patients of RT-PCR tests chest CTs conferred that Chest CTs can be examined as a primary tool with high sensitivity (Tao Ai MD et al.) [16]. A survey of different pre-trained model's architecture performance was proposed by different researchers and concluded that VGG19 has obtained 98% accuracy in the detection of COVD-19 (Muhammad llyas et al.) [17].

A method for screening coronavirus disease by concatenating traditional ResNet50 network with location attention mechanism was suggested by Xiaowei Xu et al. [18] which obtained an accuracy of 86.7%. A method for classification of patients with coronavirus using chest X-ray radiographs by a multi-objective differential evolution (MODE) model for convolutional neural network model hyperparameter tuning by Dilbag Singh et al. [19] obtained better performance than traditional methodologies. A method for separating N data points having n-dimensions with at least one hyperplane using non-iterative KE Sieve Neural Network to diagnose COVID-19 with chest X-rays achieved 98% accuracy (S Sai Thejeshwar et al.) [20]. The support vector machine classifier fed with the features extracted from a convolutional neural network architecture by Khan et al. [21] showcased that the model yielded good results than the other state-of-the-art machine learning techniques. An accuracy of 89.5% was obtained using inception transfer-learning to predict coronavirus using CT images (Shuai et al.) [22]. For respiratory pattern classification with improved gated recurrent unit (GRU) network with the addition of bidirectional and attention mechanism by Yunlu Wang et al. [23] achieved an accuracy of 94.5%.

As per the literature, many traditional [24–29] and machine learning [30–33] techniques were proposed as an alternative method for the detection of coronavirus, and the researchers found that X-ray images can also be used to detect coronavirus. This paper is concentrated on an improved deep learning model based on convolutional neural network architecture and a support vector machine for performance improvement of the model to detect COVID-19.

3   Methodology

In a coronavirus pandemic situation, the rate at which the coronavirus-positive patients are more when compared to the number of tests being conducted, and the test kits used for one person cannot be used for another person. As the tests are analyzed manually in the laboratory, the time taken for the results is high. Hence, this paper proposes an alternative efficient and reusable methodology using low-cost chest X-ray radiographs to detect coronavirus.

The proposed model system architecture is highlighted in Fig. 1. The dataset is fractionated into 80% training and 20% testing data. Preprocessing techniques such as image size conversion into 256×256, data augmentation with rotation range of 250, shift range of 0.1 in the vertical and horizontal direction, horizontal flip with 50%, and a shear range of 0.2 in the horizontal direction are applied for preprocessing the data.

The proposed hybrid convolutional neural network model is highlighted in Fig. 2. The hybrid model is built up with an input layer, three hidden layers made up of Conv2D layers with (32, 64, 128) filters having kernel sizes of (3×3, 3×3, 5×5) with pooling size of 2×2 each, one fully connected layer having 256 filters, and an output layer which is a support vector machine for output classification. ReLU activation function is used in all the layers except for the SVM layer.

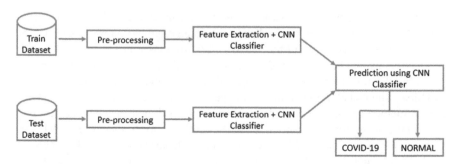

Fig. 1 System architecture

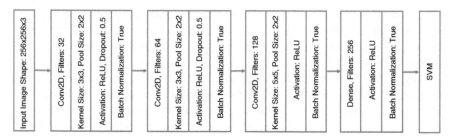

Fig. 2 Neural network model

$$\text{ReLU} : f\left(h_\theta\left(x\right)\right) = h_\theta\left(x\right)^+ = \max\left(0, h_\theta\left(x\right)\right)$$

The hybrid convolutional neural network model is trained by passing the preprocessed training set through the model where the features from the images are extracted on passing through the hidden layers if the network and the images are classified using SVM layer with the extracted features from layers of CNN. The unseen images are predicted using trained hybrid model.

4 Environmental Setup

The entire experiment was carried out in a system which is configured with Windows 10 operating system (64-bit) with Intel® Core™ i5-8250 *CPU* @ 1.80 *GHz* processor, 8 *GB* ram, and 2 *TB HDD* installed with Anaconda, Python platform with supporting keras packages, and Tensorflow as back end.

The overall experiment was performed on the Kaggle dataset [34] containing chest X-ray radiographs for two classes, namely, *NORMAL* class with 1341 images and *COVID*-19 class with 219 images. The distribution of dataset among training and testing sets is described in Table 1 and sample images from the dataset are shown in Figs. 3 and 4.

Table 1 Description of dataset distribution

Description	Normal	COVID-19
Training set	1073	176
Testing set	268	43

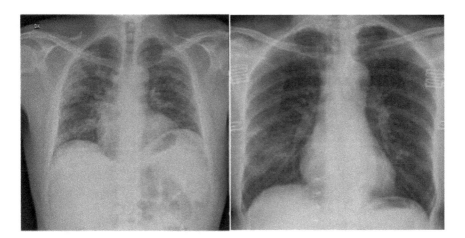

Fig. 3 Chest X-rays of a *COVID*-19 patient

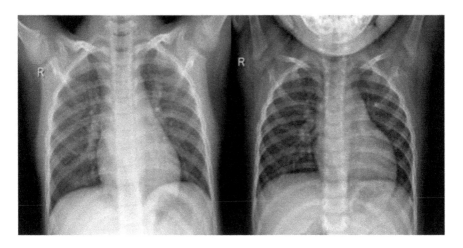

Fig. 4 Chest X-rays of a *NORMAL* patient

5   Evaluation Metrics and Result

The proposed hybrid neural network model is evaluated for its performance by considering several evaluation metrics such as precision, recall, F score, RMSE, MSE, and accuracy, which are defined as follows:

$$\text{Precision} = TP \, / \, (FP + TP)$$

$$\text{Recall} = TP \, / \, (FN + TP)$$

$$\text{F1 score} = (2 * \text{Recall} * \text{Precision}) \, / \, (\text{Recall} + \text{Precision})$$

$$\text{RMSE} = \sqrt{(TP \, / \, (TP + FP))}$$

$$\text{MSE} = TP + (FP + TP)$$

$$\text{Accuracy} = (TP + TN) \, / \, (TP + FP + FN + TN)$$

where TP = true positive, FP = false positive, FN = false negative, TN = true negative.

The proposed CNN model is compared with VGG19, mobile net, Inception, Xception, and ResNet V2 models which are proposed by Ioannis et al. [35] using transfer-learning techniques, with a dataset comprising of 728 X-ray images out of which 504 images belonging to the NORMAL class and 224 images belonging to COVID-19 class, and the observed results are as follows.

From Table 2, it can be inferred that the accuracies of VGG19 and the proposed hybrid CNN model are approximately equal. So, instead of using a neural network model with more layers such as VGG19, the proposed hybrid four-layered architecture with SVM can be used as an alternative by producing results in less time with minimum resources being utilized while maintaining better performance. Graph 1 represents the accuracy comparison of different models with the proposed hybrid model, Table 3 describes the classification metrics of the proposed model for the two classes, Graph 2 indicates the evaluation metrics of the proposed CNN model and Fig. 5 depicts the confusion matrix for the proposed hybrid neural network model.

Table 2 Accuracy comparison for different networks

Network	Accuracy
VGG19	98.75
Mobile net	97.40
Inception	86.13
Xception	85.57
ResNet V2	84.38
Proposed CNN + SVM model	98.07

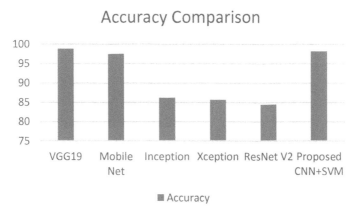

Graph 1 Accuracy comparison for different networks

Table 3 Classification metrics of proposed CNN model

Description	Precision	Recall	F1 score
Normal	98	100	99
COVID-19	100	85	92

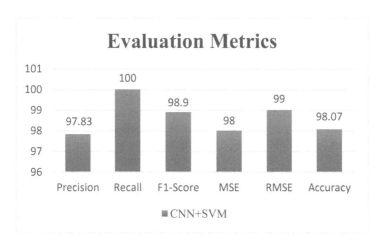

Graph 2 Evaluation metrics of proposed CNN model

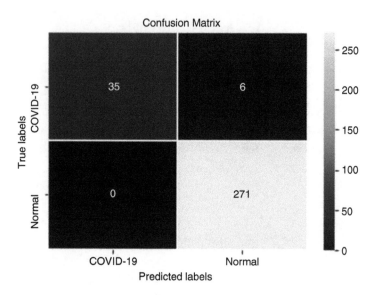

Fig. 5 Confusion matrix for proposed CNN model

6   Conclusion and Future Work

In this paper, a hybrid method using a convolutional neural network architecture combined with a support vector machine is presented to define a relationship between chest X-ray radiographs and COVID-19 detection. The results have shown that COVID-19 can be detected using chest X-ray radiographs with minimum time than the current manual laboratory testing methodology. On comparison of the proposed model whose accuracy is 98.07% with different deep learning models, it can be inferred that better performance can be obtained by using four-layered hybrid neural network with SVM instead of going for more numbered layered architectures. As COVID-19 is a new disease, the data available is minimum, and different deep learning architectures with hybrid methods can be considered for feature extraction and classification processes which can be considered as for the future task for the performance improvement of the proposed hybrid neural network model.

References

1. https://www.who.int/health-topics/coronavirus
2. Bernard Stoecklin Sibylle, Rolland Patrick, Silue Yassoungo, Mailles Alexandra, Campese Christine, Simondon Anne, Mechain Matthieu, Meurice Laure, Nguyen Mathieu, Bassi Clément, Yamani Estelle, Behillil Sylvie, Ismael Sophie, Nguyen Duc, Malvy Denis, Lescure François Xavier, Georges Scarlett, Lazarus Clément, Tabaï Anouk, Stempfelet Morgane, Enouf Vincent, Coignard Bruno, Levy-Bruhl Daniel, Investigation team, "First cases of coronavirus

disease 2019 (COVID-19) in France: surveillance, investigations and control measures", Euro Surveill, Vol. 25: No. 6, 2020.

3. Khan S., Ng ML., Tan YJ. "Expression of the Severe Acute Respiratory Syndrome Coronavirus 3a Protein and the Assembly of Coronavirus-Like Particles in the Baculovirus Expression System." Sugrue R.J. (eds) Glycovirology Protocols. Methods in Molecular Biology, Humana Press, vol 379, 2007.

4. https://www.who.int/westernpacific/emergencies/covid-19

5. Abdirizak, F., Lewis, R. & Chowell, G. "Evaluating the potential impact of targeted vaccination strategies against severe acute respiratory syndrome coronavirus (SARS-CoV) and Middle East respiratory syndrome coronavirus (MERS-CoV) outbreaks in the healthcare setting". Theor Biol Med Model. 16; 16 (2019).

6. Al Ghamdi, M., Alghamdi, K.M., Ghandoora, Y, Ameera A. "Treatment outcome for patients with Middle Eastern Respiratory Syndrome Coronavirus (MERS CoV) infection at a coronavirus referral center in the Kingdom of Saudi Arabia". BMC Infect Dis. 16; 174 (2016).

7. Corver, J., Broer, R., van Kasteren, P, Willy Span. "Mutagenesis of the transmembrane domain of the SARS coronavirus spike glycoprotein: refinement of the requirements for SARS coronavirus cell entry". Virol J 2009. 6; 230 (2009).

8. https://www.worldometers.info/coronavirus/

9. H. Li. "Application and Development of Automation Technology in Novel Coronavirus (2019-nCoV) Outbreak". Proceedings of the International Conference on E-Commerce and Internet Technology (ECIT), 2020 Apr 22-24, Zhangjiajie, China, 2020, pp. 296-298.

10. F. Gao, K. Deng, C. Hu. Construction of TCM Health Management Model for Patients with Convalescence of Coronavirus Disease Based on Artificial Intelligence. Proceedings of the International Conference on Big Data and Informatization Education (ICBDIE), 2020 Apr 23-25, Zhangjiajie, China, 2020, pp. 417-420.

11. T.V. Madhusudhana Rao, P Srinivasa Rao, P.S. Latha Kalyampudi, "Iridology based Vital Organs Malfunctioning identification using Machine learning Techniques", International Journal of Advanced Science and Technology, Volume: 29, No. 5, PP: 5544 – 5554, 2020.

12. X. Gao, Y. Zhang. "Online Case Intelligent Interaction System based on Virtual Reality Technology Under the Background of Novel Coronavirus". Proceedings of the 4th International Conference on Trends in Electronics and Informatics (ICOEI), 2020 Jun 15-17, Tirunelveli, India, 2020, pp. 862-865.

13. Nanshan Chen, Min Zhou, Xuan D., J. Qu, F. Gong, Y. Han, Y. Qiu, J. Wang, Y. Liu, Y. Wei, J. Xia, T. Yu, X. Zhang, Li Z, "Epidemiological and clinical characteristics of 99 cases of 2019 novel coronavirus pneumonia in Wuhan, China: a descriptive study", Lancet, 395: 507-13, 2020.

14. Quin Li, Xuhua. G, Peng Wu, Xiaoye. W, Lei Zhou, Y. Tong, Ruiqi Ren, Kathy. S. M. L, Eric. H. Y. Lau, Jessica Y. Wong, Xuesen Xing, Nijuan Xiang, Yang Wu, Chao Li, Qi. Chen, Dan Li, Tian Liu, Jing Zhao, Man Liu, W, Tu, Chuding Chen, L. Jin, Rui Yang, Qi Wang, Suhua Zhou, Rui Wang, Hui Liu, Yinbo Luo, Yuan Liu, Ge Shao, Huan Li, Zhongfa Tao, Yang Yang, Zhiqiang Deng, Boxi Liu, Zhitao Ma, Yanping Zhang, Guoqing Shi, Tommy T. Y. Lam, Joseph T. Wu, George F. Gao, Benjamin J. Cowling, Bo Yang, Gabriel M. Leung, Zijian Feng, "Early Transmission Dynamics in Wuhan, China, of Novel Coronavirus – Infected Pneumonia", The New England Journal of Medicine, Vol. 382: No.13, 2020.

15. Ali Narin, Ceren Kaya, Ziynet Pamuk, "Automatic Detection of Coronavirus Disease (COVID-19) Using X-ray Images and Deep Convolutional Neural Networks" [White Paper], Cornell University, https://arxiv.org/abs/2003.10849, 2020.

16. Tao Ai MD, Zhenlu Yang MD, H. Hou, C. Zhan, C. Chen, Wenzhi Lv, Q. Tao, Z. Sun, L. Xia, "Correlation of Chest CT and RT-PCR Testing in Coronavirus Disease 2019 (COVID-19) in China: A Report of 1014 Cases", Radiology, 2020.

17. Muhammad llyas, Hina Rehman, Amine Nait-ali, "Detection of Covid-19 From Chest X-ray Images Using Artificial Intelligence: An Early Review" [White Paper], Cornell University, https://arxiv.org/abs/2004.05436, 2020.

18. Xiaowei Xu, Xiangao Jiang, C. Ma, P. Du, X. Li, S. Lv, L. Yu, Y. Chen, J. Su, G. Lang, Y. Li, Hong Zhao, K. Xu, L. Ruan, Wei Wu, "Deep Learning System to Screen Coronavirus Disease 2019 Pneumonia" [White Paper], Cornell University, https://arxiv.org/abs/2002.09334, 2020.

19. Dilbag Singh, Vijay Kumar, Vaishali, Manjit Kaur, "Classification of COVID-19 patients from chest CT images using multi-objective differential evolution-based convolutional neural networks", European Journal of Clinical Microbiology & Infectious Disease, vol. 1: Issue. 11, 2020.

20. S Sai Thejeshwar, Chaitanya Chokkareddy, Dr. K Eswaran, "Precise Prediction of COVID-19 in Chest X-Ray Images Using KE Sieve Algorithm" [White Paper], ResearchGate, https://www.researchgate.net/publication/340870379, 2020.

21. Saddam Hussain Khan, Anabia Sohail, Muhammad Mohsin Zafar, Asifullah Khan, "Coronavirus Disease Analysis using Chest X-ray Images and a Novel Deep Convolutional Neural Network" [White Paper], ResearchGate, https://www.researchgate.net/publication/340574359, 2020.

22. Shuai Wang, Bo Kang, Jinlu Ma, Xianjun Zeng, Mingming Xiao, Jia Guo, Mengjiao Caim Jingyi Yang, Yaodong Li, Xiangfei Meng, Bo Xu, "A deep learning algorithm using CT images to screen for Corona Virus Disease (COVID-19)" [White Paper], medRxiv, https://www.medrxiv.org/content/10.1101/2020.02.14.20023028v5, 2020.

23. Yunlu Wang, Menghan Hu, Qingli Li, Xiao-Ping Zhang, Guangtao Zhai, Nan Yao, "Abnormal Respiratory patterns classifier may contribute to large-scale screening of people infected with COVID-19 in an accurate and unobtrusive manner" [White Paper], Cornell University, https://arxiv.org/abs/2002.05534, 2020.

24. P Srinivasa Rao, Krishna Prasad, M.H.M., Thammi Reddy, K, "An Efficient Data Integration Framework in Hadoop Using MapReduce" Published in Computational Intelligence Techniques for Comparative Genomics, Springer Briefs in Applied Sciences and Technology, ISSN:2191-530X, PP 129-137, October 2014.

25. Vidya sagar Appaji setti, P Srinivasa Rao, "A Novel Scheme for Red Eye Removal with Image Matching", Journal of Advanced Research in Dynamical & Control Systems, Vol. 10, 13-Special Issue, 2018. url: http://www.jardcs.org/backissues/abstract.php?archiveid=6088.

26. P Srinivasa Rao, MHM Krishna Prasad,K Thammi Reddy, "A Novel Approach For Identification Of Hadoop Cloud Temporal Patterns Using Map Reduce" Published In IJITCS (MECS) Vol. 6, No. 4,Pp:37-42, March 2014.

27. P Srinivasa Rao, Krishna Prasad, P.E.S.N, "A Secure and Efficient Temporal Features Based Framework for Cloud Using MapReduce", springer, 17th International Conference on Intelligent Systems Design and Applications (ISDA 2017), Volume:736, pp:114-123, ISSN 2194-5357 Held in Delhi, India, December 14–16, 2017.

28. S. Vidya sagar Appaji, P. V. Lakshmi, P. Srinivasa Rao, "Maximizing Joint Probability in Visual Question Answering Models", International Journal of Advanced Science and Technology Vol. 29, No. 3, pp. 3914 – 3923,2020.

29. P Srinivasa Rao, S Satyanarayana, "Privacy-Preserving Data Publishing Based On Sensitivity in Context of Big Data Using Hive", Journal of Bigdata (Springer), Volume:5, Issue:20, ISSN: 2196-1115, July 2018. [scopus]

30. P. S. Latha Kalyampudi, P. Srinivasa Rao, and D. Swapna, "An Efficient Digit Recognition System with an Improved Preprocessing Technique", Springer Nature Singapore, ICICCT 2019 – System Reliability, Quality Control, Safety, Maintenance and Management, pp. 312–321, 2019.

31. Madhusudhana Rao, T.V., P. Srinivasa Rao, Srinivas, Y, "A Secure Framework For Cloud Using Map Reduce", Journal Of Advanced Research In Dynamical And Control Systems (IJARDCS), Volume:9, Sp-14, Pp:1850-1861, ISSN:1943-023x, Dec, 2017.

32. P Srinivasa Rao, MHM Krishna Prasad,K Thammi Reddy, "A Novel And Efficient Method For Protecting Internet Usage From Unauthorized Access Using Map Reduce" Published In IJITCS (MECS) Vol. 5, No. 3,Pp:49-55,February 2013.

33. P Srinivasa Rao, MHM Krishna Prasad, K Thammi Reddy, "An Efficient Semantic Ranked Keyword Search Of Big Data Using Map Reduce", IJDTA, Vol.8, No.6, Pp.47-56,2015.
34. https://www.kaggle.com/tawsifurrahman/covid19-radiography-database
35. Apostolopoulos I. D., Bessiana T., "Covid-19: Automatic detection from X-Ray images utilizing Transfer Learning with Convolutional Neural Networks" [White Paper], Cornell University, https://arxiv.org/abs/2003.11617, 2020.

Feature Extraction Using GLSM for DDSM Mammogram Images

Neha S. Shahare and D. M. Yadav

Abstract One of the worst illnesses for women is breast cancer. Around 2.1 million women have this cancer per year. The prevalence of breast cancer ranges across nations, but in most instances, the second cause of death for the female population is this form of cancer. Mammography research, which shapes the experts' auto-exploration and manual exploration, is the most powerful technology for the early diagnosis of breast cancer. In the detection of calcifications and masses in the mammography photograph, there is a considerable research effort, apart from other potential anomalies, since these two forms of artefacts are the best markers of a possible early stage of breast cancer. Microcalcifications present in the optical mammograms as subtle and light spots from 0.3 mm and 1 mm in scale. The naked eye is not possible to observe since the thick breast tissue covering it renders suspicious regions nearly opaque. If cancer is diagnosed early by using breast self-examination (BSE) and clinical breast examination (CBE) at 40–49 years of age, the survival rate of breast cancer reaches 100 per cent. New strategies named CAD (computer-assisted diagnosis) programmes for early detection utilising multiple mammogram datasets, such as mini-Mias, DDSM, etc., have been discovered by several researchers. As mammography appears to be deemed a unique screening technique for breast lesion identification and evaluation, it uses lower radiation doses than ordinary chest X-rays. In this paper, DDSM dataset is used. The aim of this system is to extract features to differentiate between different categories of images like normal, benign and malignant. Dataset has tags and extra component which is not useful for processing, so all unnecessary components are removed by global thresholding method. Wavelet transform is the most popular transform with the combination of wavelet and GLCM eight significant features are extracted from mammogram images. It is observed that from features, it is possible to differentiate between normal, benign and malignant images. These features can further apply to best machine learning algorithm to check the accuracy of the system.

N. S. Shahare (✉)
Department of E&TC, SITS, Pune, India

D. M. Yadav
G.H.RCOE & M, Pune, India

© The Author(s), under exclusive license to Springer
Nature Switzerland AG 2021
A. K. Manocha et al. (eds.), *Computational Intelligence in Healthcare*, Health
Information Science, https://doi.org/10.1007/978-3-030-68723-6_17

Keywords BSE · CBE · CAD · DDSM (Digital Data Screening Mammography) · GLCM · Mammograms · Microcalcification

1 Introduction

Breast cancer is the utmost dangerous disease in women all across the globe. The increasingly prevalent illness in American women is breast cancer; it appears to be a significant public health issue in the United States. This occurs in 11% of women throughout their lives. If the disease is diagnosed at an early point, the breast cancer survival rate reaches 100 per cent. In the literature review, several techniques for automated digital mammography processing have been studied to deal with this problem. We are addressing breast cancer and associated scientific literature in this article. As per [5], Ingvar, Debra and Sophia observed that ductal carcinoma in situ (DCIS) and broad components of invasive ductal carcinoma (IDC) produced cancer marked by phenomorphic calcification, while the graded portion was shown, due to lack of edge characteristics or attenuation variation, the noncalcified broad invasive part could not be defined. Steve Mcoy submitted a thesis on breast density assessment utilising mammogram photos in [6]. Steven notes that two types of images are generated from the digital mammography machine, the raw picture, obtained from the imaging sensor, and proceed picture comprising visual enhancement property technique; currently automated algorithms of breast density rely on using the row image when radiologist used visual inspection image to proceed. Then, the extracted picture is placed in the medical history of the patient. The literature on early-stage tumour detection in Mammogram is provided by Pawar BV and Sushmal Patil. Pawar provides a technique for detecting breast tumours. The tumours identified are circular. Pixel-based mass detection is the method used to identify tumours. It uses the technique of template matching [7]. These templates are characterised by the form and luminosity of the mass of the tumour. The median filtering increases the mammogram images before template matching. The edges are improved by high-pass filtering, and then edge detection is used to identify the tumour's outline. Only circular tumours, which are often early-stage tumours, are identified if the tumour is malignant. The criterion for the measured values of cross-correlation is established in this prototype matching. Then, to establish a global threshold for each video, the percentile approach is used.

As per [8] Sheshadri HS reported in the 2005 Cancer Journal, Vol 1, Issue 4, he suggested the diagnosis by mammogram picture segmentation of breast cancer. Quantifying the substance of its framework is a fundamental approach to understanding an area. The segmentation, based on the texture function, will identify the tissue of the breast into separate categories. The algorithm assesses the properties of the mammogram picture in the area and thereby classifies the picture into significant parts. Mini-MIAS database photos (Mammogram Image Processing Society

(UK) database) are considered. The confirmation of this work was achieved by a specialist radiologist's visual examination of the segmented image.

In [9] Ayman Abubaker, reported in the 2005 International Journal of Biological and Life Sciences, Ayman suggested two algorithms to reduce mammogram image storage requirements. The picture goes through a shrinking phase that, using a pixel-depth conversion algorithm accompanied by an enhancement process, transforms the 16-bit images to 8 bits. The algorithm's output is critically and subjectively measured. With no loss of critical data in the breast area, a 50 per cent reduction in size is accomplished. A method for the identification of mammographic calcification is suggested in [10] S.A Hojjatoleslamic. The picture is first segmented into alleged regions of calcification and then labelled as calcification or regular context for each observed area. New local thresholding and area increasing techniques ideal for the identification of tiny blobs in a textured context are exploited by the segmentation process. The outcome of the experimental analysis utilising a series of 20 mammographic images indicates that in mammographic images, the proposed method has a strong capacity to identify calcifications.

In [11], F. L Valverde proposed deformable model for image segmentation. Deformable model-based segmentation approaches can solve some of the conventional image processing techniques limitations. Deformable models, currently created, will cope with holes and other entity boundary irregularities. It can segment objects in noisy images by defining a new energy function associated with image noise and avoiding the tendency of contour points to bunch up. For vessel segmentation on mammograms, the specification is validated.

2 Motivation

Today, breast cancer is the most prevalent type of cancer in women, especially in western nations. It is also the leading cause of mortality per year in women. It is a condition in which cells in the tissues of the breast grow irregular, and these abnormal cells shape too much tissue and become cancer. Any individual has a chance of developing breast cancer. Early warning is the only guarantee that life can be spared. The most accessible approach to discover breast cancer early is to get a mammogram until a tumour in the breast is found. Radiologists, however, find it challenging to offer a precise and reliable analysis of the enormous number of mammograms produced by widespread screening. It is essential to identify microcalcification at an early stage such that adequate care can be administered effectively. It is possible to examine and operate the patient more accurately by utilising fuzzy shell clustering in mammography.

3   Problem Definition

As per the literature study, it was found that it is difficult for radiologists to have correct mammogram picture detail. Since mammograms use lower doses of radiation than ordinary chest X-rays, it is also complicated to view them accurately. The best method of preventing breast cancer is early diagnosis. In early breast cancer, microcalcifications are the sole mammographic symbol. This method aims to isolate features that play an essential role in categorising multiple types of breast cancer.

4   Methodology

The CAD system includes preprocessing stage, segmentation and feature extraction stage with wavelet transform. Figure 1 shows block diagram of proposed system.

Input mammogram images are used for this system is DDSM (digital data screening mammogram). These images are available for scholars and researchers. The DDSM is a database of 2620 scanned mammography film. It contains useful cases of mammogram images with proper verified pathology information. Mammogram images are low-intensity X-ray, and hence it is very important to enhance these intensity values of mammogram images. Many techniques are developed to enhance the image [1, 2]. In this system mammogram images are preprocessed. Database includes tags and black column which is not useful for extracting the features; therefore it has been removed by applying threshold to the system [3, 4]. These images processed for filtering. Median filter is very popular filter used to remove unwanted noise. DWT (discrete wavelet transform) deals with horizontal, vertical, diagonal and approximate components. Approximate component carries maximum information, and hence this information provide to GLCM (grey-level co-occurrence matrix). GLCM works for four angles and extracts eight important features of mammogram images. These features can be used to train any neural network to differentiate between different stages of cancer.

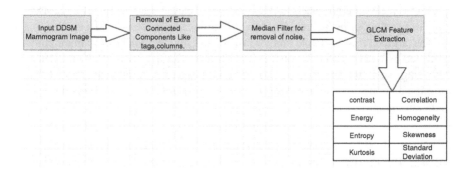

Fig. 1   Block diagram for feature extraction of the CAD system

5   Results and Observations

As seen in Figs. 2, 3, 4, 5, 6 and 7, the regular, benign and malignant picture groups are distinct. The DDSM is a database containing mammographic images, these images are available for research purposes. Feature extraction requires simplifying the volume of data used to reflect a wide range of data correctly. For the analysis of complex data, a significant amount of memory and computing is needed. If the derived features provide the necessary details from the input data, then a reduced data representation will be used to accomplish the desired purpose. The critical characteristics of a picture are colour, texture and form. Wavelet is a mathematical image processing technique that has recently been intensively researched. They were successfully extended to the study of image denoising, coding and texture. The wavelet transformation's central concept is to decompose a picture into a collection of images of many specifics and a low-quality image [12]. The low-resolution picture is obtained by smoothing (or blurring) the picture iteratively until there is no detail, but the coarse contours remain. Detailed photographs, which include the required details to restore the original image, recover the details lost during this process. After the blurring process decreases the image size, the depiction of an image is sometimes referred to as a multi-resolution (multiscale) depiction owing to its low-resolution and intricate images. All these photographs are preprocessed with the global threshold technique considered.

Wavelet transform is best tool for detection of cancer values. Wavelet transform is well-known for textural features extraction. Mammogram images are then applied to wavelet transform and grey level co-occurrence matrix.

The wavelet combination with GLCM utilises textural and predictive picture properties to diagnose and identify breast cancer in the mammogram. GLCM [13] tests image properties correlated with the statistics of the second degree. The statistical features derived from MR images are often referred to as the Grey-Level Spatial Dependency Matrix (GLSDM) using the grey-level co-occurrence matrix (GLCM). The grey-level co-occurrence matrix is known as a widespread tool for extracting textural features. The frequency of variations of these calculated pixel brightness values is calculated by the GLCM. That is, it reflects the pixel pairs'

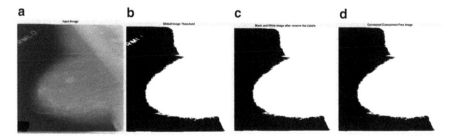

Fig. 2 Benign mammogram image B_100 (**a**) input image, (**b**) global image threshold, (**c**) black column-free image, (**d**) connected component-free image

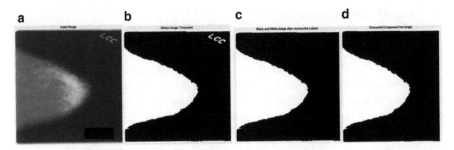

Fig. 3 Benign mammogram image B_089 (**a**) input image, (**b**) global image threshold, (**c**) black column-free image, (**d**) connected component-free image

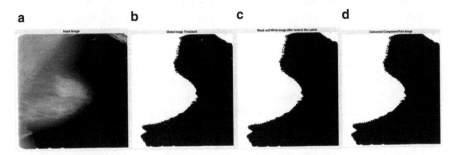

Fig. 4 Normal mammogram image N_210 (**a**) input image, (**b**) global image threshold, (**c**) black column-free image, (**d**) connected component-free image

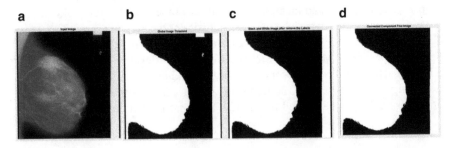

Fig. 5 Normal mammogram image N_230 (**a**) input image, (**b**) global image threshold, (**c**) black column-free image, (**d**) connected component-free image

frequency forming. The image's GLCM properties are represented as a matrix with the same number of rows and columns as the image's grey values. The elements of this matrix depend on the frequency of the two pixels that have been defined. Based on their neighbourhood, all pixel pairs will differ. These matrix elements include, based on the grey colour of the rows and columns, second-order statistical

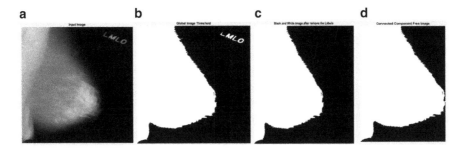

Fig. 6 Malignant mammogram image M_180 (**a**) input image, (**b**) global image threshold, (**c**) black column-free image, (**d**) connected component-free image

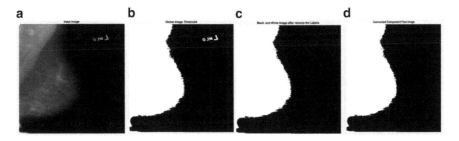

Fig. 7 Malignant mammogram image M_101 (**a**) input image, (**b**) global image threshold, (**c**) black column-free image, (**d**) connected component-free image

likelihood values. The transient matrix is very big if the intensity values are broad. This generates a process load that takes time. A GLCM is a matrix in which the number of rows and columns in the image is equivalent to the number of various levels of grey or pixels. The co-occurrence matrix is centred on two parameters, which are known to be the relative distance determined in pixel number between the pixel pairs and its corresponding orientation. It is often quantified in four directions (e.g. 00, 45 0, 900 and 135 0), but it might be necessary to combine various other variations.

Table 1 shows GLCM feature extraction from DDSM images. GLCM eight features are contrast, correlation, energy, homogeneity, entropy, skewness, kurtosis and standard deviation. It is observed that malignant image values are different than benign and normal images. From this we can conclude that malignant image pixel values are higher and completely different than other classes of images. These features can be trained to ANN (artificial neural network) to check the accuracy of the system.

Table 1 GLCM feature extractions of DDSM images

Sr.no.	Image type	Contrast	Correlation	Energy	Homogeneity	Entropy	Skewness	Kurtosis	Standard deviation
1	B_100	0.0701	0.1189	0.9009	0.9869	2.1625	1.0235	19.1969	0.0424
2	B_089	0.05	0.1117	0.9254	0.9871	2.0922	1.4217	33.3147	0.0424
3	M_101	0.0916	0.0801	0.953	0.974	1.5992	2.0662	57.0377	0.0552
4	M_180	0.089	0.0611	0.9511	0.9797	1.9377	1.9464	51.8926	0.05
5	N_210	0.0536	0.0793	0.9475	0.9859	2.1087	1.3121	32.0658	0.0424
6	N_230	0.0595	0.1049	0.9463	0.9857	2.1708	1.5321	32.1974	0.0429

6   Conclusion

Mammogram images are low-contrast images using proper filter and enhancement technique; the visuality of the image can be improved. Mini-MIAS and DDSM are the standard databases which are available for researchers. Proposed CAD system used DDSM images. Three types are used normal, benign and malignant. Median filter is the popular filter for mammogram images. These filtered images are then processed through wavelet transform. Wavelet transform extracts four components horizontal, vertical, diagonal and approximate, respectively. Approximate components contain data which is very useful for feature extractions of the mammogram. This component values is given to grey-level co-occurrence matrix to extract features which can be used to train the machine. GLCM works in four directions and extracts eight features, respectively. It has been observed that malignant feature values are higher and completely different than benign and normal images. Malignant images can be identified from extracting these features. Hence this system can be used to train any neural network to differentiate different stages of cancer.

References

1. Neha N. Ganvir, D.M. Yadav, "Filtering Method for Pre-processing Mammogram Images for Breast Cancer Detection", International Journal of Engineering and Advanced Technology. ISSN: 2249 – 8958, Volume 9, Issue 1, (pp. 4222–4229), Oct 2019.
2. Neha N. Ganvir, D.M. Yadav, "Clustered Micro-Calcifications Extraction From Mammogram Images Using Cellular Automata Segmentation With Anisotropic Diffusion Filtering", International Journal of Scientific & Technology Research. ISSN 2277-8616, Volume 9, Issue 04, (pp. 1217–1221), April 2020.
3. Xiaolong Liu, Zhidong Deng, Yuhan Yang. Recent progress in semantic image segmentation. Artificial Intelligence Review, Springer, 2018.
4. Abdulkadir Sengur, Erkan Tanyildizi. A survey on neutrosophic medical image segmentation. Neutrosophic Set in Medical Image Analysis; 2019.
5. Ingval Anderson, Debra M Ikeda, "Breast tomosynthesis & digital mammography: A comparison of breast cancer visibility and BIRDS classification in a population of cancer with subtle mammographic findings", European Society of Radiology 2018.
6. Steven M. McAoy, "Feasibility of determining breast density using processed mammogram images", thesis submitted in Univ. of Columbia, April 2010.
7. Pawar B.V, Sushma Patil,"Early stage detection of tumors in mammogram".
8. Sheshadri HS, "Detection of breast cancer by mammogram image segmentation", Cancer Journal, Vol 1, issue 4, Dec 2005.
9. Ayman Abubakar, Mushtaq Aquel, Maohammed Saleh, "Mammogram image size reduction using 16-8 bit conversion technique", International Journal of Biological and Life Science, Vol 1, issue 2, 2005.
10. S.A. Hojjatoleslami, J. Kittler, "Automatic detection of calcification in mammogram", IEEE, 6 July 1995.
11. F.L Valverde, N.Guil,J.Mulnoz,K.Doi," A deformable model for image segmentation in noisy medical images", IEEE 2001.
12. http://hdl.handle.net/10603/196911.
13. Mari Partio, Bogdan Cramariuc, Moncef Gabbouj and Ari Visa, "Rock texture retrieval using gray level cooccurrence matrix", Journal of Theoretical and Applied Information Technology, vol. 33. no. 2, pp. 155–164, 2011.

Deep Learning-Based Techniques to Identify COVID-19 Patients Using Medical Image Segmentation

Rachna Jain ⓓ, Shreyansh Singh, Surykant Swami, and Sanjeev kumar

Abstract Artificial intelligence (AI) has been able to solve the problems effectively in our day-to-day life in today's world. Year 2020 has seen worldwide pandemic COVID-19 which has thrown normal life out of gear. Social distancing and sanitization are new norms of life. Robot with AI techniques will help to solve the problems associated with it. This paper highlights use of deep learning-based techniques to predict the disease. It takes a lot of time in lab almost 2–3 days to diagnose the covid patients with the help of gold-standard real-time reverse transcription polymerase chain reaction (rRT-PCR). Another major diagnostic tool is radio imaging; however, with the help of artificial intelligence (AI)-based deep learning methods, it is much easier to diagnose the disease. Computer vision is a scientific field that deals with how computers can be made to gain high-level understanding of the real world from digital images or videos. In terms of engineering, it seeks to automate tasks that the human vision system can do. This paper is based on one specific task in computer vision called as image segmentation. Even though researchers have come up with various methods to solve this problem, in this work it will be working with architecture named U-NET a type of encoder-decoder network along with ResNet-34.

Keywords Artificial intelligence (AI) · Computer vision · COVID-19 · Image segmentation · Pandemic · Deep learning · Computer tomography (CT) · Spatiotemporal features · U-NET encoder-decoder

R. Jain (✉) · S. Singh · S. Swami · S. kumar
JSS Academy of Technical Education, Noida, India
e-mail: rachnajain@jssaten.ac.in

© The Author(s), under exclusive license to Springer
Nature Switzerland AG 2021
A. K. Manocha et al. (eds.), *Computational Intelligence in Healthcare*, Health
Information Science, https://doi.org/10.1007/978-3-030-68723-6_18

1   Introduction

Computer vision and pattern recognition problems are categorized into three major categories of problems.

1. Image Classification: Image classification is that the process of categorizing and labelling groups of pixels or vectors within a picture supported specific rules.
2. Image Detection: Image or object detection may be a technology that processes the image and detects objects in it.
3. Image Segmentation: This is often the toughest and doubtless the foremost useful class of problem among the three (Fig. 1).

Input image can be divided into various parts called segments in the output map. It's not an excellent idea to process the whole image at an equivalent time as there'll be regions within the image which don't contain any information. By dividing the image into segments, we will make use of the important segments for processing the image. That is how image segmentation works. Image segmentation [31] techniques are subclassified into two types:

1. Semantic segmentation
2. Instance aware segmentation

Consider the following images (Fig. 2):
In image 1, every pixel belongs to a specific class (either background or person). Also, all the pixels belonging to a specific class are represented by an equivalent color (background as black and person as pink). This is often an example of semantic segmentation.

Image 2 has also assigned a specific class to every pixel of the image. However, different objects of an equivalent class have different colors (Person 1 as red, Person 2 as green, background as black, etc.). This is often an example of instance segmentation.

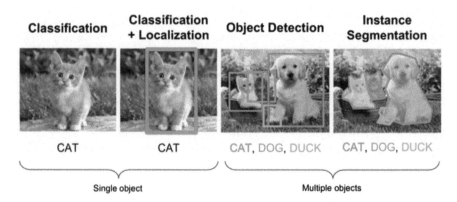

Fig. 1 Image classification and segmentation. (Source: https://www.kdnuggets.com/2018/09/object-detection-image-classification-yolo.html)

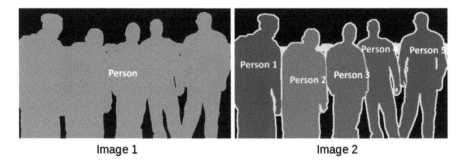

Fig. 2 Images with semantic and instance segmentation. (Source: https://www.analyticsvidhya.com/blog/2019/04/introduction-image-segmentation-techniques-python)

Image segmentation helps us understand the content of the image and should be an important topic in image processing and computer vision [33]. It has many applications like compression, scene understanding, locating objects in satellite images, etc. Over time, many algorithms have been developed for image segmentation, but with the arrival of deep learning in computer vision, many deep learning models for image segmentation have also emerged. These days even cloud based services are used for medical image segmentation [25]. Some authors have elucidated semi-supervised image segmentation also which further alleviates the reconstruction of unsupervised objects [28].

Medical image segmentation has an important role in computer-aided diagnosis systems in several applications [5, 21]. The vast investment and development of medical imaging modalities like microscopy, X-ray, ultrasound, computerized tomography (CT), resonance imaging (MRI) segmentation [32], and positron emission tomography attract researchers to implement new medical image-processing algorithms. Image segmentation is considered the foremost essential medical imaging process because it extracts the region of interest (ROI) through a semiautomatic or automatic process. It divides a picture into areas supported a specified description, like segmenting body organs/tissues within the medical applications for border detection, tumor detection/segmentation, and mass detection. COVID-19 has changed the way of life of a normal human being. Large number of deaths has been there in the entire world due to novel coronavirus. Governments of different countries have adopted strenuous measures to control the spread of virus. Science and technology have immense contribution in implementing government policies such as online classes, treating patients in hospitals with the help of robot. Coronavirus pandemic has emerged as biggest problem in this century. Symptoms of coronavirus patient include difficulty in breathing, sore throat, dry cough, and high fever as shown in Fig. 3. Some of the symptoms such as high fever is common with dengue, malaria, etc. It is very important to diagnose covid patients from other diseases. Computer tomography (CT) imaging helps in diagnosing the patients suffering from deadly virus as shown in Fig. 4. The number of available kits for corona testing

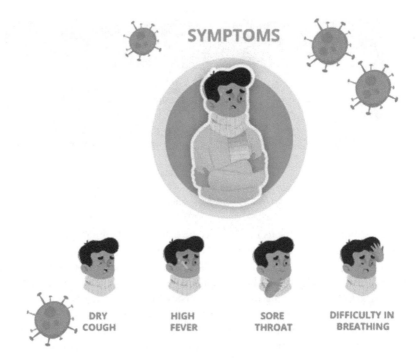

Fig. 3 Coronavirus symptoms. (Source: https://www.mygov.in/covid-19)

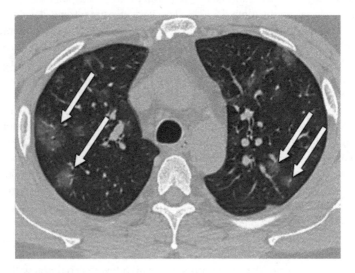

Fig. 4 CT image of a patient with axial view (Bernheim, A. et al.)

Fig. 5 Deep learning model with hidden abstraction layers between input and output

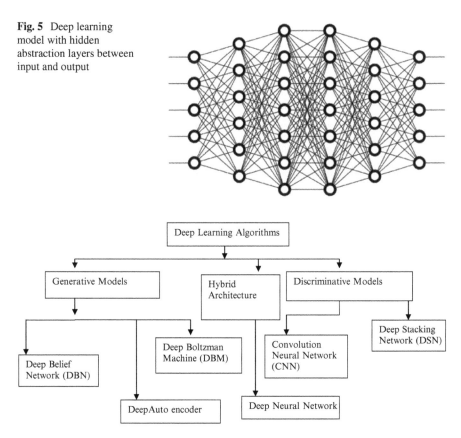

Fig. 6 Classification of deep learning algorithms

is limited; hence there is need of some automatic techniques which help in early detection [29].

Another method involves use of AI-based deep learning [3] techniques which are also useful in early detection and treatment of the patients which will reduce the burden of healthcare staff and doctors [30]. Deep learning models involve hidden layers representing abstraction levels as shown in Fig. 5. Deep learning algorithms are further classified as either unsupervised learning or supervised learning. Unsupervised mathematical model has to be formulated from dataset using inputs only. Generative models where input variables play the primary role such as density estimation fall under the category of unsupervised models. It is further subclassified as Deep Belief Network (DBN), Deep Autoencoder models and Deep Boltzmann Machine (DBM). In the case of supervised learning, models are built using inputs and already known outputs. Discriminative models fall under this category which is further divided as Convolutional Neural Network (CNN) and Deep Stacking Network (DSN) as shown in Fig. 6.

2 Classification of Deep Learning Algorithms

Deep learning algorithms can be broadly classified into two main categories as shown in Fig. 6:

(i) Unsupervised Algorithm: In this category a mathematical model has to be formulated with the help of inputs only. Generative models fall under this category. Deep Belief Network (DBN), Deep Boltzmann Machine (DBM), and Deep Autoencoder are popular examples of it.
(ii) Supervised Algorithm: In this category a mathematical model has to be formulated with the help of inputs and outputs. Convolutional Neural Network (CNN) models and Deep Stacking Networks are popular examples.
(iii) Hybrid Architecture: It takes the advantage of both above mentioned categories. Deep Neural Network is example of it.

3 Literature Survey

Paper [1] has emphasized on stronghold of AI techniques in combating battle against novel coronavirus. In this paper survey has been nicely categorized as use of deep learning models for image processing in medical field, data science methods for predicting future pandemics, and use of AI-based techniques in field of medicine. Paper [2] has exploited CT imaging feature of 21 patients to highlight some key findings. The author has found that around 71% patients have two lobes in CT of chest.

In paper [3] author has developed a model, which is made according to deep learning techniques to identify covid patients from pneumonia patients in early stages of infection. The authors have developed Convolutional Neural Network (CNN)-based models to identify the covid patients. Samples were collected from three hospitals at China. Proposed model has shown accuracy of 86.7%. Paper [4] has explored different deep learning methods to distinguish between patients suffering from pneumonia and chest infection due to covid. In the proposed methodology, the author has developed a fully automatic framework to identify covid with the help of chest CT and to measure performance parameters. Results have shown sensitivity of 87% and specificity of 92%.

In paper [5] author has summarized deep learning techniques to combat this outbreak. In this paper with the help of X-ray imaging, automatic covid detection model is proposed. The proposed methodology works for binary classifiers between no findings and covid as well as multi-classifier between no finding, pneumonia, and covid. Proposed model is made available on cloud via GitHub platform to help in fast screening of the patients. Paper [6] has exploited AI techniques to differentiate between pneumonia and covid with the help of CT images. Proposed technique has been implemented in 16 hospitals near Wuhan and Beijing. Results have shown good accuracy with sensitivity around 0.974 and specificity 0.922 approximately.

Paper [7] has highlighted the role of upcoming technologies in budding areas like big data, AI, and role of IoT in upcoming healthcare sector. The author has declared that literature survey has been done on Google Scholar and Scopus using keywords such as covid and artificial intelligence. The author has claimed that AI-based technology will help to predict in detecting covid clusters. In paper [8] author has tried to establish a relationship with infection duration. One hundred and twenty-one patients with various symptoms have been studied from 4 different geographic locations of China. Source [9] displays the graph showing active cases in India.

In paper [10] authors have developed deep learning-based framework to quantify infectious region with respect to the entire lungs using CT scan. The authors have exemplified VB Net neural network and validated their model on 300 new patients. Dice similarity coefficient (DSC) is used to measure the performance of the proposed model. In this paper, deep learning-based segmentation scheme is devised to estimate region of interest with respect to lungs volume. The authors have examined CT scan of 300 patients and by inculcating human in loop strategy iteration time have been reduced by 4 minutes. In the proposed paper, dice similarity coefficient (DSC) displays 91.6% similarity between manual and automatic segmentation techniques.

Paper [11] highlights deep learning-based model, spatiotemporal residual network (ST-ResNet) with the help of machine learning techniques to predict traffic flow in an urban scenario. Deep learning-based models help to predict the urban transportation data, emergency healthcare solutions, and public safety solutions. In this paper dynamic spatiotemporal data chosen is referenced as a case study. The author has predicted the traffic flow using five different techniques labelled as deep learning-based, machine learning-based, reinforcement learning-based, statistical methods, and transfer learning methods. Paper [12] exemplifies deep learning-based spatiotemporal residual net (St-ResNet) to predict the flow of traffic from every corner of the city. In this paper author highlighted different temporal properties such as closeness, trend, and period of the traffic. These residual units are assigned weights which are summed together with external factor to predict the traffic flow. In paper [13] Convolutional Neural Network (CNN) framework is proposed to differentiate pneumonia from COVID-19. ResNet 50 model is proposed to reduce the training time of the model. The authors have proposed covid ResNet and accentuated the performance by resizing the input image to 128*128*3, 224*224*3, and 229*229*3 pixels. Progressive resizing techniques, discriminative learning, and cyclical rate finding help to increase the accuracy of the model by 96.23%. Hemdan et al. [14] has exemplified COVIDX-Net exploits seven different architecture models such as Visual Geometric Group (VGG) network and another version of Google MobileNet. Dataset has been 50 X-ray images which comprises of 25 normal and 25 covid images. The authors have computed training as well as testing time along with accuracy for models VGG19, DenseNet201, ResNetV2, Inception ResNet V2, Inception V3, MobileNetV2, and Xception. The authors have sketched the confusion matrix for all seven types of classifier, and it has been found that VGG19 and DenseNet201 performed the best.

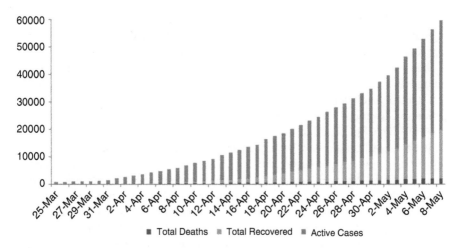

Fig. 7 Curve showing active cases in India [9]

4 Motivation Behind the Work

It has been found that there is a direct positive correlation among covid deaths and burdens faced by health workers. In order to reduce the workload of physicians, AI-based models could be a good option. Another motivation is that in large countries like India where number of cases are increasing regularly and curve has not flatten yet as shown in Fig. 7, it is almost impossible for physicians to check each and everyone showing the symptoms. So these AI-based solutions could provide a good answer to these problems.

5 Deep Learning-Based Proposed mMdel

Deep residual learning facilitates super layer structure up to 100 layers and can be extended up to 1000 layers. Forecasting the total incoming and outgoing of covid patients in any specific area, for example, 1000 square meters, is a challenging task. There are two major types of dependencies involved.

(i) Spatial dependency: Total inflow and outflow of patients with in a particular area can be maintained using geometrical coordinates of patients that can be obtained from location of mobile phone of that person.

(ii) Temporal dependency: This is the dependency with respect to time instances. There are three associated time instances classified as valid time, transaction time, and decision time. Valid time is defined as if the patient does not show any symptom after 14 days. Decision time is the time to act for hospitalization or quarantine.

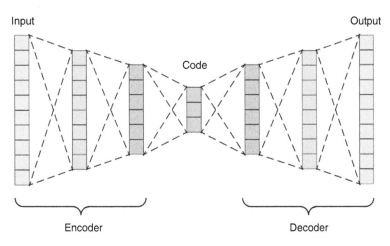

Fig. 8 Normal encoder-decoder circuit diagram

6   Normal Encoder-Decoder Network (Fig. 8)

In a normal encoder-decoder network, there is a down-sampling path known as encoder and an up-sampling path known as decoder, and there is no transfer of information from one branch to another. In an image segmentation problem, the encoder network extracts the features in the given input image, and the decoder network generates the output segmentation map from the extracted features by the encoder.

6.1   U-NET

The *U-NET* was developed by Olaf Ronneberger et al. [15] for biomedical image segmentation. U-NET is a fully convolutional encoder-decoder network. Unlike normal encoder-decoder networks, what makes U-NET special is the presence of skip connections to transfer higher semantic information from down-sampling path to the up-sampling path, thus, providing additional semantic information to the up-sampling layers. Its architecture is small and is extended to work with fewer training images and to yield more precise segmentations. It can yield good accuracy even for sparse dataset. 2D operations in U-NET proposed by Ronneberger et al. have been substituted by 3D operations [20]. Although 3D counterparts yield better results, their biggest drawback is consumption of excess memory [26]. In the following section, U-NET architecture is discussed in detail.

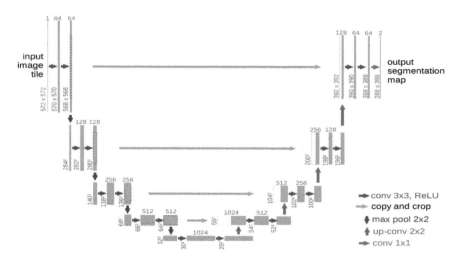

Fig. 9 U-NET architecture

6.2 U-NET Architecture

U-NET has u-shaped architecture that has a down-sampling and a similar up-sampling path yielding a u-shaped architecture (Fig. 9).

7 Attention Mechanism

Wang, K., He, J., and Zhang, L [16] have proposed a unique method of attention-based mechanism which differentiates at global and local level. Global feature extraction is at fully connected layers, whereas local extraction is at provided convolution layer. Depth of recognition in computer vision area can increase the accuracy of the proposed model [17]. Jetley et al. [18] introduced end-to-end-trainable attention module for images. In paper [27], authors have scrutinized 3D Universal U-NET model which explores universal architecture for different image segmentation processes (Fig. 10).

Attention is to give more preference to activations thus engaging the resources onto the relevant features only, providing the network with better generalization power. Essentially, the network can pay "attention" to certain parts of the image relevant to the objective instead of looking at the whole image. Attention helps in giving more priority to the features relevant to the current objective. Zhang, H [22] has presented attention mechanism-based model for generation of images.

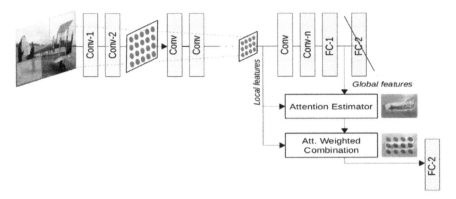

Fig. 10 Attention mechanism [18]

7.1 Types of Attention

(a) *Hard Attention:* It pays attention to the relevant features in an image by cropping the image region of interest. Hard attention can select only one area of interest in an image at a given instant of time, that is, the hard attention output can only be 0 or 1; thus it has its implications, and it is non-differentiable in nature. Since hard attention is non-differentiable, as a result, standard method of optimization of a loss function with back propagation cannot be applied with hard attention.

(b) *Soft Attention*: It works by giving weights to different parts of the image between 0 and 1. Areas of high relevance are given a larger weight, and areas of low relevance are given a smaller weight. As the model training continues, more and more focus is paid to the regions of interest by giving them higher weights. Soft attention is differentiable in natures; thus the standard method of optimization of loss function can be applied with soft attention (Fig. 11).

7.2 Transfer Learning

Transfer learning is a practice in machine learning and deep learning that focuses on elicitation of the knowledge gained while solving one problem and applying it to a different but related or similar problem. For example, knowledge gained while learning to recognize red blood cell could be applied when trying to recognize white blood cell. According to Bao, L., and Intille, S. S [19], few body activities could identify through general training data, while other activities acquire recognition through subject specific training.

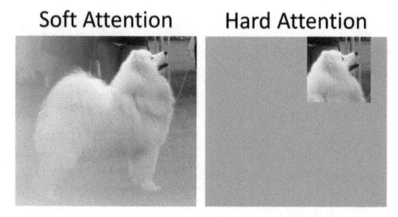

Fig. 11 Hard and soft attention. (Source: https://towardsdatascience.com/learn-to-pay-attention-trainable-visual-attention-in-cnns-87e2869f89f1)

8   Problem

In human lungs computed tomography (CT) scans with COVID-19-related findings, as well as without such findings has been studied. A small subset of studies has been annotated with binary pixel masks representing the regions of interests. The goal is to build and train deep learning model to segment the regions of interest for COVID-19-related analysis.

9   Solution Approach

Since this is an image segmentation problem as discussed above, we will be using an encoder-decoder architecture named U-NET. The base architecture will be normal U-NET with following changes in the architecture:

1. Integration of attention gates on top of the skip connections in the U-NET
2. A ResNet-34-based encoder in place of standard encoder

9.1   Attention U-NET

Segmentation performance can be achieved by integration of an attention gates on top of U-NET skip connections, without the need of training additional models. As a result, attention gates integrated into U-NET architecture can improve model sensitivity and accuracy to focus on relevant features by assigning high weights to corresponding pixels without requiring significant computation overhead. Attention

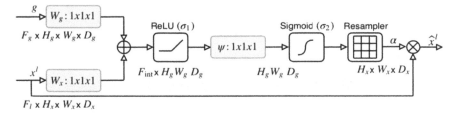

Fig. 12 Attention gate mechanism

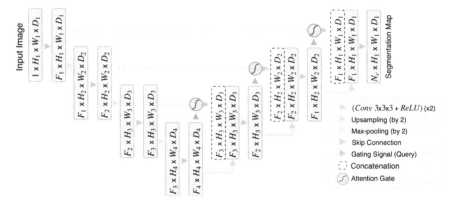

Fig. 13 Attention U-NET

gates progressively suppress irrelevant features in the image by assigning low weights to those pixels (Figs. 12 and 13).

9.2 ResNet-34

ResNet-34 is 34-layer residual neural network with skip connection from one layer to another. One of the problems ResNets solve is of the vanishing gradient. This occurs when a network is too deep; the gradients from where the loss function is calculated vanish to zero after several applications of the chained back propagation. Due to which the weights are never updating its values, and, therefore, no learning is being performed by the model. With ResNets' skip connections, the gradients can flow directly through the skip connections backward from later layers to initial filters. It is also important to preserve the information that is being passed from layer to layer [23]. Although these images are from high-resolution spaces, even low-resolution images can provide satisfactory results [24] (Fig. 14).

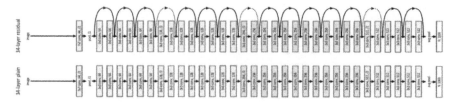

Fig. 14 ResNet-34 architecture

10 Conclusion

Many image diagnosis tasks require initial data for identifying abnormalities, quantifying measurements, and the absolute changes over time. The automated image analysis tools based on ML algorithms are used to improve the quality of image diagnosis and interpretation by facilitating by efficient identification of findings. Deep learning is one of the extensively applied machine learning techniques that provide a suitable accuracy and precision. It opened new approaches in medical image analysis that weren't possible before. Several applications of deep learning in healthcare cover a wide range of problems ranging from cancer screening and disease monitoring to personalized treatment suggestions. Various sources of data today such as radiological imaging (X-ray, MRI scans, CT), pathology imaging, and most recently genomic sequences have brought an immense amount of data at the disposal. But we are still short of tools to convert all this data to useful information. Though, deep learning is used for medical imaging, but the list is by no means complete; however, it provides an indication of the long-ranging deep learning impact in the medical imaging industry today.

Conflicts of Interest/Competing Interests Not applicable

FundingNot applicable

References

1. Nguyen, T.T., 2020. Artificial intelligence in the battle against coronavirus (COVID-19): a survey and Future research directions. *Preprint, DOI*, https://doi.org/10.13140/ RG.2.2.36491.23846.
2. Chung, M., Bernheim, A., Mei, X., Zhang, N., Huang, M., Zeng, X. ... and Jacobi, A. (2020). CT imaging features of 2019 novel coronavirus (2019-nCoV). Radiology, 200230.
3. Xu, X., Jiang, X., Ma, C., Du, P., Li, X., Lv, S., ... and Li, Y. (2020). Deep learning system to screen coronavirus disease 2019 pneumonia. arXiv preprint arXiv:2002.09334.
4. Li, L., Qin, L., Xu, Z., Yin, Y., Wang, X., Kong, B., ... and Cao, K. (2020). Artificial intelligence distinguishes COVID-19 from community acquired pneumonia on chest CT. Radiology, 200905.
5. Wang, S., Kang, B., Ma, J., Zeng, X., Xiao, M., Guo, J., ... and Xu, B. (2020). A deep learning algorithm using CT images to screen for corona virus disease (COVID-19). medRxiv, doi: https://doi.org/10.1101/2020.02.14.20023028.

6. Jin, S., Wang, B., Xu, H., Luo, C., Wei, L., Zhao, W., and Sun, W. (2020). AI-assisted CT imaging analysis for COVID-19 screening: Building and deploying a medical AI system in four weeks. medRxiv, doi: https://doi.org/10.1101/2020.03.19.20039354.

7. Vaishya, R., Javaid, M., Khan, I.H. and Haleem, A., 2020. Artificial Intelligence (AI) applications for COVID-19 pandemic. *Diabetes & Metabolic Syndrome: Clinical Research & Reviews.*

8. Bernheim, A., Mei, X., Huang, M., Yang, Y., Fayad, Z.A., Zhang, N., Diao, K., Lin, B., Zhu, X., Li, K. and Li, S., 2020. Chest CT findings in coronavirus disease-19 (COVID-19): relationship to duration of infection. *Radiology*, p.200463.

9. https://timesofindia.indiatimes.com/blogs/tastefully-contemporary/covid-india-what-is-the-trend-and-forecast-till-june-7-2020

10. Shan, F., Gao, Y., Wang, J., Shi, W., Shi, N., Han, M., Xue, Z. and Shi, Y., 2020. Lung infection quantification of covid-19 in ct images with deep learning. *arXiv preprint arXiv:2003.04655.*

11. Xie, P., Li, T., Liu, J., Du, S., Yang, X. and Zhang, J., 2020. Urban flow prediction from spatio-temporal data using machine learning: A survey. *Information Fusion*, *59*,pp.1–12. https://doi.org/10.1016/j.inffus.2020.01.002

12. Zhang, J., Zheng, Y. and Qi, D., 2016. Deep spatio-temporal residual networks for citywide crowd flows prediction. *arXiv preprint arXiv:1610.00081.*

13. Farooq, M., & Hafeez, A. (2020). Covid-resnet: A deep learning framework for screening of covid19 from radiographs. *arXiv preprint arXiv:2003.14395.*

14. Hemdan, E. E. D., Shouman, M. A., & Karar, M. E. (2020). Covidx-net: A framework of deep learning classifiers to diagnose covid-19 in x-ray images. *arXiv preprint arXiv:2003.11055.*

15. Ronneberger, O., Fischer, P. and Brox, T., 2015, October. U-net: Convolutional networks for biomedical image segmentation. In *International Conference on Medical image computing and computer-assisted intervention* (pp. 234–241). Springer, Cham.

16. Wang, K., He, J. and Zhang, L., 2019. Attention-based convolutional neural network for weakly labeled human activities' recognition with wearable sensors. *IEEE Sensors Journal*, *19*(17), pp.7598–7604.

17. He, K., Zhang, X., Ren, S., & Sun, J. (2016). Deep residual learning for image recognition. In *Proceedings of the IEEE conference on computer vision and pattern recognition* (pp. 770–778).

18. S. Jetley, N. A. Lord, N. Lee and P. H. Torr, "Learn to pay attention" in arXiv:1804.02391, 2018, [online] Available: https://arxiv.org/abs/1804.02391.

19. Bao, L., & Intille, S. S. (2004, April). Activity recognition from user-annotated acceleration data. In *International conference on pervasive computing* (pp. 1–17). Springer, Berlin, Heidelberg.

20. Çiçek, Ö., Abdulkadir, A., Lienkamp, S. S., Brox, T., & Ronneberger, O. (2016, October). 3D U-Net: learning dense volumetric segmentation from sparse annotation. In *International conference on medical image computing and computer-assisted intervention* (pp. 424–432). Springer, Cham.

21. Schlemper, J., Castro, D. C., Bai, W., Qin, C., Oktay, O., Duan, J., ... & Rueckert, D. (2018, September). Bayesian deep learning for accelerated MR image reconstruction. In *International Workshop on Machine Learning for Medical Image Reconstruction* (pp. 64–71). Springer, Cham.

22. Zhang, H., Goodfellow, I., Metaxas, D., & Odena, A. (2019, May). Self-attention generative adversarial networks. In *International Conference on Machine Learning* (pp. 7354–7363). PMLR.

23. Ronao, C. A., & Cho, S. B. (2015, November). Deep convolutional neural networks for human activity recognition with smartphone sensors. In *International Conference on Neural Information Processing* (pp. 46–53). Springer, Cham.

24. Shi, W., Caballero, J., Huszár, F., Totz, J., Aitken, A. P., Bishop, R., ... & Wang, Z. (2016). Real-time single image and video super-resolution using an efficient sub-pixel convolutional neural network. In *Proceedings of the IEEE conference on computer vision and pattern recognition* (pp. 1874–1883).

25. Liu, Z., Li, S., Chen, Y. K., Liu, T., Liu, Q., Xu, X., ... & Wen, W. (2020, October). Orchestrating Medical Image Compression and Remote Segmentation Networks. In *International Conference on Medical Image Computing and Computer-Assisted Intervention* (pp. 406–416). Springer, Cham.

26. Brügger, R., Baumgartner, C. F., & Konukoglu, E. (2019, October). A partially reversible U-Net for memory-efficient volumetric image segmentation. In *International Conference on Medical Image Computing and Computer-Assisted Intervention* (pp. 429–437). Springer, Cham.

27. Huang, C., Han, H., Yao, Q., Zhu, S., & Zhou, S. K. (2019, October). A 3D Universal U-Net for Multi-domain Medical Image Segmentation. In *International Conference on Medical Image Computing and Computer-Assisted Intervention* (pp. 291–299). Springer, Cham.

28. Chen, S., Bortsova, G., Juárez, A. G. U., van Tulder, G., & de Bruijne, M. (2019, October). Multi-task attention-based semi-supervised learning for medical image segmentation. In *International Conference on Medical Image Computing and Computer-Assisted Intervention* (pp. 457–465). Springer, Cham.

29. Narin, A., Kaya, C., & Pamuk, Z. (2020). Automatic detection of coronavirus disease (covid-19) using x-ray images and deep convolutional neural networks. *arXiv preprint arXiv:2003.10849.*

30. Ardakani, A. A., Kanafi, A. R., Acharya, U. R., Khadem, N., & Mohammadi, A. (2020). Application of deep learning technique to manage COVID-19 in routine clinical practice using CT images: Results of 10 convolutional neural networks. *Computers in Biology and Medicine*, 103795.

31. Pal, N. R., & Pal, S. K. (1993). A review on image segmentation techniques. *Pattern recognition*, 26(9), 1277–1294.

32. Bezdek, J. C., Hall, L. O., & Clarke, L. (1993). Review of MR image segmentation techniques using pattern recognition. *MEDICAL PHYSICS-LANCASTER PA-*, 20, 1033–1033.

33. Haralick, R. M., & Shapiro, L. G. (1985). Image segmentation techniques. *Computer vision, graphics, and image processing*, 29(1), 100–132.

Emerging Trends of Bioinformatics in Health Informatics

Mahi Sharma, Shuvhra Mondal, Sudeshna Bhattacharjee, and Neetu Jabalia

Abstract In the era of digital world, due to constantly evolving computational technology, bioinformatics propelled out of research labs into our everyday lives. Emerging advances in bioinformatics enable home computers to have powerful supercomputers, reducing the research expense, enhancing scientific efficiency, and accelerating novel discoveries. Bioinformatics can simply be understood as a field of data science based on the amalgamation of computers and biology. Nowadays, one of the major obstacles for humans is to attain a health system in which each patient could have a personalized medicine, as each patient possesses a unique genome, proteome, and metabolome. Hence, to understand complexity underlying diseases and its mechanism, bioinformatics can be a fundamental approach. One of the objectives of chapter is to present a comprehensive overview of bioinformatics, various omics tools and its applications, health informatics, and healthcare system. Big data technologies and their role in biomedical research is briefly addressed. The later dimension focuses on bioinformatics resources towards personalized medicine. The last section highlights the key commercial platforms for healthcare data analytics and challenges along with future prospects of bioinformatics in healthcare, which will help the readers to effectively use the information for their research endeavours.

Keywords Bioinformatics · Big data · Health informatics · Personalized medicine

1 Introduction

Medical science and public health are growing areas of concern with each pandemic and increase in vulnerable populations. With major breakthroughs "bioinformatics" has proved its efficacy in all research disciplines [37]. Targeting synonymous

M. Sharma · S. Mondal · S. Bhattacharjee
Amity Institute of Virology and Immunology, Noida, Uttar Pradesh, India
e-mail: njabalia@amity.edu

N. Jabalia (✉)
Amity Institute of Biotechnology, Amity university, Noida, Uttar Pradesh, India

© The Author(s), under exclusive license to Springer
Nature Switzerland AG 2021
A. K. Manocha et al. (eds.), *Computational Intelligence in Healthcare*, Health
Information Science, https://doi.org/10.1007/978-3-030-68723-6_19

343

research with human genome project to new generation sequencing, gene therapy, drug designing, and branching off to personalized medicine. Healthcare informatics emphasize on patient-driven therapeutics personalized on genetic, metabolomic, proteomic, and transcriptomic level [15]. The role of bioinformatics during virus outbreaks and medicine has undeniably been the frontline contributing to dry lab research. With the ongoing pandemic of COVID-19, a turmoil on global health has resurfaced. Various proteomics and similarity search databases not only deduced the structure and genome of SARS-Cov-2 but contributed towards diagnosis, identification of the antigenic property, proteins essential for virus assembly, and vaccine development.

Artificial intelligence (AI) contributes to big database analysis and medical research. Significant contributions of AI include screening biomarkers for rare cancer types, their diagnosis, drug repurposing, and healthcare applications [67]. AI as a backbone for future medicine will help cut down costs for healthcare and allow medicine within reach [40]. Various healthcare tools equipped with AI have sourced the market during the COVID-19 crises. Haptik by Reliance Industries is a start-up for conversational health advice and information on medical insurance (https://haptik.ai/blog/conversational-ai-healthcare-use-cases/). The present chapter discusses a comprehensive overview of bioinformatics, tools and applications. The next section focuses on healthcare informatics, big data technology, and their role in biomedical research. The later section focuses on the purpose of bioinformatics in personalized medicine. Further, it highlights the dynamics of bioinformatics and the healthcare system along with challenges and prospects.

2 Defining Bioinformatics

Bioinformatics is an emerging and multidisciplinary field, in which it uses computational tools to analyse, visualize, organize, and store information allied with biological macromolecules [52]. It is greatly focused on attaining biologically oriented data, for example, DNA/RNA, protein sequences, structures, functions, pathways, and interaction between them, that are organized to form a database [18]. Bioinformatics produces huge data collected from computational analysis, system biology, and computer-aided drug discovery to OMIC's studies such as genomics, transcriptomics, proteomics, metabolomics, molecular biology, statistics, chemistry, computational biology, computer science, structure prediction, and phylogenetics (Fig. 1). Recent studies have suggested that in 2025 human genomes up to 2 billion will be sequenced which will take up 2–40 petabytes of storage [81, 87].

It has also been used for in silico analysis of biological data mainly using mathematics and statistical approaches [63]. The availability and affordability of these bioinformatics tools have resulted in the generation of a lot of data that needs to be stored, integrated, and analysed most effectively with help of data science [83]. Bioinformatics majorly consist of four aims (Table 1)

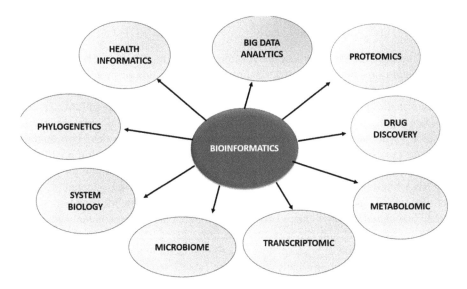

Fig. 1 Bioinformatics and its associated fields

Table 1 Major aims of bioinformatics

S. no	Aim	Description
1.	Data acquisition	Accessing and storing data from the biological studies and research, these sequences are retrieved in proper format and then linked to the stored DNA information, and this data is ordered and new entries are produced, such as in NCBI (for genomic data) and PDB (for 3D macromolecular structures)
2.	Tools and database development	It helps in aiding the analysis of the data. These tools and databases help to see whether the sequenced protein is of interest and differentiate with the already collected information of sequences, such as in FASTA and PSI-BLAST
3.	Data analysis	After the use of the tools and databases to analyse the data in a biologically meaningful way. The efficient analysis of data is possible when the database is equally efficient to provide the necessary information to the user. Languages such as C++, Java, PERL, C, and Visual Basic are useful in this area
4.	Data integration	After the analysis of the data, the data need to integrate with the data from other databases. The kind of researches that require to link between the different databases helps us to present and store the information. The key to effective data integration is knowing architecture and relationships with the various databases

2.1 Tools of Bioinformatics

Tools and database development are considered most important as it helps to analyse function or structural characterization of the nucleotide or protein sequences, genetic expression, and high-throughput screening of the generated compound data. Bioinformatics tools and webservers are classified into various types (Table 2)

Data-mining databases help in retrieving the data from genomic sequence databases and with the help of the visualization tools to analyse and retrieve information from the proteomic database. Zhang and Ding [53] developed a multimodal DBN trained on CLIP-sequence (crosslinking immunoprecipitation) database for predicting RNA-binding protein targets within the genome by taking into account the protein structural specificities [10]. SignalP is a Neural Network-based tool for predicting signal peptides trained on three non-identical data sets, namely, eukaryotes, Gram-negative, and Gram-positive bacteria [43]. CENTIPEDE computes the subsequent likelihood of binding of a transcription factor to a genomic region-given data from other epigenomic analyses [39, 70]. Table 3 shows the database and tools used for various sequential data-mining analysis.

2.2 Applications of Bioinformatics

There are many applications of bioinformatics and can be applied to several fields of research as well as medicine, environment, and agriculture as well. Some of such fields are mentioned below:

2.2.1 Medicine

Drug discovery started when the 3D structures of proteins were found out, first by the X-ray crystallography method [7]. Gene therapy is done by gene addition or removal of the risky gene by ribosomes and controlling the gene expression inside the body. BiMFG is the tool and an integrated database for marine and freshwater genomics [18]. Personalized medicine tailored to match with genetics, proteomics, and metabolomics of patients adding new standards to healthcare informatics. Preventive medicine is the medicines used to prevent a disease rather than curing or treating the symptoms caused by the disease in an individual.

2.2.2 Research

In bioinformatics, biotechnology has great use in identifying various organisms that can be useful in various fields for human use such as the dairy and food industries. The artificial cultures of the *Lactococcus lactis* and many non-pathogenic rod-shaped

Table 2 List of classified tools in bioinformatics

S.no.	Approach	Tool	Link
1.	Database retrieval tool	Entrez	http://www.ncbi.nlm.nih.gov/Entrez/
		BankIt	https://www.ncbi.nlm.nih.gov/WebSub/
		Sequin	http://www.ncbi.nlm.nih.gov/Sequin/index.html
2.	Specialized tools	ORF Finder	https://www.ncbi.nlm.nih.gov/orffinder/
		E-PCR	www.ncbi.nlm.nih.gov/sutils/e-pcr
		Spidey	https://www.ncbi.nlm.nih.gov/sutils/splign/splign.cgi
3.	Data deposition tools	ADIT (Auto Dep Input Tool)	https://www.rcsb.org /
		Pdb_extract	https://pdb-extract.wwpdb.org/
		Ligand Depot	http://ligand-expo.rcsb.org/
		Validation Server	https://validate.wwpdb.org/
4.	Pairwise sequence alignment tool	ALIGN	https://www.uniprot.org/align/
		FASTA	https://www.ebi.ac.uk/Tools/sss/fasta/
		LAGAN	http://lagan.stanford.edu/
		LALIGN	https://www.ebi.ac.uk/Tools/psa/lalign/
		SCAN2	https://gt-scan.csiro.au/
		Par-wise FLAG	http://www.bioinformatics.itri.org.tw/prflag/prflag.php
5.	Multiple sequence alignment tool	MATCH-BOX	http://www.fundp.ac.be/sciences/biologie/bms/matchbox_submit.shtml
		Muscle	http://cbcsrv.watson.ibm.com/Tmsa.html
		T-Coffee	http://www.ch.embnet.org/software/TCoffee.html
6.	Alignment analysis tool	AMAS	http://barton.ebi.ac.uk/servers/amas_server.html
		ESPript	http://prodes.toulouse.inra.fr/ESPript/
		CINEMA	http://130.88.97.239/CINEMA/#:~:text=CINEMA%20is%20a%20Colour%20INteractive,the%20use%20of%20of%20%22pluglets%22

Table 3 List of databases and tools for data mining of sequences

S.no.	Tools/database	Link
1.	NCBI (National Center for Biotechnology Information)	https://www.ncbi.nlm.nih.gov/
2.	BLAST (basic local alignment search tool)	https://blast.ncbi.nlm.nih.gov/Blast.cgi
3.	Bioedit	https://bioedit.software.informer.com/
4.	*PROSITE*	https://prosite.expasy.org/
5.	CLUSTALW	https://www.genome.jp/tools-bin/clustalw
6.	GOAL (*Logical Gene Ontology Annotations*)	https://goal-gene-ontology-annotative-listing.soft112.com/
7.	Wolfpsort	https://www.genscript.com/wolf-psort.html
8.	TMHMM Server	http://www.cbs.dtu.dk/services/TMHMM/
9.	Jalview	http://www.jalview.org/getdown/release/
10.	HIPPIE v2.2	http://cbdm-01.zdv.uni-mainz.de/~mschaefer/hippie/
11.	Cytoscape	https://cytoscape.org/
12.	Geneious	https://www.geneious.com/download/
13.	RAxML (Randomized Axelerated Maximum Likelihood)	https://raxml-ng.vital-it.ch/
14.	Simplot	https://sray.med.som.jhmi.edu/SCRoftware/simplot/

bacteria are greatly used in dairy industries. These bacteria have shown great use in fermentation in beer, pickled foods, bread, etc. In the healthcare sector, many artificially engineered organisms are used to deliver drugs. In veterinary science many sequencing projects on farm animals are being conducted such as cows, pigs, goats, and sheep to know about the organism, production, and how can we improve the livestock and the nutrition provided by these animals. Comparative studies are done to compare the biochemical functions of the gene with the bioinformatics tools to experimentally compare the similarity between species.

2.2.3 Agriculture

The genetic improvements of the crops were seen in the twentieth century, and the comparative analysis was done of the plant genomes which showed that the genes have remained conserved over evolution. The complete genome of the plant is available such as *Oryza sativa* and *Arabidopsis thaliana*. Bioinformatics is used to study the genomic sequences and the phenotype which tells us a lot about the plant and how to improve the crop field. Insect resistance of some genes can help in controlling pests mainly into cotton, maize, and potato, and that organism is *Bacillus thuringiensis* which is an insecticidal bacterium. Foodborne diseases have come up and have resulted in causing illness due to microbial and chemical contaminations in the food. Bioinformatics has been used to shape this sector by bioengineering and medical sciences to understand the toxins and to modify the food.

3   Healthcare and Healthcare Informatics

Healthcare is one of the most well-known and yet a complicated industry where the common ritual of paying for the services by the customer is not observed, instead, a third party here as in insurance companies pay on behalf of the customer after negotiating the type of services and the amount with the service providers. Data trades can be tormented by horde designs, caught, and put away in an assortment of storehouses. These trades present further complexities as 'vocabularies' or as such the coding dialects that are needed to recognize sorts of administrations that change significantly from payer to payer, state to state, and administration type to support type [66]. Also, information originates from a huge number of various specialty frameworks and is introduced from multiple points of view and should be coordinated and introduced to a guardian or expert predictably and lucidly [28, 41]. The healthcare sectors are producing a lot of data, i.e. the patient history, reports, treatment planning, bills, and insurance.

Clinical informaticians use their knowledge into determining thought which they got together with their understanding of informatics, methodologies, and prosperity informatics contraptions to assess information and data needs of clinical administration specialists, patients, and their families [7]. It assists with depicting, evaluating, and refining clinical cycles likewise making, executing, and refining clinical decisions through genuinely steady organizations and leading or taking an enthusiasm inside the procurement, customization, and headway of clinical information systems [77].

The structures and terminating paces of engine unit activity possibilities (MUAPs) in an electromyographic signal are a key factor for diagnosing neuromuscular illnesses [58]. mSplicer is a help vector machine-based classifier intended to mimic the natural cycles which produce and develop mRNA from un-spliced premRNA. GeneMark-Genesis is a Markov AI model that predicts the protein-coding and non-coding locales in obscure bacterial genome groupings by distinguishing long ORFs and recovering their boundaries [6]. Cuckoo search is a meta-heuristic calculation proposed by Yang and Deb intended to arrange four paired class data sets, Breast Cancer, Diabetes, Bupa, and Hepatitis. It was improved by joining extraordinary learning calculation to upgrade the exactness and consistency of cuckoo search [1, 14, 17, 69, 78]. Outspread premise work (RBF) neural organization is a managed learning model dependent on the feedforward organization that was applied by Venkatesan et al. to analyse diabetes mellitus dependent on hazard factors, for example, weight file, age, plasma glucose fixation, cholesterol, and lipid levels. This model was successful in anticipating 97% of cases effectively [74].

4   Healthcare Informatics and Bioinformatics

Healthcare informatics as discussed above centres its goal towards collecting accurate data and information followed by thorough analysis. Bioinformatics is a discipline where different modern tools and techniques are used to study and process

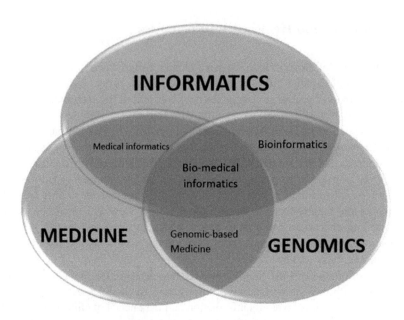

Fig. 2 Role of bioinformatics in healthcare

huge biological databases and lead research to grasp the working of genetics and proteomics by using the data from healthcare informatics. The main target is on preparing genomics and proteomics information for essential science research, yet additionally medication, drug revelation, and related regions [56]. Medical informatics or information analytics is capable of medical care improvement, a decrease in cost, and wellbeing of lives-based medicine, genomics, and bioinformatics (Fig. 2). Science and medication in this manner have advanced from the bench-based on computer-based science [23]. Huge improvement in shared exploration just as the improvement of cutting-edge and inventive apparatuses and advances to help the patient is accomplished by the reconciliation of data at the subatomic, cell, tissue, and individual level [37].

With the completion of the human genome and ongoing progressive appearance of high-throughput sequencing (HTS) and genome-wide connection examinations of single-nucleotide polymorphic living creatures, the fields of nuclear bioinformatics, bio-experiences, quantifiable inherited characteristics, and clinical informatics are joining into the rising field of translational bioinformatics [9].

Omics for drugs disclosure and repurposing is a major traumatic brain injury (TBI) subdomain – the repurposing of the medication is an engaging thought that permits the drug organizations to offer a previously endorsed medication to treat an alternate condition/infection that the medication was not at first affirmed for by the FDA [42]. The perception of subatomic marks in ailment and contrast those with marks saw in cells focuses on the chance of a medication capacity to fix and additionally assuage the side effects of a disease [5].

In the USA, few organizations offer direct-to-purchaser (DTC) hereditary customized genomic testing. The organization that plays out most of the testing is called 23andMe. Using hereditary testing in medical services raises numerous moral, lawful, and social concerns; one of the primary inquiries is whether the medical care suppliers are prepared to incorporate patient-provided genomic data while giving consideration that is unprejudiced and high calibre; hence the role of bioinformatics and healthcare system is emphasized [60].

5   Big Data Technologies

Big data is applied to characterize information with titanic volume or confusion which can't be taken care of by conventional information handling procedures. It is recognized that the highlights of large information are characterized by three significant properties that are normally known as the 3Vs: volume, assortment, and velocity. First and preeminent is the volume of information that is developing quickly in the biomedical informatics fields. The subsequent element is the assorted variety in information types and structures. The third particular component of enormous information is speed, which alludes to producing and taking care of the information [44]. Big data arrangement is a system, which involves huge parts including Hadoop (hadoop.apache.org), greatly equal handling, NoSQL information bases that are utilized for big data stockpiling, preparing, and examination [79].

Hadoop (hadoop.apache.org) a major information examination stage that is exceptionally powerful for preparing naturally relevant information sizes when considering figuring hours for both split and unsplit data sets [34]. Apache Hadoop has packages like Cloudburst, MapReduce, Eoulsan, Crossbow, Contrail, Myrna, DistMap, and Seal that can accomplish several NGS applications, such as quality checking, de novo assembly, adapter trimming, read mapping, quantification, variant analysis, expression analysis, and annotation [80]. The discussion is still on for the genuine definitions and impediments of enormous information in wellbeing and advantages of wellbeing related to large information [83].

5.1   Impact of Big Data in Bioinformatics

Big information science is a rising zone that has supplemented computational methods (Fig. 3) and the utilization of contemporary elite structures that incorporate CPU groups, mists, illustration handling units, and field-programmable entryway clusters. Next-Gen Sequencing examination needs figuring all pairwise read arrangements or all pairwise read-genome planning using virtual products like BLAST which are computationally infeasible either because of the enormous size of question information or the virtual products are not intended for that particular errand [32], this is were big data play significant role. Cloudburst is a parallel com-

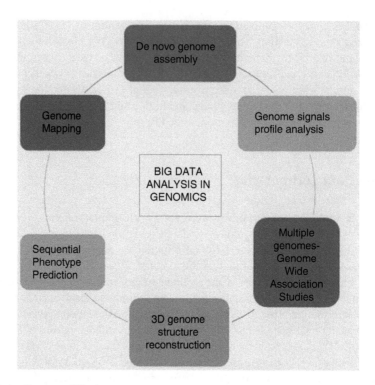

Fig. 3 Applications of big data

puting model that allows sequenced genomes to be mapped by utilizing short-read mapping that enhances the scalability of sequencing data [85].

Natural information bases assume a vital part in putting away enormous information. Organic databases, for example, the harmfulness factor information base http://www.mgc.ac.cn/VFs/ give extensive data about destructiveness variables of microbes that are therapeutically demonstrated to be pathogenic. Jagga et al. created three administered learning-based arrangement models with quick relationship determination highlight to make a qualification between various phases of clear cell renal cell carcinoma (ccRCC) because of their quality articulation in RNAseq tests, obtained from the Cancer Genome Atlas. The irregular wood model had the most noteworthy affectability (89%) and will assist oncologists with recognizing the sub-atomic apparatus behind infection progression (stage) and identify ccRCC prognostic components at a quicker movement [86]. A profound put-together system worked for Faster Region-Based Convolutional Neural Network endeavours to computerize the way towards distinguishing and measuring jungle fever and permits wellbeing specialists to consider tainted cells and characterize their stage [89].

Mobile health (m-health) is the term of checking the wellbeing utilizing cell phones and patient-observing gadgets, and large information investigations have been applied inside the m-wellbeing for giving a successful medical care framework

[23]. Different kinds of information, for example, electronic health records (EHRs), clinical pictures, and convoluted content which are expanded, ineffectively deciphered, and broadly chaotic, have been utilized in the cutting-edge clinical exploration [88]. The utilization of artificial intelligence and enormous information examination provides experiences to the clients and empowering them to design, utilizing the assets particularly for the difficulties in m-wellbeing [87]. The use of artificial intelligence for quickening drug repurposing or repositioning, for which computer-based intelligence approaches, is considered as well as is likewise vital.

The artificial intelligence models are applied in accuracy medication and, for instance, how computer-based intelligence models can quicken coronavirus drug repurposing. This gives a solid method of reasoning to utilizing computer-based intelligence-based assistive devices for drug repurposing prescriptions for human infection, including during the coronavirus pandemic [84]. Polypharmacy is a key test in medical services, particularly in more established and multimorbid patients. eHealth arrangements are progressively suggested in medical care, with huge information examination procedures as a significant part. There are existing big data analytics methods that can assist with recognizing patients devouring various medications and to aid the decrease of polypharmacy in patients [82].

The rampant increase in biological databases – genome sequences, protein sequence, image informatics, and electronic health records –requires an efficient storing, retrieving, exploring, and imaging of the data [64]. The data scientist is an emerging profession for people in expertise in managing big data. Various tools in the era of data science have appeared for the scalability and cloud-computing network for convenient data sharing [35]. The big data market accounts for the growth of about 20.6% in upcoming years with a business turnover of $40 billion in 2023. It is very promising to see how big data and tools will shape healthcare with broad applications in global health outlook [61]. Big data analysis plays an essential role in genome analysis (Fig. 3).

A blend of big data and bioinformatics is perfect and makes them stun benefits in fields of the genomic succession, protein arrangement, DNA registering, and so on. This creating innovation has likewise made the information section very simple for specialists [20, 54]. For personalized medicines, the long exploration information on genomes, proteomics, and metabolomics alongside the information from the clinical preliminaries makes it possible for specialists to mine the information and completely comprehend the structure of the ailment (Table 4). This information helps the analysts to create drugs having the quickest and most exact distinguishing proof and approval of targets [72].

In gene sequencing scientists have made a considerable amount of accomplishments in quality sequencing likewise assist with shielding babies from certain infections that have run down in a family for ages [46]. Moreover, in the healthcare area, there has been an enormous assortment of patients' information to track patients and screen the wellbeing of the patient. This gives quicker recognizable proof and treatment of sickness fundamentally lessening costs and giving better medical services of the patient simultaneously [45].

Table 4 Bioinformatics-based tools for big data

S. no.	Tools	Links
1	BART(bioinformatics array research tool)	http://igc1.salk.edu:3838/bart/
2	STRING-EMBL	https://string-db.org/
3	BioGRID	https://thebiogrid.org/
4	SparkSeq	http://spark.apache.org/streaming
5	ArrayExpress	https://www.ebi.ac.uk/arrayexpress/
6	Database of interacting proteins	https://dip.doe-mbi.ucla.edu/dip/Main.cgi
7	Stanford microarray database	http://smd.princeton.edu./
8	DNA data bank of Japan	https://www.ddbj.nig.ac.jp/index-e.html
9	Database for modern applications	https://www.mongodb.com/
10	RDP database	http://rdp.cme.msu.edu./
11	MiRNA database	http://www.mirbase.org./
12	CouchDB relax	https://couchdb.apache.org/
13	Apache Hadoop	http://hadoop.apache.org/
14	SeqMonk	https://www.bioinformatics.babraham.ac.uk/projects/seqmonk/
15	OrientDB	https://www.orientdb.org/
16	Illumina microarray	https://sapac.illumina.com/techniques/microarrays/array-data-analysis-experimental-design.html
17	Apache Giraph	http://giraph.apache.org/
18	Apache Hama	https://hama.apache.org/

6 Bioinformatics Resources for Metabolomics

Metabolomics is the advanced term for the field of little particle research in science and natural chemistry. At present, metabolomics is going through a change where the exemplary diagnostic science is joined with current cheminformatics and bioinformatics strategies, making ready for huge scope information analysis (Table 5). In the most recent 20 years, a great deal of progress has been made in the number of metabolites that can be distinguished, bringing down of the constraints of discovery with present-day investigative advancements, and the expanded throughput of tests that can be handled [43].

Today, mass spectrometry is a key innovation for metabolomics research. Because of gigantic innovative advances in mass spectrometry throughout the most recent years, the sum and intricacy of the information created have been developing rapidly. Accordingly, MetFrag was additionally upgraded to give a methodological interface to inquiry various information bases and join the data brought into the distinguishing proof cycle [21, 22]. Dale et al. established a tool called PathoLogic, for automated construction of a Pathway/Genome Database (PGDB) that describes metabolic pathways of an organism [73]. PathoLogic, a machine learning model, is built on the hypothesis that experimentally proved that metabolic pathways are

Table 5 List of tools/databases for metabolomics

S. no.	Metabolomics approaches	Tools/database	Links
1.	Metabolite	Human Metabolome Database	http://www.hmdb.ca/
		KEGG LIGAND Database	http://www.genome.jp/ligand/
		KNApSACK	http://kanaya.naist.jp/KNApSAcK_Family/
		MassBank	http://www.massbank.jp/index.html?lang=en
		MetaCyc	http://metacyc.org/
		Lipid Maps	http://www.lipidmaps.org/
		Metlin	https://metlin.scripps.edu/index.php
2.	Regulatory and signalling network	BioGrid	http://thebiogrid.org/
		DAVID	https://david.ncifcrf.gov/
		KEGG Pathway	http://www.kegg.jp/kegg/pathway.html
		Path Guide	http://www.pathguide.org/
		Pathway Commons	http://www.pathwaycommons.org/
		PhosphoSitePlus	http://www.phosphosite.org/homeAction.action

conserved among organisms and utilizes MetaCyc [29], a reference pathway database like a stencil to predict the metabolism cycles in freshly sequenced organisms [57].

7   Bioinformatics Resources Towards Personalized Medicine

In the recent decade, science has made numerous advances to profit medication, including the Human Genome Venture. Single-nucleotide polymorphisms (SNPs) are presently perceived as the fundamental driver of human hereditary diseases and are now an important asset for planning complex genetic attributes. A large number of DNA variations have been distinguished that are related to maladies and qualities. By joining these various gene relationships with phenotypes and medication reactions, personalized medication will tailor medicines to the patients' particular genotype. Bioinformatics is gainful in customized medication. Two techniques stick out, the randomized calculation and computer-aided drug design (CADD).

Bioinformatics pipelines had been made to handle information from HTS with CADD strategies, particularly to survey common compound of products (Fig. 4). Another guide of bioinformatics in drug revelation is distinguishing proof of potential medication targets given genomics, epigenetics, proteomics, furthermore, and transcriptomics contemplates [11]. A portion of these transformations can cause

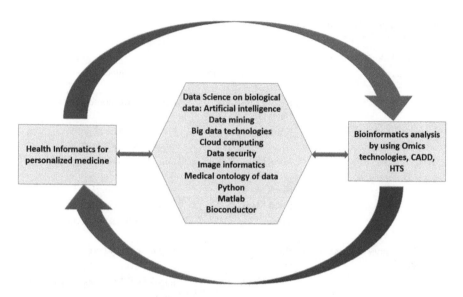

Data Science on biological
data: Artificial intelligence
Data mining
Big data technologies
Cloud computing
Data security
Image informatics
Medical ontology of data
Python
Matlab
Bioconductor

Health Informatics for
personalized medicine

Bioinformatics analysis
by using Omics
technologies, CADD,
HTS

Fig. 4 Bioinformatics in personalized medicine

infection and might be utilized as medication targets, while others are related to the qualities that actuated related to the infection. Bioinformatics devices, for example, position weight grid can be utilized to check genome examples to decide whether its change has a significant effect on quality function. The appearance of bioinformatics has reformed organic exploration and permitted specialists to reduce down expenses and time spent on their studies. Advances in bioinformatics subfields, genomics, and epigenetics extraordinarily help drug disclosure and different other clinical fields [76]. While a portion of the innovations, for example, probabilistic master thinking, norms advancement, and jargon improvement, are evolved in medical informatics or health informatics which are based on bioinformatics data set that can be utilized by clinical informaticists. Genomic medication is required to utilize such innovations progressively to improve and upgrade medical services, including customized treatments, preventive medication, and subatomic medication [27].

There are several challenges faced while making personalized medicine, and these challenges have been addressed by many scientific societies. One of the major issues in this area is approving of hereditary relationships and recognizing its significance. The clinical approval of participants and their genetic markers are developing at a very slow rate and the working of these specific genes may or may not have similar functionality for all individuals. Also, the process of collection of data before analysis such as collecting and storing the bio-specimens plays as a crucial factor and can alter the results. The collection of this data also raises different legal, privacy, and ethical concerns. The next challenge faced is importing to the correct educating and learnings to the patients and medical care suppliers. Though there are a few challenges, personalized medicine has been successful in showing its bright future perspective with the help of big data technologies if used efficiently [31].

7.1 Hardware and Software

Recent studies are done with the making of personalized medicines by the effective use of high-throughput studies that include next-generation sequencing, imaging assays, MS, and scans [54, 55]. Nowadays many diseases are based on data-intensive applications by managing the biological and clinical data as per the requirement of the patient [34]. Nowadays, high-performance resources such as multicore computing [75], GPU computing, cloud computing, and high-performance computing, are utilized for obtaining a full capability in personalized medicines. Mass spectrometry (MS)-based assays are used in studies under proteomics and metabolomics research to produce the raw data by NGS assays. To get the peptide sequence in MS is a major challenge that can be accomplished by similar spectra against known sequences in a large database [83]. Hydra is a Hadoop application that is capable to perform such scalable peptide database search.

Along with the developed devices for experimentation helping with high-throughput experimental data, the development of software is necessary. For biomedical researches, Bioconductor or R packages, Python, and MATLAB are also used that are the tools for the analysis and comprehension of low- and high-throughput genomic data. Many xenograft models with KRAS mutations have also been formed by this technology.

Many approaches were taken to condense the biological knowledge that resulted in the generation of Pathway databases which includes the biological knowledge within the biomolecular reactions and interactions in the data collection. Some of such databases are systems biology markup language [68], BioNetGen language [50], BioModels database, and COPASI.

7.2 Natural Language Processing

The natural language processing (NLP) requires simple text that will help to extract the data showing the various relationships between elements such as DNA-DNA interactions, protein-protein interactions, drug interactions, and many more. These data are used to construct a database, a network, an online service, and a predictive model of study. NLP algorithm helps to generate available databases for the formation of predictive models based on the patient-specific information.

7.3 Imaging Informatics

Imaging informatics or medical imaging informatics (MII) is a subdiscipline of biomedical research comprising of radiology, magnetic resonance imaging (MRI), CT scans, computational algorithms, and deep learning using artificial intelligence [24]. Imaging informatics concerns to extract clinically relevant information for the diagnosis, prognosis, therapy planning, and precision medicine. Healthcare big data processed using statistical tools and algorithms by specialists allows to source of electronic healthcare records (EHRs) for easy access to clinicians and patients [12].

Radiomic is categorized into two features traditional or handcrafted radiomics and deep learning radiomics [24]. Traditional or handcrafted radiomics has been used extensively for image biomarkers for detection of cancer prognosis and uses manual image splitting of the area of interest (e.g. lung tumour localization), feature extraction, and quantification describing tumour characteristics and involves machine learning to give clinical outcome. Although machine learning processes low data sets as compared to AI coupled radiomics [3].

Cloud computing in image informatics allows increasing data of medical records and images to be stored under it for easy access to clinicians. The efforts were put to use computational tools for the organization and data sharing for convenient access [66]. PACS (picture archiving and communication systems) is a cloud-computing technology that allows sharing, retrieving, and storage of medical images in a universal format known as DICOM (Digital Imaging and Communications in Medicine) [30].

Tools for image informatics facilitate image characterization, resolution, storing clinical data from patients, and clinical trials that provide robustness in the biomedical research network (Table 6). Various web interface tools, software packages, open-source libraries, and collective shared image data are available to reproduce multidimensional images, quantitative imaging, digital mammography image data set, and tumour biomarker validation [38]. Good classification results were obtained on images of multiple cells that mark a convenient future for the classification of subcellular patterns obtained by tissue imaging [90].

Image informatics and AI have contributed to medical science tremendously, from multidimensional imaging of colorectal cancer, analysing DNA damage biomarkers for forensics and cancer research [38], digital breast cancer mammography [51], studying cell proliferation in cancer prognosis, solid tumour prognosis using radiomics, and treatment selection [62].

Table 6 Tools of image bioinformatics

S. no.	Tool	Description
1.	ImageJ	This is a Java-based programme used for generating high-quality processed images
2.	CytoPaq	This is a web interface, a publicly available online service to produce multidimensional cell images that provide different configurations including optical and time-lapse [16, 19]
3.	CellProfiler	It is an open-source interface used to measure phenotypes quantitatively
4.	Foci Counter	A user-friendly, stand-alone, simple programme for the qualitative and quantitative analysis, useful for foci determination which depends on the brightness between the background and foci

7.4   Computer-Aided Drug Design

Designing and discovery of drugs are arduous processes requiring the identification of potential drugs, target receptors, preclinical trials, clinical trials, and approval for clinical purposes. CADD also is known as in silico analysis directs drug discovery into easy homology modelling, molecular docking, development of pharmacophore, and structure−/ligand-based drug designing [71]. There are various steps to be followed for lead optimization in the drug discovery process (Fig. 5).

CADD integrates biologists, a medicinal chemist, and computational scientist for screening and discovery of novel drugs. Few benefits associated with computer-aided drug discovery include an economically feasible process reducing traditional research and accelerate the drug discovery process [77]. Numerous tools and databases are used from target identification to complex (receptor-ligand) validation (Table 7) [33].

CADD has real-time applications with successful drugs available. Drug classification ranges from bacterial, parasitic, and viral infections. It is emerging as next-generation immune-oncology therapies, for structural interpretation and development of small molecules as immune modulators [26]. Screening of anti-TB drug for *Mycobacterium tuberculosis* infection was performed to design chalcone derivatives against multiple drug-resistant MTB infection. Five 5-nitro-substituted heteroaryl chalcones were identified to be more potent than standard drug isoniazid in inhibiting MTB infection [8]. For reoccurring influenza epidemics, anti-influenza drug screening resulted in nine neuraminidase inhibitors exhibiting potency at low concentrations. HIV infections and CADD-mediated virtual screening identified two chemotypes useful in inhibiting HIV infection [8]. Several tumour

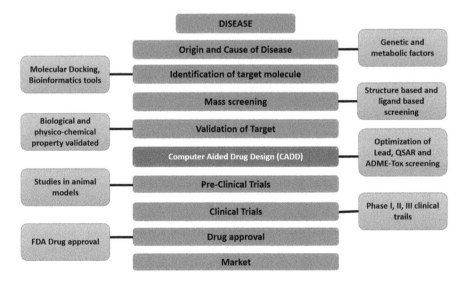

Fig. 5 Steps of CADD

Table 7 CADD tools and database

S. no.	Tools	Description
1	PubMed	Free search engine for biomedicine and life sciences
2	PubChem	Free database for chemistry molecules and their activity
3	PDB	Protein Data Bank for proteins and nucleic acids
4	BLAST	The basic local alignment search tool, used for similarity search
5	ChemSketch	Molecular modelling programme to create chemical structures
6	Modeller	Used for 3D homology modelling and comparative studies
7	AutoDock	Protein-ligand docking modelling software
8	ZINCPharmer	Virtual pharmacophore screening software
9	SwissADME	Free tool for pharmacokinetic evaluation of drug
10	Swissmodel	The basic local alignment search tool, used for similarity search
11	Protein Data Bank	Protein Data Bank archive information about the 3D shapes of proteins, nucleic acids
12	UCSF -Chimera	for the interactive visualization and analysis of molecular structures
13	SwissADME	ADME parameters, pharmacokinetic properties, drug-like nature
14	Glide (v.8.2)	Use of combinatorial chemistry and high-throughput screening (HTS)
15	pkCSM	A novel approach to the prediction of pharmacokinetic properties
16	MolSoft	High-quality molecular graphics and 3D molecules
17	SwissDock	Free protein-ligand docking web service
18	PyRx	Open-source software for computer-aided drug design
19	ZINC	A curated collection of commercially available chemical compounds
20	Gaussian	Computer-aided drug design *software*, databases, and web services
21	Accura-CADD	The draw is an accurate computer-aided design and drafting software that allows Portable Document Format's (PDF) modification
22	Chimera	Interactive visualization and analysis of molecular structures and related data
23	PyMOL	The open-source molecular visualization system
24	ModWeb	Predicted protein complexes; modelling leverage calculations
25	VMD	Molecular modelling and visualization computer programme
26	Biodesigner	BI tools for data analysis and visualization
27	XtalView	For solving a macromolecular crystal structure by isomorphous replacement

microenvironment regulators have been identified and studied for their inhibition and effector mechanism in retracting tumours and the development of cancer immunotherapies [26]. With the availability of big data in chemical biology, high-throughput screening allows us to generate virtual drugs and test for their potency and predicted using prediction of activity spectra for substances (PASS) to develop novel drugs. (http://www.way2drug.com/Projects.php) [59].

The recent pandemic COVID-19 and high mortality across the globe serve major concern for public health and the deteriorating economy due to lockdowns and travel bans. The spread of the virus concerned medical fields for the development of diagnostic kits, drugs, and vaccines. CADD has contributed fairly in the structural modelling of SARS-Cov-2 using MODELLER [47]. The ligand-based drug design software was used to determine antigenic sequences, which was further extended to drug repurposing screening for existing drugs such as hydroxychloroquine and remdesivir as an anti-viral therapy [70]. The global market of CADD rose during COVID-19, with constant growth of 16.9%. Research analysts anticipate the reach of computer-aided drug designing, in post-COVID to approximately USD 2143 billion (https://www.researchdive.com/covid-19-insights/208/global-computer-aided-drug-discovery-market).

8 Commercial Platforms for Healthcare

Innovation in healthcare using bioinformatics tools and artificial intelligence has revolutionized medical management and diverged towards more patient-centric medication [13]. The past medicine ideology of one size fits all has been curated to fit customized medicine and medical assistance. With an emphasis on healthcare, numerous commercial healthcare platforms are emerging, e.g. digital healthcare platforms in diagnosis, telemedicine, oncology screenings, and genome sequencing.

Some pioneers in the commercial healthcare platforms (Table 8) are IBM corporation which has its roots in cancer research, AI-oriented partnered with Pfizer (leading biopharmaceutical company) to provide cost-effective treatment, and targeting global health (https://www.ibm.com/in-en/industries/healthcare) [65]. IBM Watson health oncology solutions combine data centralized to the patient and allow clinicians to provide speedy treatment within their expertise. Google provides cloud storage as a one-stop for patient data, management, image informatics and builds a digital health platform. Partnered with Accenture, Google is now patient-centric with growing research and development as patient service and development of drugs (https://cloud.google.com/solutions/healthcare-life-sciences).

9 Challenges and Future of Bioinformatics in Healthcare

Bioinformatics is transforming healthcare today, envisioned to contribute to society through personalized medicine, imaging informatics, and drug designing. High-throughput data from patients and technological upgrades increases chances of coherent therapeutic approaches [34]. Progressive application of big data in precision medicine and healthcare is constantly bridging opportunities for upcoming tools and commercial platforms. It can be visualized as a new healthcare ground for patient care and clinical flexibility of patients instead of their treatment [67]. Challenges associated with big data constitute the security of patient records, technical barriers in image processing, and data sharing. These challenges can be overcome to elevate the downsides of data sharing [65].

Table 8 Commercial healthcare platforms

S. no.	Commercial platforms	Tools and description
1	Cloud computing	Google Cloud in healthcare and life sciences
2	Cancer care	IBM Watson for Oncology
3	Telemedicine	Practo – online consultation tool
4	Genomics	MedGenome – liquid biopsy screening in cancer
5	Diagnostic	Portea – remote diagnosis
6	Medical devices	SensArs – neuroprosthetics
7	Patient care	Piedmont Healthcare
8	Technology	Accenture Life Sciences
9	Biopharma	Vyome Therapeutics
10	Healthcare data	Innovaccer
11	Musculoskeletal care	Hinge Health
12	Psychological counselling	Village MD
13	Microbiome	Seres Therapeutics
14	Medical device	Siemens Healthineers
15	Genome profiling	Foundation Medicine

Despite the augmentation of the role of bioinformatics in healthcare, certain factor remains unstinted. Omics in medicine requires combinatorial education to understand basic biology, translational biology, and computational knowledge to standardize the data [4]. Future perspective of bedside medicine does require experimental data alongside omics tools. Various omics data such as transcriptomics and proteomics do not have overlapping function due to post-translational modification in eukaryotes; hence making sense out of data in an integrated way is one set back, developing networks to study protein-DNA reciprocity [4]. Challenges in image informatics, i.e. radiomics for personalized medicine include the reliability of imaging data for disease detection, data sharing among communities, and coherent amalgamation of bioinformatics and medical informatics.

Big data advancements are progressively employed for biomedical and medical care research. Heaps of natural and clinical information has been produced and gathered at an extraordinary momentum and scale. For example, the new age of sequencing advances legitimizes the preparation of billions of DNA succession data every day, and making use of electronic wellbeing records (EHRs) is archiving a lot of patient information [48]. The digitization of health records encourages and unlocks additional opportunities for science and exploration, and they ought to be presently gathered and made do because of this point [35]. The expense of procuring and dissecting biomedical information is relied upon to diminish drastically with the assistance of innovation updates [49]. Huge information applications in the present scenario bring chances to find a new information and make novel techniques to enhance the nature of medical care [25]. The key difficulties in utilizing big data lie, indeed, in discovering methods of managing heterogeneity, assorted variety, and unpredictability of the data, while its magnitude and speed obstruct arrangements are accessible for littler data sets, for example, physical curation or information warehousing. The improvement of metadata for organic database on semantic web norms can be viewed as a promising methodology for a semantic-based joining of natural data [34].

Therefore, there is still a struggle between socio-economic status, which does question if personalized healthcare will be for everyone [2]. The bioinformatics approach leaps in healthcare, a decade ago, and presently can be fully utilized in accelerating the healthcare system. Hence, in pandemic COVID-19, omics techniques contributed significantly to the detection of the viral genome and possible mutations using phylogenetic analysis. Global health crises with an increase in death rate and susceptible populations bioinformatics have demonstrated its competence in healthcare [36]. The artificial intelligence such as the revolution of digital and deep learning in precision medicine will expand enormously in near future with big data technologies.

References

1. A, T. (2010). Best Practices for QSAR Model Development, Validation, and Exploitation. *Molecular Informatic*, 476–488. https://doi.org/10.1002/minf.201000061
2. Abraham, I. (2018). Socio-economics of Personalized Medicine in Asia. East Asian Science. In I. Abraham, *Socio-economics of Personalized Medicine in Asia. East Asian Science* (pp. 551–554). taiwan: East Asian Science, Technology and Society. https://doi.org/10.1215/18752160-4207524
3. Ahmed Hosny, H. J. (2019). Handcrafted versus deep learning radiomics for prediction of cancer therapy response. *The lancet-Digital health, 1*, 106–107. Retrieved from https://www.thelancet.com/pdfs/journals/landig/PIIS2589-7500(19)30062-7.pdf
4. Akram Alyass, M. T. (2015). From big data analysis to personalized medicine for all: challenges and opportunities. *BMC medical genomics*, 1–12. https://doi.org/10.1186/s12920-015-0108-y
5. Atul J Butte, R. C. (2006). Finding Disease-Related Genomic Experiments Within an International Repository: First Steps in Translational Bioinformatics. *AMIA Annual Symposium Proceedings*, 106–110. Retrieved from https://www.ncbi.nlm.nih.gov/pmc/articles/PMC1839582/
6. Aurélien Grosdidier, V. (2011). SwissDock, a protein-small molecule docking web service based on EADock DSS. *Nucleic Acids Res*, W270–W277. https://doi.org/10.1093/nar/gkr366
7. Aziz, H. (2016). A review of the role of public health informatics in healthcare. *Journal of Taibah University Medical Sciences*, 1–5. https://doi.org/10.1016/j.jtumed.2016.08.011
8. Bruno J. Neves, R.-F. (2018). QSAR-Based Virtual Screening: Advances and Applications in Drug Discovery. *Frontiers in pharmacology*, 1–7. https://doi.org/10.3389/fphar.2018.01275
9. Cantor, M. N. (2011). Translational informatics: an industry perspective. *Journal of American Medical Informatics Association*, 1–3. https://doi.org/10.1136/amiajnl-2011-000588
10. Cascella M, R. M. (2020). *Features, Evaluation and Treatment Coronavirus (COVID-19)*. Florida: StatPearls Publishing. Retrieved from https://europepmc.org/article/NBK/NBK554776
11. Casey Lynnette Overby, a.-H. (2013). Personalized medicine: challenges and opportunities for translational bioinformatics. *Future Medicine*, 453–462. https://doi.org/10.2217/pme.13.30
12. Catalyst, N. (2018). Healthcare Big Data and the Promise of Value-Based Care. *NEJM*, 00–00. Retrieved from https://catalyst.nejm.org/doi/full/10.1056/CAT.18.0290
13. Christopher J Kelly, A. J. (2017). Promoting innovation in healthcare. *Future Healthcare Journal*, 121–125. https://doi.org/10.7861/futurehosp.4-2-121

14. Corwin Hansch, S. D. (1977). Substituent constants for correlation analysis. *J.Med Chem*, 304–306. https://doi.org/10.1021/jm00212a024
15. Cosimo Tuena, M. S.-Á. (2020). Predictive Precision Medicine: Towards the Computational Challenge. In M. S.-Á. Cosimo Tuena, *P5 eHealth: An Agenda for the Health Technologies* (pp. 71–86). Switzerland: Springer Open. Retrieved from https://doi.org/10.1007/978-3-030-27994-3
16. CytoPacq: a web-interface for simulating multi-dimensional cell imaging. (2019). *Oxford University Press. Bioimage informatics*, 1–3. https://doi.org/10.1093/bioinformatics/btz417
17. Dallakyan, S. &. (2015). Small-molecule library screening by docking with PyRx. *Methods Mol Biol*, 243–250. https://doi.org/10.1007/978-1-4939-2269-7_19
18. David Edwards, J. S. (2009). *Bioinformatics tools and applications*. New York: Springer, New York, NY. https://doi.org/10.1007/978-0-387-92738-1
19. David Wiesner, D. S. (2019). CytoPacq: a web-interface for simulating multi-dimensional cell imaging. In D. S. David Wiesner, *Bioinformatics* (pp. 4531–4533). UK: Oxford University Press. https://doi.org/10.1093/bioinformatics/btz417
20. Divya Kumari, ravi kumar. 2014. "Impact of Biological Big Data in Bioinformatics." *International Journal of Computer Applications* 22–24. https://citeseerx.ist.psu.edu/viewdoc/download?doi=10.1.1.800.2587&rep=rep1&type=pdf.
21. Enis Afgan, D. (2016). The Galaxy platform for accessible, reproducible and collaborative biomedical analyses: 2016 update. *Nucleic acids research*, 3–10. https://doi.org/10.1093/nar/gkw343
22. EscheriaFrancesco, F. R.-A.-B. (2015). Future water quality monitoring — Adapting tools to deal with mixtures of pollutants in water resource management. *Science of The Total Environment*, 540–551. https://doi.org/10.1016/j.scitotenv.2014.12.057
23. FMartin-Sancheza, I. G.-F. (2004). Synergy between medical informatics and bioinformatics: facilitating genomic medicine for future health care. *Journal of Biomedical informatics*, 30–42. https://doi.org/10.1016/j.jbi.2003.09.003
24. Gatta, R. D. (2020). Integrating radiomics into holomics for personalised oncology: from algorithms to bedside. *European Radiology Experimental*, 1–11. https://doi.org/10.1186/s41747-019-0143-0
25. Grifantini, R. L. (2018). Big Data: Challenge and Opportunity for Translational and Industrial Research in Healthcare. *frontiers in Digital Humanities*, 1–13. https://doi.org/10.3389/fdigh.2018.00013
26. Guedes, R. C.-F. (2018). Computer-aided drug design in new druggable targets for the next generation of immune-oncology therapies. *Wiley Online Library*, 1–27. https://doi.org/10.1002/wcms.1397
27. Guy Haskin Fernald, E. C. (2011). Bioinformatics challenges for personalized medicine. *Oxford Journals*, 1741–1748. https://doi.org/10.1093/bioinformatics/btr295
28. Hamed Nadri, B. R. (2017). The Top 100 Articles in the Medical Informatics: a Bibliometric Analysis. *journal of Medical Systems*, 1–12. https://doi.org/10.1007/s10916-017-0794-4
29. Helen M. Berman, J. W. (2000). The Protein Data Bank. *Nucleic acids research*, 235–242. Retrieved from https://doi.org/10.1093/nar/28.1.235
30. Huang, H. K. (2010). *PACS and imaging informatics: Basic principles and Applications*. Hong kong: Wiley, 2010. Retrieved from https://books.google.co.in/books/about/PACS_and_Imaging_Informatics.html?id=Pjjkyae_55oC&source=kp_book_description&redir_esc=y
31. Hudis, C. A. (2007). Trastuzumab — Mechanism of Action and Use in Clinical Practice. *N Engl J Med*, 39–51. https://doi.org/10.1056/NEJMra043186
32. Ibrahim IM, A. D. (2020). COVID-19 spike-host cell receptor GRP78 binding site prediction. *J Infect.*, 554–562. https://doi.org/10.1016/j.jinf.2020.02.026
33. Israel Ehizuelen Ebhohimen, L. E. (2020). In L. E. Israel Ehizuelen Ebhohimen, *Phytochemicals as Lead Compounds for New Drug Discovery* (pp. 25–37). Uganda: Elsevier. Retrieved from https://doi.org/10.1016/B978-0-12-817890-4.00003-2

34. Ivan Merelli, H.-S. (2014). Managing, Analysing, and Integrating Big Data in Medical Bioinformatics: Open Problems and Future Perspectives. *BioMed Research International*, 1–13. Retrieved from https://doi.org/10.1155/2014/134023

35. Jake Luo, M. W. (2016). Big Data Application in Biomedical Research and Health Care: A Literature Review. *Biomedical Informatics Insights*, 1–11. Retrieved from https://doi.org/10.4137/BII.S31559

36. Jason Kim, J. Z. (2020). Advanced bioinformatics rapidly identifies existing therapeutics for patients with coronavirus disease-2019 (COVID-19). *Journal of Translational Medicine*, 1–9. https://doi.org/10.1186/s12967-020-02430-9

37. Jelili Oyelade, J. S. (2015). Bioinformatics, Healthcare Informatics and Analytics: An Imperative for Improved Healthcare System. *International Journal of Applied Information Systems, 8*, 1–16. https://doi.org/10.5120/ijais15-451318

38. Jens Schneider, R. W. (2019). Open source bioimage informatics tools for the analysis of DNA damage and associated biomarkers. *Journal of Laboratory and Precision Medicine.*, 1–28. https://doi.org/10.21037/jlpm.2019.04.05

39. Kai Y Wong, A. G. (2014). QSAR analysis on tacrine-related acetylcholinesterase inhibitors. *Journal of Biomedical Science*, 21, 84. https://doi.org/10.1186/s12929-014-0084-0

40. Kalakota, T. D. (2019). The potential for artificial intelligence in healthcare. *Future Healthcare Journal*, 94–98. https://doi.org/10.7861/futurehosp.6-2-94

41. Kudyba, S. P. (2018). *Healthcare Informatics: Improving Efficiency through Technology, Analytics, and Management.* Florida: CRC Press. Retrieved from https://books.google.co.in/books/about/Healthcare_Informatics.html?id=gu4bDAAAQBAJ&redir_esc=y

42. Kuznetsov, V. L.-S. (2013). How bioinformatics influences health informatics: usage of biomolecular sequences, expression profiles and automated microscopic image analyses for clinical needs and public health. *Health Inf Sci Syst*, 1–18. Retrieved from https://doi.org/10.1186/2047-2501-1-2

43. RenéMeiera, C. (2017). Bioinformatics can boost metabolomics research. *Journal of Biotechnology*, 137–141. https://doi.org/10.1016/j.jbiotec.2017.05.018

44. Lu Chen, J. K.-C. (2012). From laptop to benchtop to bedside: Structure-based Drug Design on Protein Targets. *Curr Pharm Des*, 1217–1239. Retrieved from https://www.ncbi.nlm.nih.gov/pmc/articles/PMC3820560/

45. Mann, R. A. (2003). Mass spectrometry-based proteomics. *Nature*, 198–207. https://doi.org/10.1038/nature01511

46. Mariamena Arbitrio, M. T. (2016). Identification of polymorphic variants associated with erlotinib-related skin toxicity in advanced non-small cell lung cancer patients by DMET microarray analysis. *Cancer Chemotherapy Pharmacology*, 205–209. https://doi.org/10.1007/s00280-015-2916-3

47. Mayya Sedova, L. J. (2020). Coronavirus3D: 3D structural visualization of COVID-19 genomic divergence. *Structural bioinformatics*, 1–3. https://doi.org/10.1093/bioinformatics/btaa550

48. Metzker, M. L. (2010). Sequencing technologies — the next generation. *Nature Reviews Genetics*, 31–46. https://doi.org/10.1038/nrg2626

49. Michael R Stratton, P. J. (2009). The cancer genome. *Nature*, 719–724. https://doi.org/10.1038/nature07943

50. Michael W Sneddon, J. R. (2011). Efficient modeling, simulation and coarse-graining of biological complexity with NFsim. *Nature Methods*, 77–83. https://doi.org/10.1038/nmeth.1546

51. Morteza Heidari, S. M. (2020). Development and Assessment of a New Global Mammographic Image Feature Analysis Scheme to Predict Likelihood of Malignant Cases. *IEEE Transactions on Medical Imaging*, 1235–1244. https://doi.org/10.1109/TMI.2019.2946490

52. N M Luscombe, D. G. (2001). What is bioinformatics? A proposed definition and overview of the field. *Methods Inf Med.*, 40(4):346–58. Retrieved from https://pubmed.ncbi.nlm.nih.gov/11552348/

53. Nan Zhang& Shifei Ding &. (2018). Multimodal correlation deep belief networks for multi-view classification. *Applied Intelligence- Springer nature*, 1–12. https://doi.org/10.1007/s10489-018-1379-8

54. Nazipova, N. N. (2018). Big Data in Bioinformatics. *Mathematical Biology and Bioinformatics*, 1–17. https://doi.org/10.17537/2018.13.t1

55. Pankaj Agarwal. (2015). Next Generation Distributed Computing for Cancer Research. *Cancer Informatics*, 1–13. https://doi.org/10.4137/CIN.S16344

56. Perry L. Miller. (2000). Opportunities at the Intersection of Bioinformatics and Health Informatics: A Case Study. *Journal of the American Medical Informatics Association*, 431–438. Retrieved from https://doi.org/10.1136/jamia.2000.0070431

57. Pettersen EF, G. T. (2004). UCSF Chimera--a visualization system for exploratory research and analysis. *J Comput Chem*, 1605–1612. https://doi.org/10.1002/jcc.20084

58. Pires DE, B. T. (2015). pkCSM: Predicting Small-Molecule Pharmacokinetic and Toxicity Properties Using Graph-Based Signatures. *J Med Chem*, 4066–4072. https://doi.org/10.1021/acs.jmedchem.5b00104

59. Poroikov, V. V. (2020). Computer-Aided Drug Design: from Discovery of Novel Pharmaceutical Agents to Systems Pharmacology. *Biochemistry (Moscow), Supplement Series B: Biomedical Chemistry,SpringerLink*, 216–227. https://doi.org/10.1134/S1990750820030117

60. Prerna Sethi, K. T. (2009). Translational Bioinformatics and Healthcare Informatics: Computational and Ethical Challenges. *Perspectives Health Information Management*, 16;6(Fall):1h. Retrieved from https://pubmed.ncbi.nlm.nih.gov/20169020/

61. Richard A. Friesner, J. L. (2004). Glide: A New Approach for Rapid, Accurate Docking and Scoring. 1. Method and Assessment of Docking Accuracy. *ACS Publications*, 1739–1749. https://doi.org/10.1021/jm0306430

62. Roberto Gatta, A. D. (2020). Integrating radiomics into holomics for personalised oncology: from algorithms to bedside. *European Radiology Experimental*, 1–9. https://doi.org/10.1186/s41747-019-0143-0

63. Runxin Guo, Y. (2018). Bioinformatics applications on Apache Spark. *Giga Science*, 1–10. https://doi.org/10.1093/gigascience/giy098

64. Russ B Altman, J. M. (2003). Defining bioinformatics and structural bioinformatics. *Methods Biochem Analysis*, 44:3–14. Retrieved from https://pubmed.ncbi.nlm.nih.gov/12647379/

65. Sabyasachi Dash, S. K. (2019). Big data in healthcare: management, analysis and future prospects. *Journal of Big data*, 1–25. Retrieved from https://doi.org/10.1186/s40537-019-0217-0

66. Sahoo, S. K. (2019). Secure Big Data Computing in Cloud: An Overview. *Encyclopedia of Big Data Technologies*, 25–32. https://doi.org/10.1007/978-3-319-77525-8_233

67. Samiddha Mukherjee, R. S. (2016). Big Data – Concepts, Applications, Challenges and Future Scope. *International Journal of Advanced Research in Computer and Communication Engineering*, 66–74. https://doi.org/10.17148/IJARCCE.2016.5215

68. Sarah M Keating, N. L. (2013). Supporting SBML as a model exchange format in software applications. In S. M. Novère, *Methods in Molecular Biology* (pp. 201–225). Totowa: Humana Press, Totowa, NJ. https://doi.org/10.1007/978-1-62703-450-0_11

69. Schork, N. J. (2019). *Artificial Intelligence and Personalized Medicine*. USA: Springer, Cham. https://doi.org/10.1007/978-3-030-16391-4_11

70. Shruti Mishra, P. (2020). Bioinformatics Approach for COVID-19 (Coronavirus) Disease Prevention Treatment and Drug Validation. *EJMO*, 234–238. https://doi.org/10.14744/ejmo.2020.97358

71. Singh, N. B. (2018). Role of computer aided drug design in drug development and drug discovery. *International journal of pharmaceutical sciences and research*, 1405–1415. https://doi.org/10.13040/IJPSR.0975-8232.9(4).1405-15

72. Steve Olson, S. H. (2012). *Integrating Large-Scale Genomic Information into Clinical Practice*. washington: National Academies Press (US). Retrieved from https://www.ncbi.nlm.nih.gov/books/NBK91500/

73. Torsten Schwede, J. K. (2003). SWISS-MODEL: an automated protein homology-modeling server. *Nucleic Acids research*, 3381–3385. Retrieved from https://doi.org/10.1093/nar/gkg520

74. Truong, H.-L. S. (2010). Cloud computing for small research groups in computational science and engineering: Current status and outlook. *Researchgate*, 76–91. https://doi.org/10.1007/s00607-010-0120-1

75. Vajda, A. (2011). *Programming Many-Core Chips*. US: Springer US. https://doi.org/10.1007/978-1-4419-9739-5

76. Valeska, M. D. (2019). The Role of Bioinformatics in Personalized Medicine: Your Future Medical Treatment. *OPINI*, 1-5. Retrieved from https://www.researchgate.net/publication/337623077_The_Role_of_Bioinformatics_in_Personalized_Medicine_Your_Future_Medical_Treatment

77. VartikaTomar, M. K. (2018). Small Molecule Drug Design. In M. K. VartikaTomar, *Encyclopedia of Bioinformatics and Computational Biology* (pp. 741–760). New Delhi: Elsevier Inc. https://doi.org/10.1016/B978-0-12-809633-8.20157-X

78. Vojtech Huser, D. S.-B. (2018). Data sharing platforms for de-identified data from human clinical trials. *Society for clinical trials*, 1–11. https://doi.org/10.1177/1740774518769655

79. Vreven T, B. K. (2006). Combining Quantum Mechanics Methods with Molecular Mechanics Methods in ONIOM. *J Chem Theory Comput.*, 815–826. https://doi.org/10.1021/ct050289g

80. Wadood A, Ahmed N, Shah L, Ahmad A, Hassan H, Shams S. 2013. "In-silico drug design: An approach which revolutionarised the drug discovery process." *OA Drug Design & Delivery* 1(1):3. http://www.oapublishinglondon.com/article/1119.

81. Wanbo Tai, L. (2020). Characterization of the receptor-binding domain (RBD) of 2019 novel coronavirus: implication for development of RBD protein as a viral attachment inhibitor and vaccine. *cell and Molecular biology*, 613–620. https://doi.org/10.1038/s41423-020-0400-4

82. Wang, X. (2011). Role of clinical bioinformatics in the development of network-based Biomarkers. *Journal of Clinical Bioinformatics*, 1–3. https://doi.org/10.1186/2043-9113-1-28

83. Wilm, M. M. (1994). Error-Tolerant Identification of Peptides in Sequence Databases by Peptide Sequence Tags. *ACS Publications research*, 4390–4399. https://doi.org/10.1021/ac00096a002

84. Xuebing Wu, R. (2008). Network-based global inference of human disease genes. *Molecular systems biology*, 1–11. https://doi.org/10.1038/msb.2008.27

85. Yadi Zhou, P. F. (2020). Artificial intelligence in COVID-19 drug repurposing. *The Lancet Digital Health*, 1–10. https://doi.org/10.1016/S2589-7500(20)30192-8

86. Yoshihiro Yamanishi, M. (2014). DINIES: drug–target interaction network inference engine based on supervised analysis. *Nucleic acids research*, W39–W45. Retrieved from https://doi.org/10.1093/nar/gku337

87. Yuanmei Zhu, D. Y. (2020). Design of Potent Membrane Fusion Inhibitors against SARS-CoV-2, an Emerging Coronavirus with High Fusogenic Activity. *Journal of Virology*, 1–30. https://doi.org/10.1128/JVI.00635-20

88. Z. Faizal Khan, S. R. (2020). Recent Developments in Artificial Intelligence for Consumer Healthcare Integrative Analysis. *Journal of Healthcare Engineering*, 1–15. https://doi.org/10.1155/2020/8894694

89. Zachary D. Stephens, S. (2015). Big Data: Astronomical or Genomical? *PLOS Biology*, 1–11. https://doi.org/10.1371/journal.pbio.1002195

90. Zhou, Y. H. (2020). Network-based drug repurposing for novel coronavirus 2019-nCoV/SARS-CoV-2. *Cell Discovery*, 1–18. https://doi.org/10.1038/s41421-020-0153-3

Computational Methods for Health Informatics

Jayakishan Meher

Abstract Huge volumes of biological and healthcare data have been generated and accumulated together rapidly with high scale. The exponential growth and easy availability of these data have offered a movement in research activity of healthcare data science. The traditional methods are incapable of processing and management of enormous quantity of complex with high-dimensional healthcare data in terms of volume and variety. Recently data science technologies have been increasingly used in the research of biomedical and healthcare informatics. Big data analytics applications have unlocked innovative opportunities to extract hidden knowledge and develop advanced computational approaches to provide improved healthcare. Computational health informatics has come as an emerging field that offers enormous research opportunities for development of computational techniques that are applicable in healthcare system. Bioinformatics also provides many computational tools and techniques to analyze huge biomolecular datasets to understand disease and enables by relating genetics and proteomics with healthcare data. This chapter presents a comprehensive review of the potential of utilizing existing computational methods including machine learning as well as deep learning technologies in healthcare sector. It also looks at the contribution of bioinformatics, healthcare informatics, and analytics in improving healthcare system.

Keywords Health informatics · Bioinformatics · Computational methods · Machine learning · Deep learning · Big data analytics

J. Meher (✉)
Centurion University of Technology and Management, Odisha, India

369

A. K. Manocha et al. (eds.), *Computational Intelligence in Healthcare*, Health Information Science, https://doi.org/10.1007/978-3-030-68723-6_20

1   Introduction

During the last decade, a significant increase of healthcare data due to rapid growth
of technologies has been realized. Computational methods are progressively used
for research in healthcare informatics. Computational health informatics is an
evolving research field that integrates biomedical science, information technology,
and statistics which analyzes the healthcare information to predict status of patients'
health and improves healthcare output (HCO) [1].

The electronic health records (EHRs) is detailing huge health data in exabytes
from all sources of healthcare systems and will exceed in terms of zettabyte and
yottabyte in upcoming years [2]. The major features of big data such as volume,
variety, and velocity are growing exponentially in the biomedical informatics field.
The electronic form of healthcare data in various formats obtained from various
sources like medical records and medical diagnostic images is enormous and complex in nature, etc. [3, 4]. The traditional systems find difficulties in processing
these datasets due to its high dimension and complexity. These data are not easily
analyzed by conventional systems of software and hardware. Big data analytics
perform an important role in analyzing these huge, complex, and diverse healthcare
datasets in reduced time complexity for refining the quality of healthcare output. It
enables for decreasing the healthcare cost and makes more personalized medication [4].

Bioinformatics provides an opportunity for analyzing huge biological databases
with the help of computational tools and open the genomics and proteomics research
for study of diseases and help in drug discovery [5]. It also constitutes tools for
decision-making that can help the clinical experts to make healthier decisions. This
paper reviews the recent progress of computational methods for big data analysis in
healthcare areas and discusses the potential applications of machine learning and
deep learning methods in healthcare.

2   Computational Methods for Health Informatics

Healthcare informatics analyzes information with computational methods for
improving in healthcare and biomedical research [6, 7]. This proves the right information on health status to the correct person at right time which enables them in
taking informed decisions about the treatment of the patient [8]. A computational
health informatics includes certain phases in health informatics processing pipeline
as shown in Fig. 1.

Big data types in health informatics are categorized from information various
resources and data formats as listed in Table 1 [9, 9].

Various computational analytical techniques are used to discover useful patterns
from healthcare data for producing timely and effective decisions. The main phases
of the analyzing healthcare data include feature extraction and machine learning. In

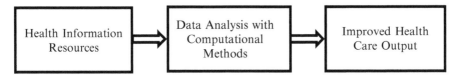

Fig. 1 Computational health informatics pipeline

Table 1 Healthcare data types and resources

Data types	Data sources	Data format
Research publications	Healthcare research papers and medical reference materials	Textual data
Diagnostic machine-produced data	Readings from various medical lab monitoring devices	Available in relational tables
Biometric-generated data	Fingerprints, heart rate, X-ray, blood pressure	Text and image formats
Social media data	Interaction data from social websites, physicians' notes, mail	Text, images, and video formats

Table 2 Feature extraction algorithms in the healthcare informatics

Healthcare diseases	Feature extraction used in healthcare systems
Diabetes, heart disease, breast cancer	PCA technique has been used in Pechenizkiy et al. 2004 and Subasi and Gursoy 2010 [10, 11]
Hepatitis diagnosis, coronary artery disease	LDA method used in Subasi and Gursoy 2010 [11]
Heart disease, genetic disease	ICA technique has been used in Subasi and Gursoy 2010 [11]
ICU readmission, EBB, and MRI datasets, predicting changes in hypertension control	Tree-based feature selection algorithm method has been used in Fialho et al. 2012 and Sun et al. 2014 [12, 13]
Breast, colon, and prostate cancer	Correlation-based feature selection (CFS) method has been used in Hall 1999 [14]

general, input data that contains redundant features, which are transformed into a small set of related features using dimensional reduction methods to make computationally less expensive with better accuracy. Hence many researchers employ feature extraction in healthcare informatics. Several feature selection algorithms have been proposed in healthcare informatics as shown in Table 2.

Machine learning algorithms allow to learn from data, extract knowledge, and identify patterns in data and make suitable inference using those patterns. Machine learning methods have been used to make advances in healthcare field and enable personalized care called precision medicine. In supervised learning used in machine learning, the labels for the known training data of number of inputs with corresponding outputs are provided to learn. This algorithm is used to predict events in the future from the past history, whereas the unsupervised learning algorithm handles unknown raw data to learns fully automatic and explore the data to draw pattern.

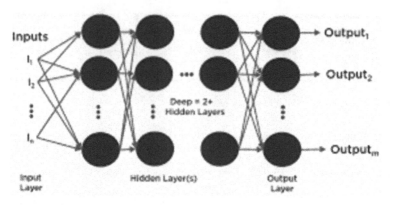

Fig. 2 Basic structure of DNNs

The supervised learning performs classification and regression problems [15]. The widely used methods to perform these problems are support vector machine, neural network, discriminant analysis, Naïve Bayes, nearest neighbor, decision tree, linear regression, ensemble methods, etc. The unsupervised learning performs clustering operation for which different methods used are K-mean clustering, neural network, Hidden Markov Model, etc.

Deep learning is a powerful tool for machine learning with its basis in artificial neural network. Deep learning is the extension of classical neural network (NN) which is built on the use of many hidden neurons with new training models to allow a deep architecture to capture the nonlinear relations [16].

The elementary structure of DNN contains of an input layer, the intermediate many hidden layers, and finally an output layer as shown in Fig. 2. The sum of the product of weight vector for each unit in the current layer with the signal produces the output expression. The output values can be calculated by applying the weighted sum through a nonlinear function such as a sigmoid, rectified linear unit, etc. [17].

Several deep learning architectures have been developed based on different methodological variants. In particular, convolutional neural networks (CNNs) have the major effect in health informatics. Other architectures for deep learning include deep Boltzmann machines (DBM), recurrent neural network (RNN), deep belief networks (DBNs), etc. [18–21].

3   Machine Learning for Health Informatics

Machine learning has been extensively used in the healthcare informatics that can help in determining effective personalized treatment [22]. Decision tree performs classification by sorting them in a tree and applying if-then rules which has been widely used in medical diagnostic [23]. Zhang et al. [24] introduced a diagnosis and prediction system based on very fast decision tree (VFDT) that can control large

Table 3 Machine learning algorithms in healthcare informatics

ML algorithms	Healthcare problems and datasets
Decision tree classifier	Brain MRI classification, medical prediction [28, 29]
SVM classifier	Image-based MR classification, children's healthcare [30]
Neural network classifier	Prediction of blood glucose level, recognition of heart rate variability, cancer disease prediction [31, 32]
Sparse	EHR count data, tumor classification, gene expression, heart beats classification [33]
Deep learning	MR brain images registration, healthcare decision-making, [34]
Ensemble	Microarray data classification, drug behavior response prediction, Alzheimer classification [28]
Partitioning clustering	Depression clustering, readmission risk prediction [35]
Hierarchical clustering	Microarray data clustering [36]
Density-based clustering	Biomedical image clustering [37]

data streams. Estella et al. [25] compared fuzzy decision tree (FDT) with other classifiers which determines the improved performance of FDT in the brain MRI classification.

SVM is a widely used method for both classification and regression by creating hyperplanes. In Zhou et al. [26], children's healthcare has been analyzed and socioeconomic status on educational fulfilment is analyzed. Vu et al. [27] presented an online three-layer NN for detection of patterns in heart rate variability (HRV) related to coronary heart disease (CHD) risk using ECG sensors. Various machine learning algorithms used to address the problems in healthcare informatics have been presented in Table 3.

4 Deep Learning for Health Informatics

Due to huge increase in healthcare multimodality data, deep learning has been used to play significant role in the analysis of health informatics big data [38]. Various deep learning architectures have been reported in area of healthcare informatics. Liang et al. [39] presented a decision-making system in healthcare using deep learning to eliminate the drawback of traditional rule-based models. The features and learning are combined in the unified model to simulate the complex producer of the human brain and thinking that has been applied successfully on healthcare datasets.

Deep learning methods have exposed the research in neuroimaging. Plis et al. [40] used deep belief networks method and restricted Boltzmann machine algorithm on functional and structural MRI data. The results have been validated by examining if the proposed methods can discover the unclear structure of large datasets. Li et al. [41] leveraged the deep learning to estimate the incomplete imaging data from

Table 4 Deep learning methods applications in health informatics

Healthcare applications	Datasets used	Deep learning methods
Cancer disease analysis, gene selection and classification, study of gene variants	Microarray gene expression datasets	DBN [42, 43], DNN [44]
Drug design	Molecule compounds	DNN [45]
Protein interaction, RNA-binding protein, DNA methylation	Protein structures, molecular compounds DNA RNA, and gene sequences	DBN [46], DNN [47, 48]
3D brain reconstruction, neural cells classification, brain tissue classification	MRI/fMRI fundus images PET scans	Deep autoencoders [49], CNN [50–53], DBN [54, 55], DNN [56]
Tissue classification, organ segmentation, cell clustering, hemorrhage detection, tumor detection	MRI image endoscopy, images microscopy, fundus images, X-ray images hyperspectral images	Convolutional DBN [57, 58], CNN [59, 60], DNN [61, 62]
Biological parameters monitoring, anomaly detection	ECG, implantable device	DBN [63, 64]
Prediction of disease, human behavior monitoring	Electronic health records, big medical dataset, blood lab tests	CNN [65], RNN [66] Convolutional DBN [67] DNN [68]

the multimodality database. They have used CNN on the Alzheimer's Disease Neuroimaging Initiative (ADNI) database. Various deep learning algorithms used to address the problems in healthcare informatics have been presented in Table 4.

5 Bioinformatics for Health Informatics

Bioinformatics helps in studies of variations in living system at molecular level. In the recent trend of personalized medication, there is growing need to examine these huge datasets within a time frame [69]. Bioinformatics targets to predict and prevent diseases with the advances in personalized treatments. The advances in biotechnology have focused on diagnostic of diseases and its treatment by investigating DNA and amino acid sequence. The genomic technologies have the capacity to progress in diagnosis and treatment of genetic diseases like cancer and accelerate in the direction of personalized medication.

The data-mining methods for genomics and proteomics have enabled to look into genetic related diseases and discovery of effective drugs. The advances in genetic research have refined the progress in personalized medicine that governs accurate medicine for the patient using the patient's genetic composition [70], and thus there is a need of inclusion of genetic information in electronic health records and create predictive models to provide personalized care in real time [71].

6 Conclusions

Computational healthcare informatics has become an indispensable platform for effective healthcare and more particularly personalized medication. Computational methods like machine learning have got significant role for handling such huge dimension and high-complexity healthcare datasets. Recently deep learning has become an important tool that is increasingly playing a significant role in machine learning and pattern recognition. In this paper, we have outlined how different machine learning and deep learning architectures have addressed various healthcare problems for effective diagnosis and treatment of patients in health informatics for diversified set of data where human interpretation is difficult. In the future advanced computational methods and deep learning architectures can be explored in health informatics to support effective personalized medication.

References

1. Matthew Herland, Taghi M. Khoshgoftaar, and Randall Wald. 2014. A review of data mining using big data in health informatics. Journal of Big Data, Springer 1, 1 (2014), 2.
2. Wullianallur Raghupathi and Viju Raghupathi. 2014. Big data analytics in healthcare: Promise and potential. Health Information Science and Systems 2, 1 (2014), 3.
3. Bonnie Feldman, Ellen M. Martin, and Tobi Skotnes. 2012. Big data in healthcare hype and hope. Technical Report, Dr. Bonnie 360 (2012).
4. Jimeng Sun and Chandan K. Reddy. 2013. Big data analytics for healthcare. In Proceedings of the 19th ACM SIGKDD International Conference on Knowledge Discovery and Data Mining (KDD'13). ACM, New York, NY, 1525–1525.
5. Jelili Oyelade, Jumoke Soyemi, Itunuoluwa Isewon and Olawole Obembe, Bioinformatics, Healthcare Informatics and Analytics: An Imperative for Improved Healthcare System, International Journal of Applied Information Systems (IJAIS) – ISSN: 2249-0868, Foundation of Computer Science FCS, New York, USA Volume 8– No.5, February 2015, pp.1-6
6. Hersh W. 2009. "A stimulus to define informatics and health information technology". BMC Med Inform Decision Making 9:24
7. In Y. C., Tae-Min K., Myung S. K., Seong K. M. and Yeun-Jun C. 2013. Perspectives on Clinical Informatics: Integrating Large-Scale Clinical, Genomic, and Health Information for Clinical Care. Genomics and Informatics. Published online by Korea Genome Organization.
8. Friedman, C. 2009. "A fundamental theorem of biomedical informatics". Journal of the American Medical Informatics Association, 16: 169-170.
9. K. Priyanka and Nagarathna Kulennavar. 2014. A survey on big data analytics in health care. International Journal of Computer Science and Information Technologies 5, 4 (2014), 5865–5868.
10. Mykola Pechenizkiy, Alexey Tsymbal, and Seppo Puuronen. 2004. PCA-based feature transformation for classification: Issues in medical diagnostics. In Proceedings of the 17th IEEE Symposium on ComputerBased Medical Systems (CBMS'04). IEEE, 535–540.
11. Abdulhamit Subasi and M. Ismail Gursoy. 2010. EEG signal classification using PCA, ICA, LDA and support vector machines. Expert Systems with Applications 37, 12 (2010), 8659–8666.

12. Andre S. Fialho, Federico Cismondi, Susana M. Vieira, Shane R. Reti, Joao M. C. Sousa, and Stan N.´ Finkelstein. 2012. Data mining using clinical physiology at discharge to predict ICU readmissions. Expert Systems with Applications 39, 18 (2012), 13158–13165.

13. Jimeng Sun, Candace D. McNaughton, Ping Zhang, Adam Perer, Aris Gkoulalas-Divanis, Joshua C. Denny, Jacqueline Kirby, Thomas Lasko, Alexander Saip, and Bradley A. Malin. 2014. Predicting changes in hypertension control using electronic health records from a chronic disease management program. Journal of the American Medical Informatics Association 21, 2 (2014), 337–344.

14. Mark A. Hall. 1999. Correlation-Based Feature Selection for Machine Learning. Ph.D. Dissertation. University of Waikato

15. M.A. Jabbar, Shirina Samreen, Rajanikanth Aluvalu, The Future of Health care: Machine Learning, International Journal of Engineering & Technology, 7 (4.6) (2018) 23–25

16. LeCun Y, Bengio Y, Hinton G. Deep learning. Nature 2015;521(7553):436–44.

17. LeCun Y, Ranzato M. Deep learning tutorial. In: Tutorials in International Conference on Machine Learning (ICML'13), 2013. Citeseer.

18. Svozil D, Kvasnicka V, Pospichal J. Introduction to multilayer feed-forward neural networks. Chemometr Intell Lab Syst 1997;39(1):43–62.

19. T.M. NAVAMANI, Efficient Deep Learning Approaches for Health Informatics, Deep Learning and Parallel Computing Environment for Bioengineering Systems. https://doi.org/10.1016/B978-0-12-816718-2.00014-2 Copyright © 2019 Elsevier Inc, 123–137.

20. Vincent P, Larochelle H, Lajoie I, et al. Stacked denoising autoencoders: learning useful representations in a deep network with a local denoising criterion. J Mach Learn Res 2010;11:33, 71–408.

21. Hinton G, Osindero S, Teh Y-W. A fast learning algorithm for deep belief nets. Neural Comput 2006;18(7):1527–54.

22. Peter C. Austin, Jack V. Tu, Jennifer E. Ho, Daniel Levy, and Douglas S. Lee. 2013. Using methods from the data-mining and machine-learning literature for disease classification and prediction: A case study examining classification of heart failure subtypes. Journal of Clinical Epidemiology 66, 4 (2013), 398–407.

23. David J. Dittman, Taghi M. Khoshgoftaar, Randall Wald, and Amri Napolitano. 2013. Simplifying the utilization of machine learning techniques for bioinformatics. In 12th International Conference on Machine Learning and Applications (ICMLA'13). Vol. 2. IEEE, 396–403.

24. Ruogu Fang, Shaoting Zhang, Tsuhan Chen, and Pina Sanelli. 2015. Robust low-dose CT perfusion deconvolution via tensor total-variation regularization. IEEE Transaction on Medical Imaging 34, 7 (2015), 1533–1548.

25. Francisco Estella, Blanca L. Delgado-Marquez, Pablo Rojas, Olga Valenzuela, Belen San Roman, and Ignacio Rojas. 2012. Advanced system for autonomously classify brain MRI in neurodegenerative disease. In International Conference on Multimedia Computing and Systems (ICMCS'12). IEEE, 250–255.

26. Xinhua Dong, Ruixuan Li, Heng He, Wanwan Zhou, Zhengyuan Xue, and Hao Wu. 2015. Secure sensitive data sharing on a big data platform. Tsinghua Science and Technology 20, 1 (2015), 72–80

27. Thi Hong Nhan Vu, Namkyu Park, Yang Koo Lee, Yongmi Lee, Jong Yun Lee, and Keun Ho Ryu. 2010. Online discovery of heart rate variability patterns in mobile healthcare services. Journal of Systems and Software 83, 10 (2010), 1930–1940.

28. Alzheimer's disease neuroimaging initiative. http://adni.loni.usc.edu/about/. (2015). Retrieved 02-15-2015-02.

29. Jinn-Yi Yeh, Tai-Hsi Wu, and Chuan-Wei Tsao. 2011. Using data mining techniques to predict hospitalization of hemodialysis patients. Decision Support Systems 50, 2 (2011), 439–448

30. Births: Data from the National Community Child Health database. http://gov.wales/statistics-and-research/births-national-community-child-health-database/?lang=en. (2014). Retrieved 02-15-2015.

31. K. Usha Rani. 2011. Analysis of heart diseases dataset using neural network approach. arXiv preprint arXiv:1110.2626 (2011).
32. Irfan Y. Khan, P. H. Zope, and S. R. Suralkar. 2013. Importance of artificial neural network in medical diagnosis disease like acute nephritis disease and heart disease. International Journal of Engineering Science and Innovative Technology (IJESIT) 2, 2 (2013), 210–217.
33. Hui Fang Huang, Guang Shu Hu, and Li Zhu. 2012. Sparse representation-based heartbeat classification using independent component analysis. Journal of Medical Systems 36, 3 (2012), 1235–1247.
34. PREDICT-HD project. https://www.predict-hd.net/. (2015). Retrieved 04-10-2015.
35. Kiyana Zolfaghar, Naren Meadem, Ankur Teredesai, Senjuti Basu Roy, Si-Chi Chin, and Brian Muckian. 2013. Big data solutions for predicting risk-of-readmission for congestive heart failure patients. In 2013 IEEE International Conference on Big Data. 64–71.
36. Hospital episode statistics. http://www.hscic.gov.uk/hes. (2012). Retrieved 02-20-2015.
37. Mehemmed Emre Celebi, Yuksel Alp Aslandogan, and Paul R. Bergstresser. 2005. Mining biomedical images with density-based clustering. In International Conference on Information Technology: Coding and Computing (ITCC'05). Vol. 1. IEEE, 163–168
38. Daniele Rav`ı, Charence Wong, Fani Deligianni, Melissa Berthelot, Javier Andreu-Perez, Benny Lo, and Guang-Zhong Yang, Deep Learning for Health Informatics, IEEE JOURNAL OF BIOMEDICAL AND HEALTH INFORMATICS, VOL. 21, NO. 1, pp.4–21, (2017)
39. Znaonui Liang, Gang Zhang, Jimmy Xiangji Huang, and Qmming Vivian Hu. 2014. Deep learning for healthcare decision making with EMRs. In 2014 IEEE International Conference on Bioinformatics and Biomedicine (BIBM'14). 556–559.
40. Sergey M. Plis, Devon R. Hjelm, Ruslan Salakhutdinov, Elena A. Allen, Henry J. Bockholt, Jeffrey D. Long, Hans J. Johnson, Jane S. Paulsen, Jessica A. Turner, and Vince D. Calhoun. 2014. Deep learning for neuroimaging: A validation study. Frontiers in Neuroscience 8 (2014).
41. Mingkui Tan, Ivor W. Tsang, and Li Wang. 2014. Towards ultrahigh dimensional feature selection for big data. Journal of Machine Learning Research 15, 1 (2014), 1371–1429.
42. R. Ibrahim, N. A. Yousri, M. A. Ismail, and N. M. El-Makky, "Multi-level gene/mirna feature selection using deep belief nets and active learning," in Proc. Eng. Med. Biol. Soc., 2014, pp. 3957–3960.
43. M. Khademi and N. S. Nedialkov, "Probabilistic graphical models and deep belief networks for prognosis of breast cancer," in Proc. IEEE 14th Int. Conf. Mach. Learn. Appl., 2015, pp. 727–732.
44. D. Quang, Y. Chen, and X. Xie, "Dann: A deep learning approach for annotating the pathogenicity of genetic variants," Bioinformatics, vol. 31, p. 761–763, 2014.
45. B. Ramsundar, S. Kearnes, P. Riley, D. Webster, D. Konerding, and V. Pande, "Massively multitask networks for drug discovery," ArXiv e-prints, Feb. 2015.
46. S. Zhang et al., "A deep learning framework for modeling structural features of rna-binding protein targets," Nucleic Acids Res., vol. 44, no. 4, pp. e32–e32, 2016.
47. K. Tian, M. Shao, S. Zhou, and J. Guan, "Boosting compound-protein interaction prediction by deep learning," in Proc. IEEE Int. Conf. Bioinformat. Biomed., 2015, pp. 29–34.
48. C. Angermueller, H. Lee, W. Reik, and O. Stegle, "Accurate prediction of single-cell dna methylation states using deep learning," bioRxiv, 2016, Art. no. 055715
49. J. Shan and L. Li, "A deep learning method for microaneurysm detection in fundus images," in Proc. IEEE Connected Health, Appl., Syst. Eng. Technol., 2016, pp. 357–358.
50. D. Nie, H. Zhang, E. Adeli, L. Liu, and D. Shen, "3d deep learning for multi-modal imaging-guided survival time prediction of brain tumor patients," in Proc. MICCAI, 2016, pp. 212–220. [Online]. Available: https://doi.org/10.1007/978-3-319-46723-8_25
51. J. Kleesiek et al., "Deep MRI brain extraction: A 3D convolutional neural network for skull stripping," NeuroImage, vol. 129, pp. 460–469, 2016.
52. B. Jiang, X. Wang, J. Luo, X. Zhang, Y. Xiong, and H. Pang, "Convolutional neural networks in automatic recognition of trans-differentiated neural progenitor cells under bright-field microscopy," in Proc. Instrum. Meas., Comput., Commun. Control, 2015, pp. 122–126.

53. M. Havaei, N. Guizard, H. Larochelle, and P. Jodoin, "Deep learning trends for focal brain pathology segmentation in MRI," CoRR, vol. abs/1607.05258, 2016. [Online]. Available: http://arxiv.org/abs/1607.05258

54. D. Kuang and L. He, "Classification on ADHD with deep learning," in Proc. Cloud Comput. Big Data, Nov. 2014, pp. 27–32.

55. F. Li, L. Tran, K. H. Thung, S. Ji, D. Shen, and J. Li, "A robust deep model for improved classification of ad/mci patients," IEEE J. Biomed. Health Inform., vol. 19, no. 5, pp. 1610–1616, Sep. 2015.

56. K. Fritscher, P. Raudaschl, P. Zaffino, M. F. Spadea, G. C. Sharp, and R. Schubert, "Deep neural networks for fast segmentation of 3d medical images," in Proc. MICCAI, 2016, pp. 158–165. [Online]. Available: https://doi.org/10.1007/978-3-319-46723-8_19

57. X. Zhen, Z. Wang, A. Islam, M. Bhaduri, I. Chan, and S. Li, "Multi-scale deep networks and regression forests for direct bi-ventricular volume estimation," Med. Image Anal., vol. 30, pp. 120–129, 2016.

58. T. Brosch et al., "Manifold learning of brain mris by deep learning," in Proc. MICCAI, 2013, pp. 633–640.

59. T. Xu, H. Zhang, X. Huang, S. Zhang, and D. N. Metaxas, "Multimodal deep learning for cervical dysplasia diagnosis," in Proc. MICCAI, 2016, pp. 115–123. [Online]. Available: https://doi.org/10.1007/978-3-319-46723-8_14

60. M. Avendi, A. Kheradvar, and H. Jafarkhani, "A combined deep-learning and deformable-model approach to fully automatic segmentation of the left ventricle in cardiac mri," Med. Image Anal., vol. 30, pp. 108–119, 2016.

61. Y. Zhou and Y. Wei, "Learning hierarchical spectral-spatial features for hyperspectral image classification," IEEE Trans. Cybern., vol. 46, no. 7, pp. 1667–1678, Jul. 2016.

62. J. Wang, J. D. MacKenzie, R. Ramachandran, and D. Z. Chen, "A deep learning approach for semantic segmentation in histology tissue images," in Proc. MICCAI, 2016, pp. 176–184. [Online]. Available: https://doi.org/10.1007/978-3-319-46723-8_21

63. Y. Yan, X. Qin, Y. Wu, N. Zhang, J. Fan, and L. Wang, "A restricted Boltzmann machine based two-lead electrocardiography classification," in Proc. 12th Int. Conf. Wearable Implantable Body Sens. Netw., Jun. 2015, pp. 1–9.

64. A. Wang, C. Song, X. Xu, F. Lin, Z. Jin, and W. Xu, "Selective and compressive sensing for energy-efficient implantable neural decoding," in Proc. Biomed. Circuits Syst. Conf., Oct. 2015, pp. 1–4

65. H. Shin, L. Lu, L. Kim, A. Seff, J. Yao, and R. M. Summers, "Interleaved text/image deep mining on a large-scale radiology database for automated image interpretation," CoRR, vol. abs/1505.00670, 2015. [Online]. Available: http://arxiv.org/abs/1505.00670

66. Z. C. Lipton, D. C. Kale, C. Elkan, and R. C. Wetzel, "Learning to diagnose with LSTM recurrent neural networks," CoRR, vol. abs/1511.03677, 2015. [Online]. Available: http://arxiv.org/abs/1511.03677

67. Z. Liang, G. Zhang, J. X. Huang, and Q. V. Hu, "Deep learning for healthcare decision making with emrs," in Proc. Int. Conf. Bioinformat. Biomed., Nov 2014, pp. 556–559.

68. E. Putin et al., "Deep biomarkers of human aging: Application of deep neural networks to biomarker development," Aging, vol. 8, no. 5, pp. 1–021, 2016.

69. Andrzej Polanski and Marek Kimmel 2007. Bioinformatics. New York: Springer Verlag Berlin Heidelberg.

70. Prerna S., and Kimberly T., 2009. "Translational Bioinformatics and Healthcare Informatics: Computational and Ethical Challenges". Online Research Journal Perspectives in Health Information Management, 6.

71. Naiem T. Issa, Stephen W. Byers, and Sivanesan Dakshanamurthy. 2014. Big data: The next frontier for innovation in therapeutics and healthcare. Expert Review of Clinical Pharmacology 7, 3 (2014), 293–298.

Computational Model of a Pacinian Corpuscle for Hybrid-Stimuli: Spike-Rate and Threshold Characteristics

V. Madhan Kumar, Venkatraman Sadanand, and M. Manivannan

Abstract Purpose: Tactile displays convey various aspects of touch through mechanical or electrical stimuli. Recent research focuses on combining these two types of stimulation (hybrid stimuli) to achieve naturalness, comfort, and reduction in the threshold, only by experiment. However, there are no computational models to study the Pacinian corpuscle's behavior under hybrid-stimuli.

Method: We developed a novel hybrid-stimuli Pacinian corpuscle model and characterized its spike-rate and threshold responses. Our model comprises biomechanical and electrical components, both of which are excited simultaneously by hybrid stimuli. We chose stimuli shape as either trapezoidal or sinusoidal, with a frequency from 5 Hz to 1600 Hz, both electrical and mechanical. We characterized the model by first considering the electrical current as an actual stimulus and mechanical vibration as a sub-threshold (magnitude less than the threshold required to produce one impulse-per-cycle response), and then the vice versa.

Results: The spike-rate characteristics exhibit a well-known phase-locking phenomenon. However, the plateaus shift toward the left as the sub-threshold stimulus amplitude increases. Furthermore, the threshold versus frequency curve shifts down. Finally, we observed a monotonic decrease in the threshold of the stimulus as the amplitude of the sub-threshold stimulus increases.

Conclusion: The shifts shown in both spike-rate and threshold characteristics indicate a significant reduction in the actual stimulus threshold. The hybrid-stimuli Pacinian corpuscle model developed and characterized in this study can be useful in improving the design of tactile displays.

Keywords Sub-threshold · Tactile displays · Electrical stimulus · Vibration perception · Electro-mechanical · Mechanical stimulus · SAIC · VAIC

V. Madhan Kumar (✉) · M. Manivannan
Touch Lab, Department of Applied Mechanics, Indian Institute of Technology Madras, Chennai, India

V. Sadanand
Department of Neurosurgery, Loma Linda University Health System, Loma Linda, CA, USA

© The Author(s), under exclusive license to Springer   379
Nature Switzerland AG 2021
A. K. Manocha et al. (eds.), *Computational Intelligence in Healthcare*, Health
Information Science, https://doi.org/10.1007/978-3-030-68723-6_21

1 Introduction

As an immersive interface to the virtual environment, tactile displays provide stimuli to the human tactile system (mechanoreceptors), which is responsible for the mechanical aspects of touch, majorly through the four channels [9, 12]. Each mechanoreceptor receives unique features of mechanical stimulation applied over the skin and produces unique neural code [22, 28]. The tactile stimulus provided over the skin surface to excite the four channels emanating from four different mechanoreceptors can be either electrical or mechanical. Mechanical stimulation replicates the surface property of the object by changing the physical amplitude and frequency of the stimulus applied over the skin surface [46]. On the other hand, application of electrical current as a stimulus, directly excites the nerves of the mechanoreceptors [25].

Electrotactile displays are considered to be advantageous than the mechanical ones in terms of size, durability, power consumption, and compatibility [24, 26]. However, in terms of naturalness of the perceived sensation, mechanical stimulus is always superior [34]. Since both possess their own advantages and disadvantages, combining them is considered as one possible solution toward achieving the better experience with a comfortable gadget. In practice, development of such gadgets can focus on the characterization of the mechanoreceptors with computational models for the improved design. Various computational models characterize the mechanoreceptors in terms of frequency, spike rate, and threshold characteristics that exist in the literature such as the works of Bensmaia [5], Saal et al. [39], Biswas et al. [7, 8] and Quindlen et al. [37].

Among the four major mechanoreceptors, Pacinian corpuscle (PC) is considered the most sensitive mechanoreceptor [13, 30, 41] since the neural activity is observed even with a mechanical stimulus of amplitude 0.01 μm [10, 11]. PC is a rapidly adapting mechanoreceptor as it exhibits wider (20 Hz to 1 kHz) frequency response [11, 40, 45]. Compared to other mechanoreceptors, they respond to high-frequency vibrations applied over the skin. Each lamellar layer of a PC acts as a mechanical band-pass filter and they are attached by tight junctions which make them electrically isolated [2].

With regard to the mechanism of mechanotransduction, there always existed a contradiction among researchers until Hamill and Martinac [20], Pawson and Bolanowski [36], Cho et al. [14], and Drew et al. [15] reported the presence of ion channels that respond to stretch and voltage, which are widely called SAIC (stretch-activated ion channel) and VAICs (voltage-activated ion channel), in the receptive area of the PC. It is because of these ion channels, the applied mechanical stimulus gets transduced into electrical signal. When the mechanical stimulus is applied, the PC deforms and produces non-propagated receptor potentials. The APs are initiated when these receptor potentials reach a threshold. Furthermore, the outer core of the PC is electrically isolated from the neurite which is responsible for the transduction of the applied stimuli by the generation of the receptor potentials [2]. The modeling of PC has been attracting researchers over the past few decades [3, 4, 6–8, 16–18, 25, 31, 32, 37, 42, 44].

PC models for a mechanical stimulus [7, 8, 31, 37] and for an electrical stimulus [25, 43] deal with separate excitation of the PC, either electrical or mechanical. Furthermore, the characteristics of the PC available in the literature are only for the excitation with single stimulus modality (either electrical or mechanical). Biswas et al. [7, 8] have modeled the PC with finer morphological details and characterized the model [7, 8] by threshold and spike-rate characteristics.

We refer to threshold here as the smallest stimulus amplitude required to initiate one impulse per cycle (ipc) response. The threshold characteristics of a PC are as follows: vibrotactile perception threshold (VTPT) curve due to mechanical stimulation and electrotactile perception threshold (ETPT) curve due to electrical stimulation are very much essential in the design and implementation of the tactile displays. Moreover, in psychophysical literature, VTPT is well known as vibration perception threshold (VPT). The threshold characteristics of a PC are well studied in the literature [7, 8, 40, 45].

A PC can be excited by either electrical or mechanical stimuli provided with suitable amplitude and frequency. Conventionally, PCs are excited by a mechanical stimulus applied over the skin. However, the PC's axon can be stimulated electrically to elicit the sensations of tactile perception [27]. The thickness of the human skin is not the same all over the human body, as it varies from fingertip to forearm and in forehead due to stratum corneum. Consequently, the amplitude requirements for an electrical display also vary to elicit the intended sensation.

The design of electrotactile displays with optimal stimulus parameters is still a challenge. Kaczmarek et al. [23] have given the list of performance criteria for the design and evaluation of optimal displays. In this list, seventh criterion mentions that there should be a maximum comfort level and a minimal variation in the sensory threshold. To reduce the required amplitude of an electrical stimulus and to increase the comfort level for the user, an additional stimulus can be provided in the sub-threshold level. Several researchers [29, 34, 48] have focused on achieving this hybrid-stimuli tactile devices in which one stimulus assists the other, electrical and mechanical. Especially, Kuroki et al. [29] mentioned that the threshold of a mechanical stimulus can be reduced by adding an electrical stimulus of required amplitude and vice versa.

Although the models available in the literature characterize PC more accurately, they all excite PC model with only one type of stimulus, either electrical or mechanical. None of the available PC model is developed for both types of stimuli simultaneously (hybrid stimuli). Therefore, to improve the design of hybrid-stimuli tactile displays, we need to (1) develop a PC model that can be excited by both mechanical and electrical stimuli simultaneously and (2) characterize the model in terms of spike-rate and threshold characteristics.

The main objective of this work is to understand the behavior of the PC excited by the hybrid stimuli. We characterize the proposed model in terms of spike rate and threshold characteristics. We propose that by applying a mechanical stimulus as a sub- threshold for a PC model excited by an electrical stimulus, or vice versa, the threshold of the stimulus amplitude reduces. We also propose that the threshold characteristics reported in this work can be utilized in the design of hybrid-stimuli tactile displays in order to reduce the amplitude required to elicit the intended sensations.

The novelties of the proposed model include (1) the computational model of a PC for hybrid stimuli and its characterization and (2) a method of reducing the amplitude requirements in hybrid stimulation using the threshold characteristics reported here.

2 Methods

The computational model of a PC excited by electrical and mechanical stimuli is described in this section. We combine and extend our previous computational modeling works on a PC [7, 8, 43] with single stimulus into a PC model to which both electrical and mechanical stimuli are applied simultaneously. The proposed model, hybrid-stimuli PC model, comprises two pathways: one is biomechanical and the other is electrical. The biomechanical pathway of the PC model is preceded by the biomechanical skin model and the electrical pathway of the PC model is preceded by the electrode-skin interface model.

2.1 Model Description

The basic block diagram of the hybrid-stimuli PC model is shown in Fig. 1a. The biomechanical pathway of the PC model consists of PC lamellae and neurite, whereas the electrical pathway of the PC model consists of only neurite. The signals emanating from these two segments are summed up to excite the first node of Ranvier.

Stimuli specifications: The two segments of the hybrid-stimuli PC model are executed simultaneously by applying two different types of stimuli: mechanical and electrical. The shape of the stimulus in both electrical and mechanical is chosen to be either trapezoidal or sinusoidal. The frequency of the both types of stimuli is varied from 5 Hz to 1600 Hz. The amplitude of the mechanical stimulus is varied from 0.1 μm to 10 μm and that of the electrical stimulus is varied from 0.02 mA to 2 mA. The duty cycle of the electrical stimulus is always 50%. The stimulus function is given as follows:

$$
e_1(t) = \begin{cases} A.\dfrac{t}{t_1}, & \text{if } 0 \le t < t_1 \\[2mm] A, & \text{if } t_1 \le t < t_2 \\[2mm] A.\dfrac{t - t_3}{t_2 - t_3}, & \text{if } t_2 \le t < t_3 \end{cases} \tag{1}
$$

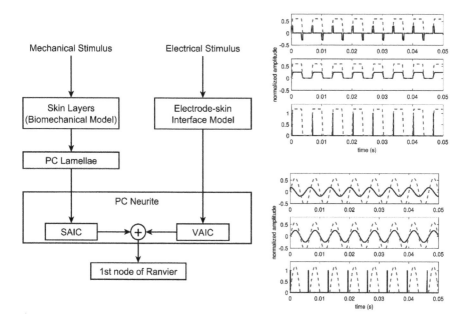

Fig. 1 (**a**) Block diagram of the hybrid-stimuli PC model depicting two separate pathways for two different stimuli, mechanical and electrical. For a mechanical stimulus, biomechanical properties of the skin and lamellae of PC are included. For an electrical stimulus, electrical properties of electrode-skin interface are included. The signal from both pathways excites the ion channels (SAIC and VAIC) in the PC neurite and then summed up to excite the first Ranvier node. Response (top row) of the electrode-skin interface, response (middle row) of the biomechanical skin transfer function, and the Spike response (bottom row) from the first node of Ranvier for trapezoidal (**b**) and sinusoidal (**c**) stimuli of frequency 150 Hz. The dashed lines in each subplot indicate the stimulus. The amplitude of the mechanical stimulus here is 0.5 μm and that of the electrical stimulus is 0.1 mA, in both the cases. This amplitude is chosen such that it lies in the one impulse per cycle plateau in the spike rate characteristics of the 150 Hz stimulus

$$e_2(t) = A.\sin(2\pi ft) \tag{2}$$

The mechanical stimulus applied over the skin gets filtered by the skin layers, PC lamellae, and then reaches the neurite. Each PC lamella acts as a band-pass filter to the applied mechanical stimulus. PC neurite comprises SAICs. Similarly, the electrical stimulus is filtered by skin layers and then directly reaches the PC's neurite. The PC's neurite introduces nonlinearity in the generation of receptor potential and it comprises VAICs. Both SAICs and VAICs are modeled as nonlinear-dependent charge sources along with their impedance and the details are described in Biswas et al. [7, 8] and Vasudevan et al. [43]. The output of the neurite is the receptor potential which is the summation of signals from mechanical and electrical segments of the hybrid-stimuli PC model. The receptor potential is then applied as the input to the first node of Ranvier which again consists of VAICs modeled as a nonlinear-dependent charge source and the associated impedance.

Since the outer core of the PC is electrically isolated from the neurite, the electrical stimulus does not reach the neurite directly through the outer core. Rather it reaches antidromically to the neurite through the axon. To support this, there are several experiments reported in the literature during the event of finding the AP initiation site. Hunt and Takeuchi [21] reported one such experiment where they excited a partially decapsulated PC antidromically. Furthermore, Ozeki and Sato [35] supported the fact that the antidromic APs can reach the terminal neurite. Our current model is based on the electrical stimulation of neurites through antidromic APs. Moreover, in the basic block diagram, the antidromic propagation is not shown explicitly since our interest is to explain the threshold variations due to the hybrid stimuli. Therefore, the basic block diagram shown in Fig. 1a is the simplified block diagram where the antidromic propagation is not shown. The filtered stimuli undergo two-stage nonlinear neural spike generation which is modeled as an adaptive relaxation pulse frequency modulator (ARPFM). Except for the lossy integrator and adaptive threshold, the modeled ARPFM stage is similar to the integrate-and-fire neuron model. It is a measure of the refractoriness of the VAICs to go for the next avalanche opening. For the spike generation, the neural noise, an additive random noise, is multiplied with the adaptive threshold. The ARPFM threshold is amplified by the threshold amplification factor in the refractory period, as found in Loewenstein and Altamirano-Orrego [33]. The experimental data have shown an exponential decay with a time constant of 0.56 ms, after the time $(t) = 2.5$ ms. The threshold amplification factor (TAF) considered for the ARPFM [7, 8] is given as follows:

$$\text{TAF} = 1 + \left(7.75 * t^{-0.16} * \exp\left(-0.56t\right)\right)$$

The transfer functions of the hybrid-stimuli PC model include Gm and Ge, which indicate transfer functions of skin for mechanical and electrical stimuli, respectively; Hm and He indicate the transfer functions pertaining to PC for mechanical and electrical stimuli, respectively.

2.2 Model Parameters and Approximations

The model parameters and approximations given in Biswas et al. [7, 8] and in Vasudevan et al. [43] apply same to the proposed hybrid-stimuli PC model. The following are the additional parameters:

t, s : time domain and Laplace domain variables, respectively.

ei (t) : stimuli with respect to time, $i = m$ indicates mechanical stimulus and $i = e$ rep- resents electrical stimulus.

ej (t) : stimuli, $j = 1$ represents sinusoidal stimulus and j=2 represents trapezoidal stimulus.

vi (*t*) : receptor potential, i=m indicates potential due to mechanical stimulus and
$i = e$ represents potential due to electrical stimulus.

*A*m : amplitude of the mechanical stimulus in microns.

*A*e : amplitude of the electrical stimulus in mA.

f: frequency of the stimulus in hertz.

2.2.1 Model Assumptions

Approximations and assumptions given in PC models for mechanical stimulus and electrical stimulus are equally applicable in this hybrid-stimuli PC model. The additional assumptions pertaining to the present model are as follows:

(a) Although PCs exists as a cluster [47] of two or three, we assume single PC beneath the skin in this model.
(b) Both electrical and mechanical stimuli are assumed to be applied in the same point over the skin so that the effect of Gaussian receptive field reported in Vasudevan et al. [44] could be neglected.
(c) Furthermore, both stimuli are applied simultaneously with respect to time.
(d) The delay between the biomechanical and electrical segments of the hybrid-stimuli PC model is assumed to be very small and neglected. The axon of the PC is assumed to be perpendicular to the direction of the stimulation.
(e) We consider only identical frequency for both the stimuli.
(f) For the simulation of the present model, the noise variations are not included, especially neural noise.

3 Simulation of the Hybrid-Stimuli PC Model

The hybrid-stimuli PC model involves (a) creating a PC model with both mechanical and electrical stimuli as input, (b) simulating the model with two different stimuli shape as given in (1) and (2), for both mechanical and electrical, (c) characterizing the model for the frequency response, and finally (d) generating various spike rate and threshold characteristics to understand the behavior of the model. All the model simulations and characterizations are implemented in MATLAB Simulation Software.

The various conditions simulated on the hybrid-stimuli PC model are as follows:

(a) Initially, we characterized the model with the frequency response and then we generated the spike response for a hybrid stimuli with a mechanical amplitude $Am = 0.5$ μm and an electrical amplitude $Ae = 0.1$ mA. Both the stimuli are maintained at a frequency of $f = 150$ Hz for this spike response. During this simulation, the responses from skin layers and the final response are recorded for observation.

(b) The simulation of spike response explained in (a) is repeated for both trapezoidal (1) and sinusoidal (2) stimuli.

(c) After the spike response, the hybrid-stimuli PC model is stimulated with variations in stimuli frequency and amplitude to obtain spike-rate characteristics. For this simulation, the various mechanical stimulus amplitudes ($Am = 0.1$ μm, 0.2 μm, and 0.5 μm) are chosen in the sub-threshold level which is slightly lower than the threshold that can elicit one impulse per cycle in the APs of the model. The electrical stimulus amplitude (Ae) is varied from 0 to 2 mA (step size: 2 μA). The model is simulated for various stimulus frequencies (f); however, the frequency of mechanical and electrical stimuli is always the same.

(d) Another simulation involves generating ETPT and VTPT curves for various stimulus frequencies (5 Hz to 800 Hz). Here, the threshold indicates the minimum amplitude of the stimulus required to elicit one impulse per cycle. In this simulation, only one stimulus is applied and the other stimulus is made zero. This is to study the behavior of the model and to correlate it with the electrical-alone [43] or mechanical-alone [7, 8, 37] stimuli models of PC.

(e) The threshold characteristics in terms of ETPT are simulated by considering various mechanical stimuli amplitude in the sub-threshold level. For various stimulus frequencies, the ETPTs obtained are recorded.

Similarly, the threshold characteristics in terms of VTPT are simulated by considering various electrical stimuli amplitude and the VTPTs are recorded for various stimulus frequencies. Results

The hybrid-stimuli PC model is simulated under various conditions to obtain spike-rate and threshold characteristics. We have used two different stimuli: electrical and mechanical, as hybrid-stimuli. Moreover, two different wave shapes are used: trapezoidal and sinusoidal. The various characteristics obtained are visualized in this section.

3.1   Spike Response

The excitation of the hybrid-stimuli PC model resulted in the spike response as shown in Fig. 1b and c. This is obtained by applying mechanical and electrical stimuli simultaneously with $f = 150$ H z, $Ae = 0.1$ mA, and $Am = 0.5$ μm. Figure 1b shows the response of the hybrid-stimuli PC model for a trapezoidal stimulus as given in (1), and Fig. 1c shows the same for a sinusoidal stimulus as given in (2). Top plots given in Fig. 1a represent the response of the electrode-skin interface model, middle plots in Fig. 1b and c indicate the response of the biomechanical skin model, and the bottom plots represent the spike response emanating from the First node of Ranvier.

3.2 Spike-Rate Characteristics

The variation in the spike rate with respect to the electrical stimulus amplitude for various levels of mechanical stimulus in the sub-threshold range is shown in Fig. 2a and b. Similarly, the variation in the spike rate with respect to the mechanical stimulus amplitude for various levels of electrical stimulus in the sub-threshold range is shown in Fig. 2c and d. Figure 2a and c represents the spike rate variations for the stimuli frequency of 100 Hz, whereas Fig. 2b and d represents the same for the stimuli frequency of 200 Hz. In Fig. 2a and b, the electrical stimulus amplitude is varied from 0 to 2 mA with a step size of 2 µA and the mechanical stimulus amplitudes are chosen as 0.1 µm, 0.2 µm, and 0.5 µm. Similarly, in Fig. 2c and d, the mechanical stimulus amplitude is varied from 0 to 10 µm with a step size of 0.01 µm and the electrical stimulus amplitudes are chosen as 2 µA and 8 µA.

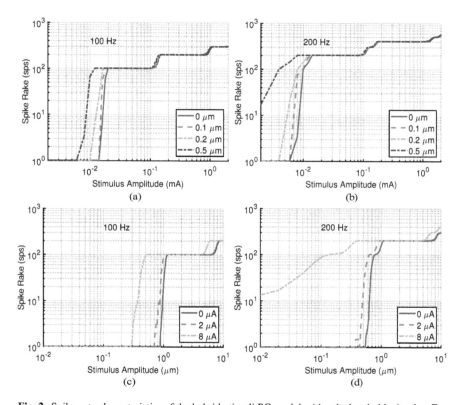

Fig. 2 Spike-rate characteristics of the hybrid-stimuli PC model with sub-threshold stimulus. For various sub-threshold mechanical stimuli, spike rate plotted for the variation in electrical stimulus amplitude with constant stimulus frequency, (**a**) 100 Hz and (**b**) 200 Hz. Similarly, (**b**) and (**d**) represent the spike-rate plot with electrical stimulus as the sub-threshold and mechanical stimulus as the actual input to the model. As in mechanical (Biswas et al. 2015) or electrical stimuli [43] models, the spike rate here plateaus at the values which are equal to the multiples of stimulus frequency

3.3   Threshold Characteristics

The variation in minimum stimulus amplitude (threshold) required to elicit one impulse per cycle for various stimulus frequencies is shown as threshold characteristics in Fig. 3a, b, and c. Both ETPT and VTPT are shown independently with separate ordinates in Fig. 3a. In this plot, threshold curves for electrical and mechanical stimuli are given under the condition of zero sub-threshold stimulus. Figure 3b represents ETPT with the sub-threshold mechanical stimulus, whereas Fig. 3c represents VTPT with the sub-threshold electrical stimulus. In both plots, electrical and mechanical stimuli are applied simultaneously to the PC model.

The variation of the actual stimulus amplitude with respect to the sub-threshold stimulus amplitude, for different stimulus frequencies, is shown in Fig. 3d and e. In Fig. 3d, the actual stimulus is electrical and the sub-threshold stimulus is mechanical, and in Fig. 3e, it is vice versa. Discussion

The primary objective of this work is to develop a novel PC model which can accept both mechanical and electrical stimuli, simultaneously. The computational model of a PC for a mechanical stimulus [7, 8] and that for an electrical stimulus [43] are combined and extended to propose this model. We have characterized the proposed model in terms of spike-rate and threshold characteristics which can be verified in future experiments.

Although there are four major mechanoreceptors beneath the skin, in the proposed model, we consider only the PC as it is responsible for the vibration perception in the somatosensory system. We consider that the locations of both stimuli are at the same point. In our future work, we will explore based on the potential distribution of the electrical stimuli and the distribution of the mechanical stimuli over the skin spatially – spatial distribution. Additionally, we assumed both stimuli are applied simultaneously with respect to time. In the experimental work reported by Gray and Malcolm [19], they suggested that both the stimuli should be within the time interval of 1.2 ms tò achieve the increased electrical excitability of the PC with sub-threshold mechanical stimulus. This 1.2 ms indicates the absolute refractory period of the PC's response to mechanical stimulus. Within the absolute refractory period, PC assumes any number of stimuli as a single stimulus. This is the reason we assumed temporal synchronization between the stimuli.

Response of the hybrid-stimuli PC model

The frequency response characteristics of the proposed model are same as that of the previously developed models of the PC for a mechanical stimulus by Biswas et al. [7, 8] and an electrical stimulus by Vasudevan et al. [43]. Therefore, in this paper, we focus only on the spike response and threshold characteristics. We observe that the skin models, both electrical and mechanical, act as band-pass filters to the stimulus applied over the skin, as shown in (top and middle plots) Fig. 1b and c. The frequency response of these models considering the skin alone is discussed in Biswas et al. [7, 8] and in Vasudevan et al. [43]. The spikes are generated by the ARPFM stage which is the modification of integrate and fire neuron model as mentioned in Section 2. The spike responses shown in the bottom plots of Fig. 1b and c

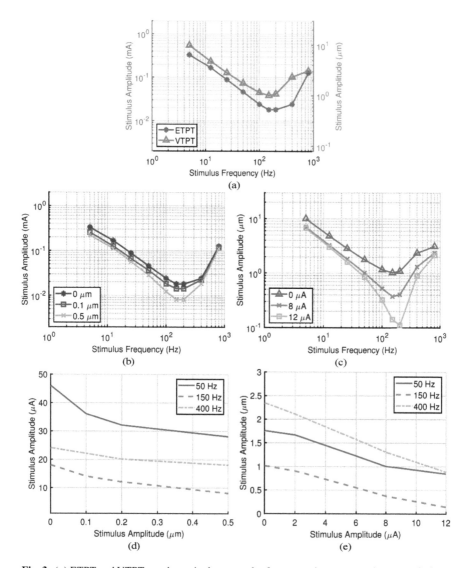

Fig. 3 (a) ETPT and VTPT are shown in the same plot for comparison purpose in terms of stimulus frequency. Both shows the lower-most threshold in the stimulus frequency range 100 Hz to 200 Hz which is the typical VPT response of a PC as mentioned in the literature [11]. The left-side ordinate indicates the electrical stimulus amplitude in mA and the right-side ordinate indicates mechanical stimulus amplitude in μm. (b) The threshold characteristics in terms of ETPT for various sub-threshold mechanical stimuli; As the mechanical stimulus amplitude is increased, the characteristics show reduction in the thresholds. (c) The threshold characteristics in terms of VTPT for various sub-threshold electrical stimuli showing shift down in the thresholds as the electrical stimulus amplitude is increased. Abscissa in both (d) and (e) indicate the sub-threshold stimulus amplitude, whereas ordinates indicate the actual stimulus amplitude. The variation in the stimulus amplitude (required to elicit one impulse per cycle) due to the increment in the sub-threshold stimulus amplitude for three different stimulus frequencies is shown here. It is clear that the required stimulus amplitude decreases monotonically as the sub-threshold stimulus amplitude increases, in both cases

are the typical one impulse per cycle (ipc) response of the hybrid-stimuli PC model. Above a certain stimulus strength, the spike rate would be shifted to 2 ipc response.

As mentioned previously, all the simulation results are due to the excitation of the model with electrical and mechanical stimuli of identical wave shapes (either trapezoidal or sinusoidal). We also simulated the model with non-identical wave shapes, for instance, trapezoidal electrical stimulus and sinusoidal mechanical stimulus and vice versa. However, since there is no effect of non-identical wave shapes on the spike-rate and threshold characteristics, we have shown only results with stimuli of identical wave shapes.

Observations on spike-rate changes:

To achieve the 2 ipc spike response, we increase the amplitude of the electrical stimuli based on the spike-rate characteristics shown in Fig. 2a and b. Figure 2a and c shows the plateaus of spike rates at 100 spikes per second (sps), 200 sps, and 300 sps for 100 Hz stimuli. Similarly, in the remaining two plots, we observe the response of spike-rate plateaus at 200 sps, 300 sps, and 400 sps. This well-known phase-locking [11] phenomenon is clearly observed in all the plots of Fig. 2 even in the presence of a sub-threshold stimulus of different type. Further- more, in Fig. 2b, we can observe 300 sps which is 1.5 ipc for a 200 Hz stimulus, but for a short span of stimulus amplitude. Although the spike-rate characteristics of our model show conventional spike-rate characteristics of a PC such as plateaus and phase-locking, there are several differences that we observe in the presence of a sub-threshold stimulus. From our results, we observe that the plateau widths are larger for the spike-rates pertaining to the 1 ipc or 2 ipc response (equal to integer multiplication of the stimulus frequency) than the 0.5 or 1.5 ipc.

In all four plots of Fig. 2, we observe that the threshold for initiating 1 ipc plateau is shifted left as we increase the sub-threshold stimulus amplitude from a zero to a next level. However, the threshold to initiate the 2 ipc plateau shows negligible change. This means that the width of the plateau increases as we increase the sub-threshold stimulus amplitude.

In Fig. 2a and b, we observe that the 2 ipc plateau shows negligible shift even for the increments in the sub-thresholdmechanical stimulus, whereas in Fig. 2c and d, 2 ipc plateau shifts substantially as we increase the sub-thresholdelectrical stimulus. However, this shift is lesser in width compared to the 1 ipc plateau shift. Therefore, we infer that the mechanical input as a sub-threshold stimulus for an electrical stimulus affects only the 1 ipc plateau and increases only the first plateau width. However, in the same conditions, if we apply electrical signal as a sub-threshold stimulus for a mechanical input, it affects the width of both first and second plateaus.

Moreover, the 1 ipc plateau shifts in Fig. 2a and b are not noticeable for the mechanical stimulus amplitudes of 0 μm, 0.1 μm, and 0.2 μm. However, the shift is noticeable for 0.5 μm. Similarly, in Fig. 2c and d, the shift in the 1 ipc plateau is noticeable only for 8 μA sub-thresholdelectrical stimulus.

The reasons for these differences in the behavior of PC model between mechanical and electrical stimuli could be due to (a) the absence of lamellae in the electrical part of the PC model and (b) differences in the absolute refractory period of APs generated with mechanical and electrical stimuli, as discussed in the subsection "possible mechanisms."

Variations in the threshold characteristics:
In Fig. 3a, the threshold curves for ETPT and VTPT are independently generated by stimulating the model with only electrical stimulus and only mechanical stimulus, respectively. The purpose of this plot is to demonstrate the basic threshold characteristics when the PC model is excited by one stimulus at a time. These curves are comparable to the characteristics reported in the literature. The threshold curve for mechanical stimuli (VTPT) can be validated from the experimental results reported by Bolanowski Jr and Zwislocki [11]; Biswas et al. [7], [8] and the ETPT is same as reported by Vasudevan et al. [43].

Shifts due to the sub-threshold amplitude
The variations in ETPT are observed for three different levels of mechanical stimulus (0 μm, 0.1 μm, and 0.5 μm) in Fig. 3b. As we clearly observe, the entire threshold curve shifts down as we increase the sub-threshold mechanical stimulus amplitude. This explains the fact that the sub-threshold mechanical stimulus amplitude, although it is not sufficient to generate 1 ipc response in the model, is assisting the actual electrical stimulus to reach the 1 ipc response with lesser amplitude. That is, the 1 ipc response is achieved with the amplitude that is lower than the threshold as shown in ETPT of Fig. 3b.

Similarly, the variations in VTPT are observed for three different levels of electrical stimulus (0 μA, 8 μA, and 12 μA) in Fig. 3c. The same observations discussed for Fig. 3b is applicable to this plot too. Major difference is that the threshold reduction for VTPT is much higher compared to that in ETPT, especially for the frequencies from 100 Hz to 200 Hz. The observed shifts in the characteristics need to be verified experimentally in future studies. Threshold values shown in the model can be tested experimentally and the various tactile perceptual experiences can be mapped to each level of a threshold and its frequencies.

Threshold Versus Sub-threshold
From Fig. 3b and c, it is evident that there is always a reduction in the threshold amplitude whenever there is an increment in the sub-threshold stimulus amplitude. However, to get better insight, we need to explain the reduction in terms of percentage or a relationship curve. One such explanation is shown in Fig. 3d and e, and it is evident from both the relationships that the threshold amplitude of an actual stimulus is monotonically decreasing. The percentage reduction varies slightly different for different levels of threshold variations. In the case of 50 Hz stimuli, the application of sub-threshold mechanical stimulus of 0.1 μm reduces the threshold of an electrical stimulus by 22%, and if we further increase the sub-threshold amplitude to 0.2 μm, then the reduction is 11%. This observation leads to the question, what happens when the sub-threshold stimulus is equal to the threshold? As we observe from Fig. 3d and e, actual stimulus amplitude approaches zero as the sub-threshold stimulus amplitude increases. It is obvious that when the sub-threshold stimulus is equal to its threshold, the model already reached its 1 ipc response and, therefore,

the required amplitude of the actual stimulus is zero. Any further increments in the amplitude will have no effect on the spike-rate plateau until the amplitude is sufficient enough to reach the 2 ipc response. This brings the response of the model into a second spike-rate plateau.

Possible Mechanisms

The proposed model is an attempt to simulate the response of a PC, when given both electrical and mechanical stimuli together, in which the threshold level for both stimuli can be substantially reduced. There are few literatures to support this statement. Gray and Malcolm [19] reported that if the afferent fiber of a PC is excited by an electrical stimulus and a sub-threshold mechanical stimulus within 1.2 ms between each other (within the absolute refractory period), then the "excitability" of the PC could be enhanced. Based on this, they have suggested that there exist non-propagated potentials capable of summation, which was later called receptor potentials. Even though the ion channels (SAICs and VAICs) in the neurite were not found until in the early 2000s, Gary and Malcolm found that there are separate pathways for the electrical and mechanical stimuli in the attempt of finding AP initiation site. Moreover, the aforementioned 1.2 ms unresponsive time is the absolute refractory period for an AP which is very much essential to determine, since the two different stimuli should be applied within this period, if not it will be not be considered as hybrid stimuli. Gray and Malcolm [19] reported the absolute refractory for a mechanical stimulus, 1.1 ms to 2.6 ms. Alvarez-Buylla and De Arellano [1] reported the absolute refractory of 1.3 ms for mechanical stimuli and that of 0.5 ms for electrical stimuli.

Furthermore, it is reported in Kuroki et al. [29] that the PC is not considered to be stimulated by electrical stimulation. However, the frequency of the electrical stimulus that they have used in their experiments is always 20 Hz. It is evident from the literature that the RA-1 resonates better in this frequency. This is the reason they have mentioned that PC would not be stimulated by electrical stimulation in their paper. Whereas in our model, we are using a wide range of frequencies up to 1 kHz. This suggests that the excitation of the PC is reported in this work, rather than RA-1, for the range of frequencies considered.

Novel Predictions and Model Applications

Three novel predictions from this work are as follows: (1) the variations in the width of the spike-rate plateaus in presence of sub-threshold stimuli, (2) the range of threshold reductions due to the application of sub-threshold stimuli for one particular stimulus frequency, using the relationship provided in Fig. 3d and e, and (3) the shifts in the entire threshold curves whenever there is an increment in the sub-threshold stimulus.

The development of the PC model as described in this paper finds its application in the design of tactile displays in which both electrical and mechanical stimuli can be used to elicit various kinds of perception by varying the combinations of amplitude and frequency of both stimuli. Moreover, such hybrid-stimuli tactile displays can also help in reducing the intensity of electrical stimulus to obtain the threshold by having mechanical stimulus in the sub-threshold level. Another application could be diagnosis and therapy for diabetic neuropathy. As PCs are the first to get affected in the peripheral neuropathy condition, development of vibrotactile device with sub-threshold electrical stimulus may help in improving the diagnosis and therapy of diabetic neuropathy. This model can also be useful to explain in vitro studies with a decapsulated PC. In this case, the terminal neurite is exposed without any electro-ionic barrier like intermediate zone and the capsule Ozeki and Sato [35].

4   Conclusion and Future Work

In this work, we proposed that the PC's threshold reduces with hybrid stimuli along with the application of a sub-threshold stimulus. We achieved this through the combination and extension of our earlier models of PC. We developed the hybrid-stimuli PC model and characterized it to observe the variations in the spike-rate and threshold responses. A substantial reduction in the threshold amplitude of the actual stimulus, when applied along with the sub-threshold, can be inferred from our spike-rate and threshold characteristics. Moreover, the monotonic decrease in the threshold suggests that the tactile displays' amplitude requirements can be reduced by invoking the method of sub-threshold stimulus reported in our characterizations.

The future works include two different aspects: computational model and experimental. The behavior of the PC model can be studied further (1) by using the cluster model [44] to add the Gaussian receptive field and study the effect of applying the hybrid stimuli in different locations over the skin, (2) by using non-identical frequencies between electrical and mechanical stimuli, and (3) by applying two or more different stimuli of the same type (mechanical or electrical), one or more in the sub-threshold level. First, it helps us understand the source localization by analyzing the effects of inter-spike delay due to hybrid stimuli. Second, although the present model can be simulated with any combination of frequencies between electrical and mechanical stimuli, we limit our study only to identical frequencies for both stimuli to observe various characteristics. Finally, the third is to improve the ergonomics of the tactile displays.

Furthermore, Kajimoto et al. [25] reported the strange uncomfortable feeling for the electrical stimulation with frequencies more than 200 Hz. One of the experimental studies conducted by our own group Rahul Kumar and Manivannan [38] suggests that the electrical stimulation of skin can lead to a vibration sensation of up to 1200 Hz. In a future study, we will explore the experimental results reported in the literature along with the computational model Vasudevan et al. [43] reported in our previous work.

In an experimental point of view, we intend to conduct psychophysical experiments to relate the characteristics reported here with different perception levels. Moreover, the changes in the perception due to non-identical combinations of stimuli frequency can also be observed experimentally.

Acknowledgments The authors would like to appreciate the suggestions given by the members of Haptics Lab for the improvement of this model.

Declaration of Interest The authors report no conflicts of interest.

References

1. Alvarez-Buylla R, De Arellano JR. 1952. Local responses in pacinian corpuscles. American Journal of Physiology-Legacy Content. 172(1):237–244.
2. Bell J, Bolanowski S, Holmes MH. 1994. The structure and function of pacinian corpuscles: a review. Progress in neurobiology. 42(1):79–128.
3. Bell J, Holmes M. 1992. Model of the dynamics of receptor potential in a mechanoreceptor. Mathematical biosciences. 110(2):139–174.
4. Bell J, Holmes MH. 1994. A note on modeling mechano-chemical transduction with an application to a skin receptor. Journal of mathematical biology. 32(3):275–285.
5. Bensmaia S. 2002. A transduction model of the meissner corpuscle. Mathematical biosciences. 176(2):203–217.
6. Biswas A, Manivannan M, Srinivasan MA. 2013. A biomechanical model of pacinian corpuscle & skin. In: In 2013 Biomedical Sciences and Engineering Conference (BSEC). IEEE. p. 1–4.
7. Biswas A, Manivannan M, Srinivasan MA. 2015. Multiscale layered biomechanical model of the pacinian corpuscle. IEEE Transactions on Haptics. 8(1):31–42.
8. Biswas A, Manivannan M, Srinivasan MA. 2015. Vibrotactile sensitivity threshold: Nonlinear stochastic mechanotransduction model of the pacinian corpuscle. IEEE transactions on haptics. 8(1):102–113.
9. Bolanowski SJ, Gescheider GA, Verrillo RT. 1994. Hairy skin: psychophysical channels and their physiological substrates. Somatosensory & motor research. 11(3):279–290.
10. Bolanowski Jr S, Zwislocki J. 1984. Intensity and frequency characteristics of pacinian corpuscles. ii. receptor potentials. Journal of neurophysiology. 51(4):793–811.
11. Bolanowski Jr S, Zwislocki JJ. 1984. Intensity and frequency characteristics of pacinian corpuscles. i. action potentials. Journal of neurophysiology. 51(4):812–830.
12. Bolanowski Jr SJ, Gescheider GA, Verrillo RT, Checkosky CM. 1988. Four channels mediate the mechanical aspects of touch. The Journal of the Acoustical society of America. 84(5):1680–1694.
13. Brisben A, Hsiao S, Johnson K. 1999. Detection of vibration transmitted through an object grasped in the hand. Journal of neurophysiology. 81(4):1548–1558.
14. Cho H, Shin J, Shin CY, Lee SY, Oh U. 2002. Mechanosensitive ion channels in cultured sensory neurons of neonatal rats. Journal of Neuroscience. 22(4):1238–1247.
15. Drew LJ, Rugiero F, Wood JN. 2007. Touch. In: Current topics in membranes. vol. 59. Elsevier; p. 425–465.
16. Freeman AW, Johnson KO. 1982. Cutaneous mechanoreceptors in macaque monkey: temporal discharge patterns evoked by vibration, and a receptor model. The Journal of physiology. 323(1):21–41.
17. Grandori F, Pedotti A. 1980. Theoretical analysis of mechano-to-neural transduction in pacinian corpuscle. IEEE Transactions on Biomedical Engineering. BME-27(10):559–565.
18. Grandori F, Pedotti A. 1982. A mathematical model of the pacinian corpuscle. Biological cybernetics. 46(1):7–16.
19. Gray JAB, Malcolm J. 1950. The initiation of nerve impulses by mesenteric pacinian corpuscles. Proceedings of the Royal Society of London Series B-Biological Sciences. 137(886):96–114.
20. Hamill OP, Martinac B. 2001. Molecular basis of mechanotransduction in living cells. Physiological reviews. 81(2):685–740.

21. Hunt C, Takeuchi A. 1962. Responses of the nerve terminal of the pacinian corpuscle. The Journal of physiology. 160(1):1.
22. Johnson KO. 2001. The roles and functions of cutaneous mechanoreceptors. Current opinion in neurobiology. 11(4):455–461.
23. Kaczmarek KA, Webster JG, Bach-y Rita P, Tompkins WJ. 1991. Electrotactile and vibrotactile displays for sensory substitution systems. IEEE transactions on biomedical engineering. 38(1):1–16.
24. Kajimoto H. 2016. Electro-tactile display: principle and hardware. In: Pervasive haptics. Springer; p. 79–96.
25. Kajimoto H, Kawakami N, Maeda T, Tachi S. 1999. Tactile feeling display using functional electrical stimulation. In: Proc. 1999 ICAT. p. 133.
26. Kajimoto H, Kawakami N, Maeda T, Tachi S. 2004. Electro-tactile display with tactile primary color approach. Graduate School of Information and Technology, The University of Tokyo.
27. Kandel E, Schwartz J, Jessell T. 1991. Principles of neural science. Elsevier. Prentice-Hall International edit.
28. Kandel E, Schwartz J, Jessell T. 1991. Principles of neural science. Elsevier. Prentice-Hall International edit.
29. Kuroki S, Kajimoto H, Nii H, Kawakami N, Tachi S. 2007. Proposal for tactile sense presentation that combines electrical and mechanical stimulus. In: Second Joint EuroHaptics Conference and Symposium on Haptic Interfaces for Virtual Environment and Teleoperator Systems (WHC'07). IEEE. p. 121–126.
30. LaMotte RH, Srinivasan MA. 1991. Surface microgeometry: Tactile perception and neural encoding. In: Information processing in the somatosensory system. Springer; p. 49–58.
31. Loewenstein W, Skalak R. 1966. Mechanical transmission in a pacinian corpuscle. an analysis and a theory. The Journal of physiology. 182(2):346–378.
32. Loewenstein WR. 1959. The generation of electric activity in a nerve ending. Annals of the New York Academy of Sciences. 81(2):367–387.
33. Loewenstein WR, Altamirano-Orrego R. 1958. The refractory state of the generator and propagated potentials in a pacinian corpuscle. The Journal of general physiology. 41(4):805–824.
34. Mizuhara R, Takahashi A, Kajimoto H. 2019. Enhancement of subjective mechanical tactile intensity via electrical stimulation. In: Proceedings of the 10th Augmented Human International Conference 2019. p. 1–5
35. Ozeki M, Sato M. 1964. Initiation of impulses at the non-myelinated nerve terminal in pacinian corpuscles. The Journal of physiology. 170(1):167.
36. Pawson L, Bolanowski SJ. 2002. Voltage-gated sodium channels are present on both the neural and capsular structures of pacinian corpuscles. Somatosensory & motor research. 19(3):231–237.
37. Quindlen JC, Stolarski HK, Johnson MD, Barocas VH. 2016. A multiphysics model of the pacinian corpuscle. Integrative Biology. 8(11):1111–1125.
38. Rahul Kumar R, Manivannan M. 2021. Spatial summation of electro-tactile displays at subthreshold level (in press). In: International Conference on Human Interaction and Emerging Technologies. Springer. p. 00–00.
39. Saal HP, Delhaye BP, Rayhaun BC, Bensmaia SJ. 2017. Simulating tactile signals from the whole hand with millisecond precision. Proceedings of the National Academy of Sciences. 114(28):E5693–E5702.
40. Sato M. 1961. Response of pacinian corpuscles to sinusoidal vibration. The Journal of physiology. 159(3):391–409.
41. Skedung L, Arvidsson M, Chung JY, Stafford CM, Berglund B, Rutland MW. 2013. Feeling small: exploring the tactile perception limits. Scientific reports. 3:2617.
42. Summers IR, Pitts-Yushchenko S, Winlove CP. 2018. Structure of the pacinian corpuscle: Insights provided by improved mechanical modeling. IEEE Transactions on Haptics. 11(1):146–150.

43. Vasudevan MK, Sadanand V, Muniyandi M, Srinivasan MA. 2020a. Coding source localiza-
    tion through inter-spike delay: modeling a cluster of pacinian corpuscles using time-division
    multiplexing approach. Somatosensory & Motor Research. 37(2):63–73.
44. Vasudevan MK, Ray RK, Muniyandi M. 2020b. Computational model of a pacinian corpuscle
    for an electrical stimulus: Spike-rate and threshold characteristics. In: International Conference
    on Human Haptic Sensing and Touch Enabled Computer Applications. Springer. p. 203–213.
45. Verrillo RT. 1966. Vibrotactile sensitivity and the frequency response of the pacinian cor-
    puscle. Psychonomic Science. 4(1):135–136.
46. Wagner CR, Lederman SJ, Howe RD. 2004. Design and performance of a tactile shape display
    using rc servomotors. Haptics-e. 3(4):1–6.
47. Wu G, Ekedahl R, Stark B, Carlstedt T, Nilsson B, Hallin RG. 1999. Clustering of pacin-
    ian corpuscle afferent fibres in the human median nerve. Experimental brain research.
    126(3):399–409.
48. Yem V, Okazaki R, Kajimoto H. 2016. Fingar: combination of electrical and mechanical
    stimulation for high-fidelity tactile presentation. In: Acm siggraph 2016 emerging technolo-
    gies. p. 1–2.

Index

A
ABCD functionality, 273
Accuracy, 92
A-consciousness, 2
Acquisition, 97
Activation function
  binary classifier, 217
  ELM, 218
  function $G(.)$, 218
  hardlim, 227, 228
  N_0, 219
  nonlinear, 216
  RBF, 216
  sigmoid, 225
  sine, 228–229, 231
Adaptive relaxation pulse frequency modulator
    (ARPFM), 384
Aggregated E-health system
  algorithmic centric, 182
  design I, 182
  design II, 184
  design III, 184
  design IV, 185
  design V, 185
AI-based deep learning, 331
AI-based models, 334
All-pole filter, 243
Alzheimer's Disease Neuroimaging Initiative
    (ADNI), 374
American Telemedicine Association (ATA), 68
Animal life, 20
Anticipatory behavioral control, 20
AP initiation site, 384
Apple Watch, 94
Application programming interface (API), 294

Arabidopsis thaliana, 348
Architecture Management Office (AMO), 298
Arithmetic coding, 48, 49
Arithmetic operations, 53, 54
AROGYASREE, 78
Artificial intelligence (AI), 9, 10, 97, 118, 215,
    344, 353
Artificial neural models, 273
Artificial neural network (ANN), 120–122,
    128, 133, 323
Attention-based mechanism
  global feature extraction, 336
  hard attention, 337
  image generation, 336
  soft attention, 337
Attention gate mechanism, 339
Attributes' dimension reduction, 220
Augmented reality (AR), 85
Aura, 6, 12
Aura photography, 3
Auto depth encoder, 136
Autoencoders, 128–131
Automated digital mammography
    processing, 318
Automated image analysis tools, 340
Automated skin lesion categorization, 276
Automatic feature learning, WHM, 149
Averaging pixel intensity, 260

B
Bacillus thuringiensis, 348
Back-propagation (BP), 216
Ballistocardiogram (BCG), 84
Band-pass (BP) filter, 259

Basal skin cancer (BSC), 271
Big data advancements, 362
Big data analytics, 353, 370
Big data technologies
    AI model, 353
    arrangement, 351
    bioinformatics, 353
    biological databases, 353
    ccRCC, 352
    Cloudburst, 351
    computational methods, 351
    conventional information handling
            procedures, 351
    gene sequencing, 353
    genome analysis, 353
    Hadoop, 351
    market, 353
    m-health, 352
    natural information, 352
    progressive application, 361
Billing Management Service, 297
BiMFG, 346
Bioelectric activities, 4
Bioelectricity, 2, 4, 22
Bioelectrograms, 11
Bioinformatics, 370, 374
    AI, 344
    aims, 344, 345
    applications fields
        agriculture, 348
        medicine, 346
        research, 346
    availability and affordability, 344
    Big data (see Big data technologies)
    computational analysis, 344
    definition, 344
    healthcare, 349–351, 361–363
    metabolomics, 354, 355
    research disciplines, 343
    resources (see Personalized medicine)
    tools, 346, 347
Biological databases, 353
Biological processes, 4
Biomedical engineering, 122
Biomedical instruments, 186
Biorthogonal wavelet transform, 46
Bits per pixel (bpp), 38, 50
Body area network (BAN), 109
Bone density/bone mineral density (BD/BMD)
    definition, 192
    evaluation, 192
    LR model, 196
    NTD, 196
    osteoporosis, 192

    T-score, 194, 196, 197
    ultrasonic transducers, 193
    X-rays, 192
Boolean kernel, 278
Box plot
    chaos attributes, 221, 226
    conventional, 219
    graphic approach representation, 219
    labeling and structure, 219
    NSR-CAD and NSR-CHF, 220
Brain and respiration, 163
Breast cancer, 318–321

C
CAD and CHF disease detection and
            classification methods, 216, 225,
            227, 229, 230
CADD-mediated virtual screening, 359
CAD system, 320, 325
Cancer Genome Atlas, 352
Capacity-building exercises, 298
Cardiac diseases (CDs), 214
Cardiovascular activities, 13, 14
Cardiovascular diseases (CVDs), 214
Carry-free adder, 62, 63
Carry-save adder (CSA), 61, 62
Categorical adversarial autoencoder
            (CatAAE), 135
Causal transfer function, 239
CENTIPEDE, 346
Chaos attributes
    CBC, 225
    CD, 222
    DFA, 223
    HE, 224
    MPE, 225
    PE, 224
    poincare plot investigation, 223
    SamEn, 223
Chest CT, 306
Chest X-ray radiographs
    classes, 308
    coronavirus detection, 306, 307, 312
    MODE, 307
Chinese cosmology, 7
Chromosome, 244
Classical neural network (NN), 372
Clear cell renal cell carcinoma (ccRCC), 352
Clinical informaticians, 349
Cloud-based HIPPA compliance, 302
Cloud-based service delivery platform, 291
Cloud-based storage, 298
Cloud-based technology, 289

Cloudburst, 351
Cloud computing, 289, 290, 358
Cloud environment, 290
Cloud Help Line Manager, 297
Cloud interoperability standards manager, 296
Cloud models, 298
Cloud Security Manager, 297
Cloud technologies, 297
CNN model, 180, 332
Codewords, 48
Coding redundancy, 36
Coefficient quantization, 241
Cognitive heart failure (CHF), 214, 215
Cohesive approach, 288
Coiflet filters, 45
Commercial healthcare platforms
    digital, 361
    IBM corporation, 361, 362
    innovation, 361
Common alerting protocol (CAP), 187
Common Service Centers (CSCs), 289
Communication, 200
Communication channel, 89
Communication methods, 186
Communication protocol, 109
Compliance Report Generator, 297
Compression, 36
Compression ratio (CR), 36
Computational health informatics
    analytical techniques, 370
    Big data, 370, 371
    deep learning, 372
    DNN, 372
    machine learning algorithms, 371
    ML, 375
    phases, 370
    selection algorithms, 371
    unsupervised learning algorithms, 371
Computer-aided drug design (CADD), 355,
        359, 360
Computer-based intelligence-based assistive
        devices, 353
Computer-based science, 350
Computer-based skin cancer detection system
    feature extraction, 275
    image enhancement, 274
    standard ABCD assessment, 272
    stripes and color patterns, 272
    SVM, 273, 275, 276
    watershed segmentation, 274
Configurable logic blocks (CLBs), 59
Confusion matrix, 169, 172
Connectome, 15

Consciousness, 2, 20
Contactless HR monitoring method
    post-processing
        FFT, 260
        zero hertz component, 260
    preprocessing
        human face detection, 258
        ROI detection/tracking, 258, 259
    signal extraction
        averaging pixel intensity, 260
        BP filtering, 259
Continuous patient monitoring (CPM), 180
Contractive autoencoder, 131
Conventional PID controller, 209
Convolutional neural network (CNN), 126,
        131–133, 136, 141–143, 148, 149,
        273, 331, 372
    accuracies, 310
    architecture, 307
    classification metrics, 311
    comparison, 310
    confusion matrix, 312
    evaluation metrics, 311
    hyperparameter tuning, 307
    pre-trained models, 306
    support vector machine, 306
    SVM, 307
Coronary artery disease (CAD)
    diagnosis methods, 214
    ECG, 214, 215
    WHO statistical details, 214
Coronary heart disease (CHD), 373
Coronavirus (COVID-19), 175, 305
    active cases, 306
    diagnosis, 306
    MERS-CoV virus, 305
    serious acute respiratory distress
        syndrome, 306
Coronavirus symptoms, 330
Correlation, 20
Correlation dimension (CD), 222
Cost-effectiveness, 298
COVID-19 pandemic, 79, 80, 360, 363
COVID-19-related findings, 338
Crossover principle, 244
C-scan ultrasonic facility ULTIMA
        200M2, 192
Cuckoo search, 349
Cumulative bi-correlation (CBC), 217, 225
Customary PSNR measures, 38
Customized Report Generators, 297
Cybersecurity, 200
Cycle crossover (CX), 246

D

Data acquisition system, 148
Data and information exporting service, 296
Data as a Service (DaaS), 292, 293
Data dictionaries, 296
Data dissection service, 295
Data distribution service, 295
Data dithering service, 295
Data mining
    anomaly detection, 117
    feature extraction, 119
    feature selection, 120
    health monitoring system, 117
    ML, 120
    modeling and learning methods, 120
    PCA, 124
    physiological data processing
        frameworks, 117
    prediction, 117
    raw data, 118, 119
    stages, 116
    wearable sensors, 118
    WHM systems, 117
Data-mining databases and tools, 346, 348
Data-mining methods, 374
Data mirroring service, 295
Data privacy, 77
Data scientists, 92
Data trades, 349
Daubechies wavelet, 40, 45
    decomposition, 166
    input signal splitting, 165
    KNN, 171
    noise removal, 165
    PCA, 165, 167, 169
    signals classification, 168, 169, 171
    statistical parameters, 167, 168
    wavelet denoising, 166
Decay, 44
Decay tree, 45
Decision fusion, 147
Decision-making system, 373
Decision support system/s, 296
Decision tree, 372
Decomposition level selection
    Daubechies wavelet, 45
    decay tree, 45
    extreme incentive, 44
    graphical representation, 45
    wavelet channels, 44
Deep autoencoder, 129, 136
Deep autoencoder encoding and decoding
        process, 130
Deep Autoencoder models, 331
Deep belief network (DBN), 128, 331, 372

Deep Boltzmann machine (DBM), 127, 128,
        331, 372
Deep convolutional neural network,
        WHM, 132
Deep learning (DL), 372
    advantage, 135
    AI, 125
    applications (see DL applications, WHM
        systems)
    architectures, 137–139
    auto depth encoder, 136
    autoencoders, 128–131
    CNN, 131–133, 136
    deep autoencoder, 136
    framework, 125, 126
    GAN, 134, 135
    human activity identification field, 125
    ML, 125
    prominent characteristics, 125
    RBM, 126–128, 136
    RNN, 133, 134, 136
    sparse coding, 131, 136
Deep learning algorithms
    classification, 331, 332
Deep learning architectures, 375
Deep learning-based segmentation
        scheme, 333
Deep learning techniques
    AI techniques, 332
    CNN-based models, 332
    covid detection model, 332
    healthcare sector, 333
    infectious region quantification, 333
    proposed mMdel, 334
    ResNet 50 model, 333
    ST-ResNet, 333
    U-NET, 335
Deep Stacking Network (DSN), 331
Deformable model-based segmentation
        approaches, 319
Denoising autoencoders, 130
Department of Electronics and IT (DeitY), 297
Dermatoscopy, 272
Dermoscopic image, 272
Detrended flunctuation analysis (DFA), 223
Dice similarity coefficient (DSC), 333
Digit QSD number, 55
Digital communication system, 35
Digital data screening mammogram
        (DDSM), 320
Digital filters
    advantages, 237
    coefficients calculation, 239, 240
    finite word length, 241
    frequency response characteristics, 238

hardware and software
    implementation, 241
implementation, 240
low-pass-type filter, 237
magnitude response, 239
performances, 237
process diagram, 237, 238
pulse transfer function, 243, 244
structure realization, 240
types, 237
z-domain, 243
Digital images, 35
Digital Imaging and Communications in
    Medicine (DICOM), 358
Digitalization, 84
Digital mammography machine, 318
Digital signal processing, 54
Direct-to-purchaser (DTC) hereditary, 351
Discrete Fourier Transform (DFT), 264
Discrete wavelet changes (DWT), 42
Discriminative models, 331
Distributed data fusion acquisition, 11
DIY medical instrumentation, 181
DL applications, WHM systems
    atrial fibrillation detection, 143
    BCI, 142
    CNN, 142, 143
    data mining, healthcare, 141
    data preprocess, 141
    DBN, 141–143
    feature acquisition, 141
    feature selection, 141
    heterogeneous devices and
        platforms, 144
    human activities, 144
    human motion analysis, 141
    human physical activity identification, 143
    multiplicate EEG sensors, 141
    neural morphological electronic
        systems, 144
    overview, 140
    RBM, 142, 143
    software packages, 144, 145
    TensorFlow, 144
    wearable sensor data, 140
DNA damage biomarkers, 358
DNN structure, 372
Documentation, 77
Dopamine, 16
Double point crossover, 246, 247
Double-slit experiment, 7
Drug-resistant MTB infection, 359
Dualism, 7
Ductal carcinoma in situ (DCIS), 318
DWT-based decomposed image, 43, 44

E
Ear accessory device, 112
Earlier time identification, 272
Early detection, 181
ECG-based cardiovascular diseases
    diagnosis, 215
ECG monitoring sensor, 100
eHealth arrangements, 353
E-healthcare business logic and rules, 187
E-healthcare data analytics monitoring, 188
E-healthcare data processing, 187
E-healthcare service interface, 186
E-health design comparison, 189
E-health framework
    advantage, 176
    COVID-19 pandemic, 176, 188, 189
    designs (*see* Aggregated E-health system)
    dominant standards, 188
    health monitoring and detection
        deep learning, 180
        issues tracking, 178
        ML, 178
        statistics, 177, 178
    online monitoring
        CPM, 180
        DIY medical instrumentation, 181
        early detection, 181
        machine learning modeling, 182
        RPM, 181
        shared data models, 181
    reliable and flexible, 176
Electrical current, 380
Electrical stimuli, 381, 382, 385
Electrical stimulus, 380–388, 390–393
Electrocardiogram (ECG), 71, 84, 98, 99, 112,
    162, 214
    CVDs diagnosis, 236
    frequency range, 235, 250
    information/recording, 235
    MATLAB software, 247, 248
    response, 255
    time intervals, 235, 236
Electrode-skin interface model, 386
Electroencephalogram (EEG), 100, 101, 162
Electromyographic signal, 349
Electronic communication system, 73
Electronic hardware, 185
Electronic health records (EHR), 77, 96,
    353, 370
Electronic tattoos, 86
Electrooculogram (EOG), 162
Electrotactile, 381
Electrotactile displays, 380
Electrotactile perception threshold (ETPT),
    381, 386, 388, 389, 391

Email-based communications, 70
Emission coefficient (EC), 12
Emotions
    brain, 162
    types, 162
Emotions detection
    respiration patterns, 172
    sensors, 161, 162
    techniques, 162
Encoding
    decomposition, 46
    Embedded Wavelet, 46
    SPIHT, 46, 47
    STW, 47
    WDR, 47
Energy, 3
    anatomy, 21
    distribution, 16
    measurement, 4
Enhanced classification AC, 229
Enthusiasm, 71
Environment sensors, 107
E-textiles, 85, 112
Eulerian Video Magnification, 263
Expensive technology, 77
Extended e-health services platform, 188
Extreme learning machine (ELM)
    box plot, 219
    chaos and nonlinear features, 216
    fundamental estimation capability, 216
    fundamentals, 218
    learning speed, 216
    OSELM, 216, 219
    phases, 218
    training phase, 216
EZW encoder, 46

F
Farcicality coefficient (FC), 12
Fast Fourier transform (FFT), 42, 260
Faster Region-Based Convolutional Neural
        Network, 352
Feature acquisition, 124
Feature extraction, 119, 148, 149, 282, 294
Feature selection, 120
Fifth-generation wireless network technology
        (5G), 149
FIR type filters
    difference equation, 243
    unique traits, 242
    unit pulse, 241, 242
Fitness, 244
Fitness trackers, 85

Foodborne diseases, 348
Format converters, 295
FPGAs
    algorithm implementation, 63
    application, 55
    data processing, 62
    enhancement, 55
    portable electronic devices, 59
    real-time processing systems, 59
    VIVADO tool, 59
Frequency response characteristics, 388, 390
Frequential DBN (FDBN), 142
Fundamental flexural-guided wave
        (FFGW), 193
Fuzzy decision tree (FDT), 373
Fuzzy shell clustering, 319

G
GA-based digital low-pass IIR type filter, 255
GA-based IIR (GAIIR) filter, 250
Galvanic skin reflex, 13
Galvanic skin resistance (GSR), 162
Gas discharge bioelectrograph, 12
Gas discharge visualization (GDV), 11, 12
Gastrointestinal (GI)
    data handling and processing, 290
    electronic documentation, 288
    procedural expertise, 288
Gated recurrent unit (GRU), 133, 307
Gating feedback RNN (GF-RNN), 134
Gaussian filter, 273
Gaussian pyramids, 264
Gayatri Mantra, 9, 22
GDV Compact Device, 13
GDV processor, 11
GDV Processor Software, 13
Gene sequencing, 353
GeneMark-Genesis, 349
General packet radio service (GPRS), 109
Generalized Discriminant Analysis (GDA)
    attributes dimension reduction, 220, 222
    classification performance, 228, 231
    formulation, 220
    OSELM, 227, 228, 231
    projections matrixs, 221
    RBF kernel function, 226
    reduction scheme, 226, 227
    space transformation technique, 217
Generative adversary network (GAN),
        134, 135
Generic system architecture, WHM
    BAN, 109
    communication protocol, 109

design, 108
GPRS, 109
mobile telecommunication
technologies, 109
offline monitoring, 110
primary features, wireless protocols,
109, 110
PU, 109
real-time monitoring, 110
Genetic algorithm (GA), 229
basic function, 244
crossover operation, 245
fitness function, 246, 247
heuristic algorithm, 255
mutation operator, 246
normalized frequency, 251
parameters, 250, 252
phase response, 252
population size, 245
random exploration approaches, 244
selection operation, 245
Genome-wide connection, 350
Genomic medication, 356
GI Cloud
applications, 298
architecture, 290
functionalities, 299
information architecture, 292
medical practices, 301
parametric model-based evaluation,
299, 300
services architecture
DaaS, 292, 293
data center assets, 291
generic services, 297
HCaaS, 296
OPEX model, 291
overview, 292
P-IaaS, 295, 296
P-SaaS, 295
SaaS, 293, 294
use cases, 299
GI environment, 299
GI-office service, 297
GitHub platform, 332
GLCM feature extraction technique
gray level picture matrix, 275
melanoma spot analysis, 283
pixel intensity variance, 275
segmented images, 283
statistical approach, 273
texture attributes, 278
vector, 275
Global feature extraction, 336

Global health crises, 363
Global positioning system (GPS), 85
Glossary manager, 296
Google, 361
Google Contact Lens, 111
Google Glass, 94
Government bodies, 78
GrabCut neural network, 272
Gravitational energy, 3
Grey-level co-occurrence matrix (GLCM)
directions, 325
feature extractions, 323
mammogram images, 320
pixel pairs, 323
textural features, 321
transient matrix, 323
Grey-Level Spatial Dependency Matrix
(GLSDM), 321
Ground truth (GT), 272, 283

H
Haar wavelet, 40
Hard attention, 337
Head-mounted devices, 85
Head systems, 15–17
Head-up displays (HUDs), 85
Health informatics
bioinformatics, 374
computational methods, 370
(see also Computational health
informatics)
deep learning, 373, 374
EHRs, 370
ML, 372, 373
Health Information Privacy and Portability Act
of the USA (HIPPA), 71, 296
Health monitoring system, 117, 185
Health sensor data management, 10
Healthcare, 349
Healthcare Delivery Organization (HDO), 200
Healthcare informatics, 349
feature extraction algorithms, 371
patient-driven therapeutics, 344
Healthcare monitoring, 107
Healthcare organizations, 9
Healthcare output (HCO), 370
Healthcare professionals, 288
Health-related computations, 177
Heart failure (HF), 229
Heart rate (HR), 98
abnormality, 257
definition, 257
measurement, 265, 266

Heart rate (HR) (*cont.*)
  monitoring (*see* Contactless HR
      monitoring method)
  physical exercise, 265, 267
  Python program, 261–264
  resting condition, 268
Heart rate variability (HRV), 13, 373
  attributes vector, 220
  bi-correlation, 225
  feature vector, 222
  ML, 215
  NN interval, 223
  role, 214
  sample analysis, 222, 223
  segmented database, 216, 217
  signal processing methods, 215
  time series, 224
Helper method, 261
Heterogeneous sensor fusion, 147
Hidden Markov Model, 372
High-pass filtering, 318
High-performance arithmetic, 53
High-speed QSD arithmetic/logic unit, 55
High-throughput data, 361
High-throughput screening, 350, 360
HIPPA compliance, 296
Historical data analyzer, 294
Huffman and arithmetic coding, 36
Huffman coding, 47
Human aura, 6
Human biosignals, 114
Human body, 5
Human computer interface management, 297
Human Computing as a Service (HCaaS), 296
Human face detection, 258
Human Genome Venture, 355
Human wearable devices
  attachable devices
      real-time health monitoring systems, 85
      smart contact lenses, 86
      wearable skin patches, 85
  implantable devices, 86
  ingestible pills, 86
  portable devices
      e-textiles, 85
      head-mounted devices, 85
      medical facilities, 84
      wrist-mounted devices, 84
Hurst exponent (HE), 224
Hybrid convolutional neural network model
  evaluation metrics, 309
  layers, 307
  preprocessed training set, 308
  Python platform, 308

Hybrid stimuli, 381
Hybrid-stimuli PC model, 382–386
  characteristics, 386
  computational model, 388
  frequency response characteristics,
      388, 390
  mechanoreceptors, 388
  spike response, 383, 386
  spike-rate changes, 390, 391
  spike-rate characteristics, 387
  sub-threshold amplitude, 391
  threshold characteristics, 388, 389, 391
  threshold *vs.* sub-threshold, 391, 392

I
IBM Watson health oncology solutions, 361
IIR-type filters
  advantages, 243
  basic GA pseudo code, 250
  coefficient vector, 249
  cost function, 249
  designing goals, 249
  difference equation, 242
  frequencies bands, 249
  GA flow chart, 251
  GA implementation procedure, 250
  impulse response, 242
  input and output relationship, 248
  preferred and actual responses, 249
  pulse transfer function, 249
  unit pulse, 241
Image comparators, 294
Image compression
  algorithms, 40
  classification, 38
  CR, 36
  lossless, 39
  medical image, 40
  model, 37
  quality measures, 38, 39
  redundancies, 36
Image enhancement, 274
Image segmentation
  algorithms, 329
  CT, 329
  image processing, 329
  instance, 328
  medical image, 329
  semantic, 328
  types, 328
  U-NET model, 336
Immune systems, 17, 18
Impulse responses, 242

In silico analysis, 344
Indian sciences, 9
Indian Space Research Organisation
    (ISRO), 78
Inertial measuring units (IMUs), 91
Infinite-impulse-response (IIR), 244
Information analysis, 354
Information and communication technology
    (ICT), 107
Infrared sensor, 163
Infusion pump control model
    drug delivery system, 202
    drug infusions, 202
    implement modeling, 203
    medical infusion system, 202
    modern infusion system, 202
    pharmacokinetics study, 202
    reference speed, 203
    sophisticated devices, 202
Infusion pumps
    categories, 201
    control parameters comparison, 207, 209
    control strategies (see Proportional integral
        derivative (PID) controller)
    definition, 201
    design, 207
    LQG, 206, 207
    MCPS-based, 200
    optimum flow rate, 209
    patient/healthcare personnel, 200
Ingestible Pills, 86
Injury tracking, 92
INSAT satellites, 78
Instance segmentation, 328
Integrated Disease Surveillance Project
    (IDSP), 78
Intermediate carry, 58
Intermediate sum, 58
International Journal of Biological and Life
    Sciences, 319
International standard ASTM, 193
Internet, 291
Internet of things (IoT), 96
Internet service providers (ISP), 184
Internet-connected devices, 11
Interoperability, 298
Inter-pixel redundancy, 37
Interquartile range (IQR), 219
Intervening carry, 58
Intervening sum, 57
Invasive ductal carcinoma (IDC), 318
IoT scenario, 11
IR-based sensors, 98
IRF530 Power MOSFET, 194
ISRO-based concept, 78

J
Jap, 21

K
Kaggle dataset, 308
Kalman gain, 207
Kinetics, 202
Kirlian camera, 14
Kirlian photography, 3, 15
K-mean clustering, 272, 372
k-means statistical models, 272
K-nearest neighbor (KNN), 106, 124,
    141–143, 169, 171, 172
Knowledge-related query manager (KQM), 297
Kriging model, 122, 123

L
Lactococcus lactis, 346
Life cycle analyzer, 294
Life cycle data handlers, 293
Linear discriminant, 169
Linear Quadratic Gaussian (LQG)
    control parameters, 206, 207
    cost function, 206
    Kalman gain, 207
    optimal controllers, 206
    Riccati equation, 207
    state feedback matrix, 206
    time response analysis, 209
Linear regression (LR) algorithm, 196, 197
Local Binary Patterns (LBP), 273
Location transparent storage, 295
Logistics, 94
Lossless compression
    arithmetic coding, 39, 48, 49
    codewords, 39
    Huffman coding, 39, 47
    proportion, 40
    reconstructed image, 47
    run-length encoding strategy, 39
    weight, 39
Lossy compression, 39
Lossy image pressure, 38
Lossy pressure, 41
Low Cost Broadband Ultrasonic Pulser-
    Receiver, 192

M
Machine learning (ML), 10, 97, 215, 307, 372
Machine learning-based approaches
    AI *vs*. DL, 118
    ANN, 121, 122

Machine learning-based approaches (*cont.*)
data mining, 120
distinct fields, 121
DL (*see* Deep learning (DL))
feature acquisition, 124
healthcare services, 120
k-NN, 124
Kriging model, 122, 123
PCA, 121, 124
state-of-the-art techniques, 120
SVM, 123
traditional artificial set feature learning
method, 125
WHM, 120, 124
Magnetic resonance imaging (MRI), 357
Mammograms
breast cancer, 319
early-stage tumour detection, 318
low-intensity X-ray, 320
median filtering, 318
photos, 318
picture segmentation, 318
wavelet transform, 321
Mantra, 22
Marine sensor network R&D centers, 299
Mass spectrometry, 354, 357
Maternal Care Project, 72
MATLAB application, 168
MATLAB Simulation Software, 385
MCPS-based devices, 200
Mean square error (MSE), 38, 251, 276
Mean standard deviation (MSD), 251
Mechanical band-pass filter, 380
Mechanical stimuli, 380–388, 390–393
Mechanoreceptors, 380, 388
Mechanotransduction
mechanism, 380
MedEx Ambulance Service, 93
Median filter, 278, 325
Medical care, 362
Medical Cyber Physical System (MCPS), 200
Medical image compression, 40
Medical image segmentation, 329
Medical images, 35
Medical imaging informatics (MII), 357
Medical imaging modalities, 329
Medical infusion systems, 202
Medication, 7
Meditation, 8
Melanin production and surface (PDT), 272
Melanoma, 271
Metabolomics, 354, 355
MetaCyc, 355
Metadata managers, 295
MetFrag, 354

Microcalcification, 319, 320
Microcontroller, 88
Micromechatronics, 107
Miners, 87
Mini-MIAS database photos, 318
Ministry of Health and Family Welfare
(MoHFW), 78
Mixed reality (MR), 85
ML algorithms, 373
ML-/DL-based WHM
challenges, 146–148
open research directions, 148, 149
MLX90614 DAA sensor, 163–165
Mobile health (m-health), 75, 352
Mobile telecommunication technologies, 109
Model system architecture, 307
MODELLER, 361
Modern infusion system, 202
Modern telemedicine, 71, 72
Motor actuation, 201
mSplicer, 349
Multilayer perceptron (MLP), 121
Multimodal data fusion-based data processing
method, 10
Multimodal unstructured data, 10
Multi-objective differential evolution
(MODE), 307
Multi-parameter multi-protocol Crypto
Service, 295
Multi-resolution (multiscale) depiction, 321
Multiscale permutation entropy (MPE), 225
Musculoskeletal systems, 18, 19
Mutation, 244

N
National Aeronautics and Space
Administration (NASA), 70
National Cancer Network (OncoNET), 78
National Data Centers (NDCs), 289
National e-Governance Plan (NeGP), 289
National e-Health Authority (NeHA), 78
National initiatives, 289
National Knowledge Network (NKN), 289
National Optical Fiber Network (NoFN), 289
Natural language processing (NLP), 357
Naturalness, 380
Net Time Delay (NTD), 194, 196
Neural network (NN), 121, 216
Neurotransmitters, 16
Next-Gen Sequencing examination, 351
Noncontact respiration rate detector
ATMega328P, 164
breathing pattern, 163
infrared sensor, 163

methods, 163
MLX90614 DAA sensor, 163, 164
Noncontact temperature sensor, 162, 172
Nondisclosure agreements (NDAs), 293
Non-disease population, 20
Nonintrusive wearable sensors, 107
Non-iterative KE Sieve Neural Network, 307
Non-melanocytic skin cancer (NMSC), 271
Non-recursive type filter, 242
Normal encoder-decoder network, 335
Norwegian Telemedicine Project, 71
NoSQL information, 351
NSR-CAD dataset, 221, 225, 226
NSR-CHF dataset, 221, 225, 226
Number-crunching encoding, 49

O
Objective function (OF), 204
Offline monitoring, 110
Offspring, 244
Om mantra, 22
OMIC's studies, 344
Online sequential extreme learning machine
    (OSELM), 216, 217
OpenCV platform, 263
OPEX model, 302
Optical head-mounted displays (OHMDs), 85
Optimal control system, 203
Optimal controllers, 206
Optimized physician schedule, 73
Order crossover (OX), 246
Organic databases, 352
Organs analysis, 15
Orthostatic test, 12
Oryza sativa, 348
OSELM analytical derivation, 219
Osteoporosis, 192, 197
Outline detectors, 294

P
Pacinian corpuscle (PC)
    applications, 392, 393
    approximations, 384, 385
    APs, 380
    characteristics, 381
    computational model, 382
    description, 382–384
    electrical stimuli, 381, 382
    electrotactile, 381
    electrotactile displays, 380
    hybrid stimuli, 381
    hybrid-stimuli PC model, 385, 386
    lamellar layer, 380

mechanical stimuli, 381, 382
mechanisms, 392
mechanoreceptors, 380
modeling, 380
naturalness, 380
novel predictions, 392, 393
parameters, 384, 385
SAIC, 380
sub-threshold mechanical stimulus, 388
tactile stimulus, 380
VAICs, 380
virtual environment, 380
VPT, 381
Partially matched crossover (PMX), 245–246
Particle Swarm Optimization (PSO)
    fitness function, 206
    infusion pump, 206
    OF computation, 204
    optimization algorithm, 205
    search efficiency, 205
    steps, 205
PathoLogic, 354
Pathway/Genome Database (PGDB), 354
Patient monitoring system, 261
Patient-physician relationship, 77
Patient-provided genomic data, 351
Patient-specific data storage, 290
Pattern recognition problems, 328
PC lamellae, 383
P-consciousness, 2
Peak signal-to-noise ratio (PSNR), 276
Pearson correlation, 178
Permutation entropy (PE), 224
Personalized medicine
    bioinformatics, 356
    CADD, 359, 361
    challenges, 356
    epigenetics, 356
    genomic medication, 356
    genotype, 355
    hardware/software, 357
    high-throughput experimental data, 357
    HTS with CADD strategies, 355
    imaging informatics, 357, 358
    NLP, 357
Personalized medicines, 353
Pharmacokinetics, 202
Photo-acoustic skeletal (FAS), 193
Photography, 3
Photoplethysmography (PPG), 162
Physical devices, 200
Picture archiving and communication systems
    (PACS), 358
Piezoelectric ultrasonic transducer, 193
Pixel, 260

Pixel intensity, 268
Pixel-depth conversion algorithm, 319
Platform as a service (PaaS), 294
Polypharmacy, 353
Pontine respiratory group, 163
Portability and Interoperability as a Services
        (P-IaaS), 295, 296
Portable unit (PU), 109
Positive prediction value (PPV), 217
Prana/ki, 4
Pranik Urja, 4, 5
Prediction, 114
Prediction of activity spectra for substances
        (PASS), 360
Preprocessing, 172, 274, 276
Primary healthcare units, 72
Principal component analysis (PCA), 119,
        121, 124, 165, 167
Privacy and Security as a Service
        (P-SaaS), 295
Private Cloud providers, 290
Proportional integral derivative (PID)
        controller
    block diagram, 203
    gain parameters, 209
    industrial control applications, 204
    mathematical representations, 204
    time response analysis, 204, 208
    transfer function, 203
    tuning, 204–206
Proposed E-health system architecture
    E-healthcare business logics/policies, 187
    E-healthcare data analytics
        monitoring, 188
    E-healthcare data processing, 187
    E-healthcare service interface, 186
    extended platform, 188
Protected Health Information (PHI), 200
Protein-DNA reciprocity, 362
ProTransport-1, 93
Provenance data handlers, 293
Psycho-visual redundancy, 37
Pulse-echo method, 193
Pulse generator, 194
Pulse rate, 98
Pulser-receivers, 192, 193
Pulse transfer function, 240
Pump actuation, 203
Python program
    BP-filters, 264
    color magnification parameters, 263
    FFT, 264
    Gaussian pyramids, 264
    helper method, 261

import keyword, 261
output display parameters, 263
output video, 263
reconstruct resulting frame, 264
webcam parameters, 263

Q
q-digit QSD information, 55
QSD adder, 57, 59
QSD cipher notation system, 54
QSD integer, 57, 58
QSD number systems, 55
Quality of service (QoS), 293
Quantitative ultrasound (QUS), 193
Quantum consciousness, 7
Quantum objects, 7
Quaternary, 55
Quaternary signed adder system, 54
Quaternary signed digit (QSD)
    adders, 54
    arithmetic units, 53
    number systems, 54
    propagation chains, 54
    subtraction/addition operation, 54

R
Radiological images, 69, 340
Radiomic, 358
Range of frequency (VLF), 14
RBF kernel function, 226
RBF neural organization, 349
Real-time interactive mode, 74
Real-time monitoring, 110
Real-time-polymerase chain reaction
        (RT-PCR), 306
Receiver circuit diagram, 194, 195
Recurrent neural network (RNN), 372
Reduced care continuity, 77
Redundancy, 36
Region of interest (ROI), 258, 259, 329
Relative cost unit (RCU), 299
ReLU activation function, 307
Remote monitoring, 74
Remote patient monitoring (RCPM), 181
Remote radio doctor, 69
Remotely controlled devices, 185
Replicator NN (RNN), 122
Research data analytic service, 297
ResNet-34, 339, 340
Respiration rate analysis (RR), 162
Restricted Boltzmann machine (RBM),
        126–129, 136, 142, 143, 149

Riccati equation, 207
Ripple carry adder (RCA), 59, 62
RNNs, 133, 134, 136
ROI detection/tracking, 258, 259
Role based security and access
    controller, 297
Roulette-wheel-selection, 245, 246
RS419 Ring Scanner, 94
Run-length encoding strategy, 39

S
Sadhus, 21
Sales personnel, 93
Sample entropy (SamEn), 223
SATCOM-based telemedicine connectivity, 73
SatelLife/HealthNet, 70
Satellite-based communications, 70, 73
Satellite communication, 185
Scalar quantization (SQ), 41
Science of Mantra, 8
Science of Yajna (Yagya), 9
Screening biomarkers, 344
Second-order system, 240, 241
Segmentation performance, 338
Segments, 328
Semantic segmentation, 328
Semi-supervised image segmentation, 329
Sensitivity (SE), 217
Service-level agreement (SLA), 293, 301
Seven chakras, 5, 19
Shared data models, 181
Short-time Fourier transform (STFT), 42
Sigmoid function, 221, 225, 226
Signal intensity, 194
Signal processing, 109
Signal to noise ratio (SNR), 196
SignalP, 346
Signed digit (2's complement form), 55, 56
Signed-integer QSD number, 54
Single transducer systems, 193
Single-hidden-layer feedforward networks
    (SLFNs), 216
Single-nucleotide polymorphisms (SNPs), 355
Single-point crossover (SPX), 246, 247
Single-stage amplifier, 194
Sinusoidal stimulus, 386
Sinusoidal wave, 13
Skin lesion classification, 273–275
Skin models, 388
Skin temperature measurement (STM), 162
Sleep pattern monitoring trackers, 92
Smart clothing, 85
Smart contact lenses, 86

Smart drug library, 201
Smart fabrics, 112
Smart infusion pumps
    design and implementation, 200
    generic block diagram, 201
    infusion set, 201
    motor control, 201
    wireless ecosystem, 200
Smart Melanoma Prediction Method, 273
Smart textile-based WHM devices, 112
Smartphone, 10
Smartwatch, 84, 92, 111
Soft attention, 337
Software as a Service (SaaS), 293, 294
Somatosensory system, 388
Sony SmartWatch, 94
Sound, 21
Space transformation technique, 217
Sparse autoencoder, 130
Sparse coding, 131, 136
Sparse version DBN (SDBN), 141
Spatial dependency, 334
Spatial orientation tree wavelet (STW), 47
Spatiotemporal residual network
    (ST-ResNet), 333
Specificity (SP), 217
SPIHT coder, 46, 47
Spike response, 383, 386
Spike-rate changes, 390, 391
Spike-rate characteristics, 387
Squamous skin cancer (SSC), 271
Standard ABCD assessment, 272
Standard of care, 77
State data centers (SDCs), 289
State Wide Area Networks (SWANs), 289
State-of-the-art machine learning
    techniques, 307
State-wide telemedicine program, 71
Statistical algorithms, 120
Stochastic universal sampling (SUS), 245
Store-and-forward mode, 73, 74
Stress psychological pressure, 21
Stretch-activated ion channel (SAIC), 380,
    383, 392
Structural similarity index (SSIM), 276
Structural similarity index measure
    (SSIM), 278
Sub-image extractors, 294
Sub-threshold, 381, 386–393
Sub-threshold amplitude, 391
Support vector machine (SVM), 106, 121,
    123, 125, 141, 142, 144, 275,
    306, 307
SVM classification system, 273

SVM classifier
    comparative representation, 276
    parameters, 283
    performance analysis, 283
    performance evaluation, 278
    PH2 database, 278
    PH2 dataset, 276
    SSIM, 278
Symlet wavelet, 45
Sympathetic component correlation, 13
Syringe pumps, 202

T
Tactile displays, 380–382, 392, 393
Tactile stimulus, 380
Tarchanoff's galvanic skin response, 13
Telecardiology, 76
Teleconsultation devices, 72
Teledentistry, 76
Teledermatology, 75
Telehealth, 68
Telemedical system, 71
Telemedicine
    advantages, 72
    architecture, 72
    categories, 75
    COVID-19 pandemic, 79, 80
    data compression technology, 71
    healthcare delivery, 69
    healthcare providers, 68
    healthcare sector, 80
    image digitization, 71
    in India, 78
    modalities, 73–75
    modern, 71
    NASA, 70
    programs, 70
    renaissance, 71
    risks, 77, 78
    technologies, 69, 80
    teledermatology, 75
    telepsychiatry, 76
    video communications, 69
Teleneurology, 76
Telenursing, 76
Telenutrition, 76
Teleophthalmology, 76
Telepathology, 75
Telepharmacy, 76
Telepsychiatry, 76
Teleradiology, 75
Telerehabilitation, 76

Telesurgery, 76
Teletrauma care, 76
Temporal dependency, 334
Tensorflow, 144, 308
Tetrodes, 112
Textile electrodes, 112
Theatro's wearable computer, 93
Threshold amplification factor (TAF), 384
Threshold characteristics, 388, 389, 391
Threshold vs. sub-threshold, 391, 392
Thumbnail generators, 294
Total harmonic distortion (THD), 195
Traditional medical solution and
        homeopathy, 12
Trained hybrid model, 308
Transfer learning, 147, 150, 337
Transient response analysis, 210
Traumatic brain injury (TBI), 350
Tree method, 171

U
Ultrasonic echoes, 192
Ultrasonic phase velocity evaluation, 192
Ultrasonic sound wave, 193
Ultrasonic technique, 192
Ultrasound, 193
U-net algorithm, 273, 283
U-NET architecture, 336
U-NET encoder-decoder
    attention U-NET, 338
    ResNet-34, 339
Unsupervised mathematical model, 331
US National Institute of Standards and
        Technology's (NIST), 289, 291

V
Value-added data handlers, 293
VB Net neural network, 333
Vector quantization (VQ), 41
Velocity and attenuation, 193
Vendor lock-in breaking service, 296
Very fast decision tree (VFDT), 372
Vibration perception, 388
Vibration perception threshold (VPT),
        381, 389
Vibrotactile perception threshold (VTPT),
        381, 386, 388, 389, 391
Village Resource Centre (VRC), 78
Viola-Jones detection method, 259
Virgin Atlantic staff, 94
Virtual environment, 380

Virtual land-based communications, 70
Virtual reality (VR), 85
Visual Geometric Group (VGG), 333
Visually lossless, 38
Vital signals, WHM
  activity applications, 114
  anomaly detection, 114
  blood glucose level, 115
  categories, 114
  clinical settings, 117
  data analysis, health monitoring
    system, 117
  data mining, 116–120
  diagnosis-based support, 114
  electrocardiography method, 115
  healthcare, 116
  home and remote monitoring
    settings, 117
  human biosignals, 114
  human health, 115
  physiological signals, 114, 116
  prediction, 114
  survey topics and restrictions, 115
  wearable sensor, 116
Voltage-activated ion channel (VAICs), 380,
  383, 384, 392

W
Watershed segmentation, 274, 278, 281, 283
Watershed transforms function, 275
Wavelet, 321
Wavelet analysis significance
  CWT, 42
  DCT, 43
  DWT, 42
  energy, 43
  examination changes, 42
  FFT, 42
  Fourier change, 42
  GWFT, 42
  LL, 43
  quantization, 44
  scale deterioration, 42
  STFT, 42
  symmetrical wavelet changes, 42
Wavelet-based image coding, 45
Wavelet changes (CWT), 42
Wavelet Difference Reduction (WDR), 47
Wavelet transform, 321, 325
  analysis significance, 42–44
  applications, 40
  image compression, 40–42

  images decomposition, 40
  strategy, 42
Wearable cameras, 92
Wearable devices
  human physical activities, 84
  quality parameters, 86
  smartphone, 84
Wearable devices with IoT
  clinical trials, 101
  ECG monitoring, 98–100
  EEG monitoring, 100, 101
  EHR, 96
  healthcare industry revolution, 96
  healthcare sector, 97
  RFID reader, 96
  transformed healthcare system, 96
  virtual signs monitoring, 98, 99
Wearable health devices, 71
Wearable health monitoring (WHM)
  data processing technologies, 106
  devices, 111, 113
  DL (see Deep learning (DL))
  environment sensors, 107
  generic system architecture (see Generic
    system architecture, WHM)
  health/healthcare monitoring, 107
  heart trackers, 113
  ICT, 107
  medical service evolution,
    micromechatronic system, 107, 108
  micromechatronics, 107
  ML (see Machine learning-based
    approaches)
  nonintrusive wearable sensors, 107
  technical designs, 106
  vital information, 106
  vital signals (see Vital signals, WHM)
  wireless communication systems, 107
Wearable skin patches, 85
Wearable smart biometric apps, 85
Wearable technology
  challenges, 102
  definition, 84
  emergency services, 92, 93
  healthcare and medicine industry, 95
  logistics, 94
  mining sectors, 87, 88, 90–91
  oil and gas industry, 95
  smart devices, 84
  sports and fitness, 89, 91, 92
  travel and hospitality industry, 93, 94
  wholesale and retail industry, 93
Web-based interface, 73

Wet electrodes, 112
WHO statistical CD details, 214, 215
Wi-Fi-enabled health management
      systems, 184
Wireless communication system, 84, 88, 107
World Health Organization (WHO), 176, 214
Wrist-mounted devices, 84

X
Xilinx code, 59

Y
Yagya and Mantra therapy applications
   chakra measurement, 19
   Kirlian captures, 19
   life energy, 20
   Pranik Urja calculations, 20
   science of Mantra, 18
Yagyas, 9, 14, 15
Yajna, 8, 9
Yin and Yang energy, 6, 7